Global Health and Geographical Imaginaries

To date, geography has not yet carved out a disciplinary niche within the diffuse domain that constitutes global health. However, the compulsion to *do* and *understand* global health emerges largely from contexts that geography has long engaged with: urbanisation, globalisation, political economy, risk, vulnerability, lifestyles, geopolitics, culture, governance, development and the environment. Moreover, global health brings with it an innate, powerful and politicising spatial logic that is only now starting to emerge as an object of enquiry.

This book aims to draw attention to and showcase the wealth of existing and emergent geographical contributions to what has recently been termed 'critical global health studies'. Geographical perspectives, this collection argues, are essential to bringing new and critical perspectives to bear on the inherent complexities and interconnectedness of global health problems and purported solutions. Thus, rather than rehearsing the frequent critique that global health is more a 'set of problems' than a coherent disciplinary approach to ameliorating the health of all and redressing global bio-inequalities; this collection seeks to explore what these problems might represent and the geographical imaginaries inherent in their constitution.

This unique volume of geographical writings on global health not only deepens social scientific engagements with health itself, but in so doing, brings forth a series of new conceptual, methodological and empirical contributions to social scientific, multidisciplinary scholarship.

Clare Herrick is a Reader in human geography at King's College London, UK. Her research critically explores the intersections of behavioural risk factors with urban environments across a variety of geographic settings.

David Reubi is a Wellcome Trust Fellow at the Department of Global Health & Social Medicine, King's College London, UK. His research explores the knowledges, socialities and material forms that undergird the politics and practices of contemporary global health and medicine. He is currently working on the biopolitics of the African smoking epidemic.

Routledge Studies in Public Health

A full list of titles in this sereis is available at:
www.routledge.com/Routledge-Studies-in-Public-Health/book-series/RSPH

Global Health and
Geographical Imaginaries

**Edited by Clare Herrick and
David Reubi**

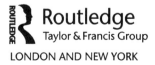

LONDON AND NEW YORK

First published 2017
by Routledge

2 Park Square, Milton Park, Abingdon, Oxfordshire OX14 4RN

52 Vanderbilt Avenue, New York, NY 10017

Routledge is an imprint of the Taylor & Francis Group, an informa business

First issued in paperback 2019

British Library Cataloguing-in-Publication Data
A catalogue record for this book is available from the British Library

Library of Congress Cataloging in Publication Data
Names: Herrick, Clare, editor. | Reubi, David, editor.
Title: Global health geographies / edited by Clare Herrick and David
   Reubi.Other titles: Routledge studies in public health.
Description: New York : Routledge, 2017. | Series: Routledge studies in
   public health | Includes bibliographical references and index.
Identifiers: LCCN 2016036638| ISBN 9781138852389 (hardback) |
   ISBN 9781315723525 (ebook)
Subjects: LCSH: World health. | Medical geography. | Economic
   development—Health aspects. | Public health—Developing countries.
Classification: LCC RA441 .G5678 2017 | DDC 362.1—dc23
LC record available at https://lccn.loc.gov/2016036638

ISBN: 978-1-138-85238-9 (hbk)
ISBN: 978-0-367-27771-0 (pbk)

Typeset in Times New Roman
by RefineCatch Limited, Bungay, Suffolk

Contents

Notes on contributors

Sarah Atkinson is Professor of Geography and Medical Humanities at Durham University. Her research is characterised by interdisciplinary encounters through which tease out and interrogate the assumptions underlying mainstream health-related policies and practices. These include the interpretation and practice of well-being and the understandings and constraints of care and responsibility. She is one of the editors of *The Edinburgh Companion to the Critical Medical Humanities* and *Wellbeing and Place*.

Jane Battersby is a senior researcher at the African Centre for Cities at the University of Cape Town, South Africa, and research coordinator of the ESRC/DFID-funded Consuming Urban Poverty Project. Her research for the past ten years has focused on urban food security and urban food systems in Africa.

Uli Beisel is Assistant Professor of Culture and Technology at Bayreuth University, Germany. She holds a Ph.D. in Human Geography from the Open University. She has worked on human–mosquito–parasite entanglements in malaria control in Ghana and Sierra Leone, and the translation of new technologies in Uganda and Rwanda. She is currently researching trust in biomedicine and healthcare infrastructures following the Ebola epidemic. She has published articles in *Science as Culture, Society and Space, Biosocieties* and *Geoforum.*

Betsey Behr Brada is Assistant Professor of Anthropology at Reed College. Her research focuses on transnational health interventions, biomedical expertise, and the postcolonial state in southern Africa. She received her Ph.D. from the University of Chicago and completed a postdoctoral fellowship in Princeton University's Program in Global Health and Health Policy.

Susan Craddock's research focuses on social and political factors shaping the experience and patterns of, as well as responses to, infectious diseases. She has published on access to AIDS drugs, non-commercial clinical trials, and the roles of poverty, gender and race in public health responses to tuberculosis. Her forthcoming book, *Compound Solutions: Pharmaceutical Alternatives for Global Health,* is on collaborative efforts to produce new tuberculosis vaccines and drugs for the first time in decades.

Caitlin Henry is a Ph.D. student in the Department of Geography and Planning at the University of Toronto. Her research focuses on the impacts of healthcare restructuring on the geographies of social reproduction, nursing and healthcare services in the USA.

Clare Herrick is a Reader in Human Geography at King's College London. Her research explores the intersections of behavioural risk factors for non-communicable disease, urban governance agendas and development. Her most recent research project critically explores the ways in which global health is increasingly being reconfigured as development in and through partnership working.

Stephen Hinchliffe is Professor of Geography at the University of Exeter. With research interests that span the human–nonhuman and microbiological interface, he has recently authored *Pathological Lives* (2017, Wiley Blackwell) and co-edited *Humans, Animals and Biopolitics* (2016, Routledge). His research has focused on relational approaches to health as a more than human condition.

Paul Jackson is an Assistant Professor of Geography at the University of Delaware. Grounded in political ecology of health, he researches how experts grapple with the interaction between humans and the environment. He focuses on those experts who presume that this interaction produces populations that are deficient, disadvantaged and/or diseased.

Nele Jensen is a trained medical doctor and Ph.D. candidate in the Department of Sociology at Goldsmiths, University of London. Her research is supported by the UK Economic and Social Research Council (ESRC) and focuses on the making and dissemination of health research evidence through evidence-informed policy networks.

Gerry Kearns is Professor of Human Geography at Maynooth University, Ireland. He works at the intersection of medical, political and historical topics in geography. He is the author of *Geopolitics and Empire: The Legacy of Halford Mackinder* (Oxford University Press, 2009) and co-editor of *Spatial Justice and the Irish Crisis* (Royal Irish Academy, 2015).

Jamie Lorimer is an Associate Professor in the School of Geography and the Environment at the University of Oxford. His research explores environmental governance in the Anthropocene, working across the micro and the macro. He is currently leading a project developing participatory approaches to engaging with the microbiome (www.goodgerms.org).

David Reubi is a Wellcome Trust Fellow at the Department of Global Health and Social Medicine, King's College London. Trained in sociology and anthropology at the London School of Economics, his work examines the politics of knowledge in the global governance of health. He is currently researching and writing on the biopolitics of the African smoking epidemic.

ories that can 'generalise findings . . . into durable intellectual frameworks that
be applied not only to distinctive health problems, but to different contexts
d future scenarios' (2010, 1518). Global heath's biomedical predilection to be
idence-based' rather than 'theory-orientated' has arguably and ironically
ited the 'emergence of an intellectually robust field' (ibid.). As Paul Farmer
d colleagues then argue, 'the process of rigorously analysing these problems,
rking to solve them, and building the field of global health into a coherent
cipline demands an interdisciplinary approach' (Farmer *et al.*, 2013, 2). This
mewhat paradoxical point is worth dwelling on, since it marks an area of
plicit) debate within the burgeoning global health field: namely is it or should
be a 'discipline' in its own right and, if so, what would it be and do? As a
nsequence, Farmer *et al.'s* contention that an interdisciplinary approach is
ded for the making of global health as a 'coherent discipline' is both common-
sical and nonsensical. From a social scientific perspective, it is obvious that a
ld as complex as global health demands multiple, critical disciplinary frame-
rks. However, the degree to which this aspiration is stymied by disciplinary
ritoriality as well as the location of most academic programmes within either
dical or public health schools also makes this pragmatically nonsensical
atheson *et al.*, 2014). Kleinman (2010, 1519) draws further attention to the
ys in which disciplinary territoriality plays out: 'Social scientists have at times
d theories simply to attack medicine, not to improve medical practice. That is
ailure of social science every bit as damaging as the profession of medicine's
lure to seriously engage with social theories.' He continues by imploring that
e time has long since come to supersede this untenable situation and to make
ial theory another instrument of improving health and reforming health care'
id.). It is this question of the appropriate *role* of disciplinary perspectives that
s allowed some to carve out distinctive analytical voices, while leaving others
uggling to gain traction.

With this context in mind and, as geographers, we continue to be struck by the
gree to which the social scientific study of global health has been largely domin-
d by two disciplines: medical anthropology (Janes and Corbett, 2009; Pfeiffer
d Nichter, 2008) and international relations (Davies *et al.*, 2014; Elbe, 2010;
cInnes and Lee, 2012). The emergent field of 'critical global health studies'
rown *et al.*, 2012) is thus often far from the harmonious interdisciplinary pursuit
visaged by Farmer *et al.* (2013). In both cases, it is not actually that the discip-
es themselves have helped advance the *enterprise* of global health, but rather
t the empirical uptake of global health has provided the foundation for challen-
g and advancing the disciplines themselves (Davies *et al.*, 2014). For medical
hropology, the field has been both legitimated and dominated by the use of
ols from medical anthropology to hone a vision of health equity and social
tice' (Farmer *et al.*, 2013, 16). For 'global apostles of health' (Fassin, 2012,
4) like Paul Farmer, Vinh-Kim Nguyen and Salmaan Keshavajee, their commit-
nts extend beyond academia and North American consulting rooms to active
vice in the Global South. And, with their dual training conferring upon them
th a biomedical authority and an anthropological ability to compellingly narrate

Introduction

As we write this introduction, global health seems to be bo[
nowhere, something and nothing. To us, it is of course every
media; newspapers; in what we read, think about and write. Y
health really is nowhere. What to us is so self-evidently *some*
nothing to the colleague who asked 'What's that?' when we t
book project over lunch. This perspectival disjuncture is nothin
health as we would similarly not always be able to locate the si
colleagues' research interests. However, what is particular is
was actually still familiar with many of the components of th
composes global health: the Bill and Melinda Gates Foundation
Organisation; GAVI; Ebola, to name but a few. This encou1
Didier Fassin's argument that the 'idea' of global health has 'ge
for granted as the best descriptor of contemporary issues in wo
all knew what it was' (2012, 96). While we might not go
MacPhail (2014) in suggesting that 'global health doesn't exist
the case that we cannot take it for granted that global health h
taken for granted'. Yet, the march of global health programmes
nerships across universities of the global north continues. This i
inexorable increase in the institutional members of the Consorti
for Global Health (CUGH), from 24 at its 2008 inception, to c
growth has been driven by the dynamics of student demand, in
inter-university competition and the attractions of global healt
And, as global health programmes in the Global North clin
number of 'strategic partnerships' with institutions in the Globa
has been an explosion in a (very particular form of) knowled
praxis, even if the very term used to describe it remains frustr
even to those familiar with it (Crane, 2011).

The nature of this ephemerality has been aptly summed up by
in his assertion that 'global health is more a bunch of problem
discipline' (2010, 1518). It is thus often the *problems* that we a
HIV/AIDS, malnutrition, TB, maternal health, malaria – rathe
a coherent discipline capable of exploring, explaining and miti;
than that, Kleinman argues, this 'bunch of problems' is despe

the lived experiences of individuals, they have made a morally inarguable case for the 'vitality of praxis' (Farmer *et al.*, 2013, 3), even if they have often and problematically 'situated whole communities within a discourse of victimization' (Panter-Brick, 2014, 439). International relations, through its concern with global health governance and diplomacy as well as the securitisation of public health, has been instrumental in drawing attention to the reconfiguration of the relationships between politics, policy and disease associated with the globalisation of unhealthy lifestyles like smoking and the re-emergence of infectious diseases, from HIV/AIDS and bird flu to Ebola (Elbe, 2010). Amid this and despite notable work by geographers within the field (Brown, 2011; Craddock, 2000, 2012; Ingram, 2005, 2009, 2013; Kearns and Reid-Henry, 2009; Sparke and Anguelov, 2012), geography seems to have allowed itself to be sidestepped in a way that may well say less about the discipline's capacity to contribute to the interdisciplinary making of global health and more about the relative paucity of those who self-identify as health/medical geographers (Herrick, 2016a).

Indeed, and perhaps without realising it, many geographers are actively engaged in global health research, especially in their analyses of the multiple upstream factors that affect the distribution and differential experiences of health and well-being. Indeed, many of geography's well-established sub-disciplines – economic, cultural, political, urban, development, historical, environmental – are actively engaged in exploring the kinds of questions and problems that also preoccupy critical scholars of global health. These include, but are in no way limited to, the influence of political economy, scientific knowledge, security and vulnerability, diplomacy, changing paradigms of aid and development assistance, socioeconomic inequity, sustainability, embodiment, social justice, governance, globalisation, rights and responsibilities, risk, resilience, urbanisation, socio-natures and the dialectical relationships between people and places. This is far from an exhaustive list, but gives a sense that in *doing geography,* many geographers are actually, already and inadvertently making significant contributions to the broad domain of global health. This collection thus aims to speak to two audiences. First, geographers who do not necessarily work on global health, because we believe, following Didier Fassin (2012, 103), that global health is a 'powerful analyser of contemporary societies'. Second, anthropologists, sociologists, political scientists and public health experts with an interest in global health, to incite reflection on what geography can bring to their discussions. We, however, need to be clear that we do not intend this collection to be a summary of existing geographical contributions to the study of global health, which has been ably done elsewhere (Brown, 2014; Brown *et al.*, 2012; Brown and Moon, 2012; Herrick, 2014). Rather, we see the chapters that comprise this collection as opening up and developing three new lines of inquiry into global health to which geography is crucial. The first, which has tended to be ignored amid almost obsessive attempts to come up with the perfect definition of global health, is to explore the multiple imaginaries that inform and make up the global health field. The second is to examine the power and politics of global health and to remember that these must be central objects of analysis for 'critical studies of global health'. The third and last of these lines of inquiry is to study how global health solutions often presage the very problems they purport to address, often with dire material consequences. In the remainder of this introduction, we will briefly attend to each of these lines of inquiry before setting out the structure and content of the collection.

Global health imaginaries

The emergence of global health has been accompanied by considerable efforts to define this 'linguistic novelty' and to give it a clear and widely accepted meaning (Fassin, 2012, 95). The CUGH has been at the forefront of these efforts. Complaining that while 'global health is fashionable' and 'frequently referenced', it is 'rarely defined' (Koplan *et al.*, 2009, 1993), an international meeting was convened in 2008 to develop a definition that was 'short, sharp and widely accepted, including by the public' (Beaglehole and Bonita, 2010, 1). The highly cited result from the meeting was the following definition:

> Global health is an area for study, research, and practice that places a priority on improving health and achieving equity in health for all people worldwide. Global health emphasises transnational health issues, determinants, and solutions; involves many disciplines within and beyond the health sciences and promotes interdisciplinary collaboration; and is a synthesis of population-based prevention with individual-level clinical care.
>
> (Koplan *et al.*, 2009, 1995)

These attempts at capturing and affixing the meaning of global health are highly problematic. They fail to realise that the power of global health to mobilise interest and resources lies precisely in the 'polysemous' nature of a concept that 'makes intuitive sense, but eludes a simple definition' (Panter-Brick, 2014, 432). It is also somewhat naïve to believe that a definition like the one drafted at the CUGH meeting can ever capture the 'obscure object of global health' (Fassin, 2012) or somehow order the 'open source anarchy' of overlapping and competing agencies, researchers, personnel and objectives that make up global health 'on the ground' (Biehl and Petryna, 2013, 376). Furthermore, while a common definition may well help coordinate existing global health institutions and efforts, it can also lead to the exclusion and de-legitimisation of those who believe in other meanings and who, unlike the CUGH, do not have the power to voice their own views.

However, instead of continuing the definition debate, here we want to explore the multiple and often conflicting *imaginaries* that inform and make up the field of global health. While the notion of imaginaries has been used widely in the political and social sciences, from Edward Said's (1977) imagined geographies of Empire, to Benedict Anderson's (1983) national imaginations and Sheila Jasanoff's (Jasanoff and Sung-Hyun, 2015) sociotechnical imaginaries, it has not yet been used in any systematic way to make sense of contemporary global health efforts. By global health imaginaries, we understand here the 'normatively loaded' and 'often complex visions of the world' that shape agendas, projects, policies and behaviours in the field (Smith, 2009, 462; cf. also Gregory, 1994; Atkinson, Chapter 4, this volume; Kearns, Chapter 1, this volume). These visions bring together and exist, through intricate constellations of moral narratives, scientific theories, administrative practices and architectural spaces that both enable and constrain thought and action. Travelling along transnational expert and advocacy networks and often informed by formal bodies of knowledge like epidemiology, development economics and public health, these global health imaginaries are necessarily multiple, co-constitutive but also often in conflict. Andrew Lakoff (2010), for example, identifies two key imaginaries at work within contemporary global health efforts: security and humanitarianism. In the securitisation imaginary, 'emerging infectious diseases' like bird flu and Ebola are 'seen to threaten wealthy countries' of the Global North (Lakoff, 2010, 59). To defend against these threats, multilateral health organisations, national security agencies and reference laboratories have come together to set up global disease surveillance systems and prepare for the next emergency with action plans, crisis centres and the stockpiling of vaccines (Keck, 2010; Weir and Mykhalovskiy, 2010). The imaginary of humanitarianism centres on suffering in poorer countries where poor public health infrastructures have left people exposed to diseases like malaria and AIDS (Fassin, 2007; Redfield, 2013). Here, we see humanitarian organisations, overseas development agencies, philanthropists and local community groups collaborate to alleviate this human suffering by 'providing access to existing medical technologies and spurring the development of new medications addressed to neglected diseases' (Lakoff, 2010, 60).

While Lakoff's work offers a useful start into the exploration of the imaginaries of global health, it is not without its limitations. Thus, his identification of security and humanitarianism as two distinct ways of envisioning global health fails to acknowledge the complex ways in which these two imaginaries intersect. An excellent illustration of such intersections is the way in which pharmaceuticals – themselves an iconic object of global health imaginaries – traverse both the securitisation of health (where drugs like Tamiflu are stockpiled by governments to guard against the next viral outbreak) and medical humanitarianism (where NGOs like Médecins Sans Frontières campaign for access to essential medicines for all) (Redfield, 2013; Elbe, 2014). Furthermore, as Lakoff (2010, 59) acknowledges himself, the two imaginaries he identifies do 'by no means exhaust the expansive field of global health', where many other visions are at work. One of these visions is the imaginary of globalisation, as Theodore Brown and others have shown (e.g. Brown *et al.*, 2006; Reubi, 2016a; Jensen, Chapter 8, this volume). Influenced by the theories on globalisation that had become so pervasive by the late twentieth century, many global health experts believe that the world has become a 'global health village' (Yach and Bettcher, 2000, 736), with developments in air travel leading to 'the microbial unification of the world' (Berlinguer, 1999, 18), and trade liberalisation allowing the transnational food, alcohol and tobacco industries to export unhealthy Western lifestyles around the world. For these experts, these new global health threats can only be addressed through new global forms of knowledge and action, from global epidemiological data like the Global Burden of Disease to global laws like the WHO Framework Convention on Tobacco Control (Reubi, 2016a; Reubi and Berridge, 2016). As contributions in this volume show, this global imaginary with its allure of 'worldliness [and] postmodernity' (Fassin, 2012, 101) stands in uneasy tension with older, uglier imperial imaginaries of race and postwar imaginaries of modernisation and development (Brada, Chapter 3, this volume; Kearns, Chapter 1, this volume; Reubi, Chapter 2, this volume). At root, however, these imaginaries are spun together by the inherently geographical nature of their constitution and deployment. It is this spatial axis that underpins this collection.

Global health, power and politics

The global health enterprise emerges from an assemblage of biomedical knowledge, technology, agendas, initiatives, objectives, data and politics. It is constituted in and through a multi-layered architecture articulated through the interconnections among nation states, international organisations, NGOs, regional trade agreements, localities, philanthropists, laypeople and experts, and through an array of projects, interventions and surveillance enterprises. Global health is thus a dynamic enterprise whose landscape and architecture is constantly shifting, but which hypothetically coalesces around the will to secure health for all, redress fundamental health inequities and tackle the mounting economic burden posed by disease and suffering (Lakoff, 2010). How, why and where these compulsions should best be deployed are questions that comprise both some of global health's most pressing concerns as well as providing the basis of its most ardent critiques (Biehl and Petryna, 2013; Nguyen and Peschard, 2003). These are also the foundations of the kinds of political questions that the biomedical framing of global health often eviscerates (Clark, 2014). In a recent editorial, Shiffman (2014) thus makes a case for critical consideration of the workings of both *structural* (our relationships with and to one another) and *productive* (the processes whereby meanings are created) power in global health. The former references the body of anthropological writing on structural violence (Farmer, 2004; Farmer *et al.*, 2006) and social suffering (Bourgois, 2003), while the latter speaks to a cadre of work within Science and Technology Studies (STS) that explores the powerful influence of categorisation, naming and counting in the context of (global) health (see MacPhail, 2015). The consideration of power advocated by Shiffman (2014) consequently draws attention to the politics involved in the creation of legitimacy, the generation of particular forms of validated knowledge and, as a result, the creation of an evidence base suitable for policy formation.

A major influence on the forms of legitimacy, knowledge and policies that dominate the global health field has been the market-based ideology of neoliberalism, as many scholars have argued (e.g. Thomas and Weber, 2004; Keshavjee, 2014; Battersby, Chapter 11, this volume; Jackson and Henry, Chapter 10, this volume). Specifically, these scholars point out that structural adjustment programmes (SAPs), which grew out of the neoliberal critique of the postwar state-led model of development and which have dominated international development from the early 1980s onwards, so often negatively impacting upon medical care and public health across the developing world (Stuckler *et al.*, 2008; Rowden, 2009). Similarly, the neoliberal *leitmotiv* of rolling back the state and opening up healthcare to market forces has led to the emergence of new forms of governance and actors from private–public partnerships and corporate social responsibility to philanthropists and NGOs, leading to the concentration of power in private hands and reduced levels of democratic accountability (Rushton and Williams, 2011; McGoey, 2015; Herrick, 2016b). For many authors, there has been a hope that international human rights and, specifically, the right to health can offer us a bulwark against neoliberalism and its detrimental impact on human vitality (e.g. Forman, 2008; Schrecker *et al.*, 2010; cf. also Mold and Reubi, 2013). However, there are dangers in working with too simple a dichotomy between a bad neoliberalism and good human rights. Indeed, as a growing number of authors show, human rights and the judicialisation of global health is not without its problems, from the failure of human rights to recognise transnational corporations like pharmaceutical companies as obligation holders, to the way in which the right to health is mostly used by middle-class patients, thus widening inequalities (Petryna, 2009; Biehl *et al.*, 2009; Reubi, 2011). Furthermore, as other authors have shown, there is more to neoliberalism than SAPs and more to the economisation of life than neoliberalism; with taxes on cigarettes, alcohol and sugar being an example of how economic strategies can help improve health (Collier, 2011; Ferguson, 2015; Reubi, 2013, 2016b).

When exploring the politics of global health, one cannot fail to mention the post-colonial tensions and power imbalances between North and South that inform the field. As Meyers and Hunt (2014) note, most global health initiatives concern themselves with particular regions of the global South (Anderson, 2014b; cf. also Brada, Chapter 3, this volume). Yet there are many spaces of exemplary healthcare facilities across the Global South, just as there are many spaces of abject neglect in the Global North (Meyers and Hunt, 2014; cf. also Jackson and Henry, Chapter 10, this volume). Furthermore, despite a pervasive rhetoric of 'collaboration', global health as a field and form of knowledge is produced through the strategic cultivation and uptake of certain types of 'valuable inequalities' (Crane, 2013, 167). In this reading, certain geographies – real and imagined – become 'fodder for profound institutional and intellectual opportunity' (ibid). In particular, Crane shows how burgeoning global health partnerships are made possible only because 'the very poverty and inequality [North American researchers] aspire to remedy is also what makes their global health programs both possible and popular' (2013, 168). Global health is therefore, in Crane's view, something that is made in and through new forms of scientific knowledge extracted from strategic sites of the Global South (often drawing upon the labour of southern health sector employees). This then flows back to the publishing houses, universities and funders of the North, whereupon the new knowledge becomes the basis for the further movement of people and resources south. These new, post-colonial forms of 'extraction' are obviously and inherently political in their reliance on the maintenance of profound socio-spatial differences (Horton, 2013, 2014a).

As Rushton (2015, 313) contends, one crucial omission when examining power relations in global health is the 'political nature of our analyses and . . . our own scholarly activity', especially given that 'our disciplines themselves are often just as elitist, hierarchical and non-transparent as the global health institutions we wish to criticise'. This reflexivity is a particularly silent realm of global health governance, but one that is all too obvious in proclamations by medical anthropologists that ethnography is solely and 'uniquely suited' to the study of global health (Pigg, 2013; Storeng and Mishra, 2014) and, as such, a favoured method to reinvigorate political debate. While much anthropological work usually involves deep reflection on the power dynamics at play in shaping the realities under study, these voices have little power and credibility in a field clearly dominated by biomedicine and public health. Indeed, the latter claim most of the funding and institutional support available, and their methods and concepts dominate the way in which problems are framed and addressed. Thus, as historian Anne-Emmanuel Birn (2005, 515–517) has noted, key global health actors like the Gates Foundation tend to privilege narrow 'medical/technical measures' such as vaccines and pharmaceuticals over 'social' solutions that address the inequalities underpinning ill-health. Similarly, as Vincanne Adams (2013b, 2016) and others (e.g. Storeng and Behague, 2013) point out, global health's infatuation with the burden of disease and cost-effectiveness metrics has meant that other, non-quantitative forms of research and advocacy like ethnography and social justice have little purchase. Many political and social scientists have reacted against the biomedical and public health domination of the field. Paul Farmer (Farmer *et al.*, 2006; cf. also Gandy, 2005), for example, has argued that global health must be a 'biosocial' enterprise in which medical problems are always and at the same time understood as problems with social origins that emanate from multiple scales, and which, therefore, demand social and political explanations and solutions across disciplines. Such an approach demands a nuanced, contextualised and situated series of analytical tools that are attuned to context, community and culture. It also ensures that narratives of blame are rendered visible, inequalities are not unintentionally reinforced through the activities of public health and, finally, that power structures are examined and laid bare (Adams, 2013b). Such an approach echoes critical ethnographic interventions which seek to provide an alternative evidence base to that generated by a metricised worldview (Adams, 2013b), by ensuring that the lives and voices of the people who are the subjects of these biomedical and epidemiological interventions are heard (Biehl and Petryna, 2014). This approach sits at a strategic nexus where geography so plainly matters and where global health, power and politics converge.

When solutions make problems

If the global health enterprise aims to improve the health of those in the Global South, then it does so through a fascination with metrics, surveillance, surveys and trials that often unfold in universes distinct from those of national and local public health systems (MacPhail, 2015). For this reason, it should come as little surprise that when global health emergencies such as Ebola strike, they become so largely because of the infrastructural inadequacies of the healthcare system (Kieny and Dovlo, 2015). They also become so because of the disproportionate sequestering of resources for HIV/AIDS which has created a two-tier health system in many countries (De Cock and El-Sadr, 2015). Indeed, as Storeng (2014) argues, one of the factors that limits global health's ability to fulfil its own aims is its antagonistic relationship with health systems strengthening, an issue and weakness that the magnitude of Ebola has laid bare. One potential reason for this is global health's tendency to use its fixation with technocratic solutions to guide the ways in which problems are framed, communicated and understood, rather than vice versa. In particular, criticism of the universal applicability of the 'Gates approach' (McGoey, 2012; Sridhar and Batniji, 2008) is mounting, especially as a profound gap is emerging between the funding priorities of 'philanthrocapitalism' and the revised concerns of the Sustainable Development Goals (SDGs) (Yamey *et al.*, 2014). The 'vertical-technical-fix approach' (Biehl and Petryna, 2013, 108) was well suited to the relatively simple targets and metrics of the Millennium Development Goals that focused on child mortality, maternal health, HIV/AIDS, malaria and TB (Kharas and Zhang, 2014). However, this 'global report card' approach is far less suited to the more complex intersections of the 'triple bottom line' of environment, economy and society that make the initial conceptual starting point for the SDGs (Sachs, 2012). It is also fundamentally inadequate in the face of the global non-communicable disease (NCD) burden, which now far outstrips that of the infectious diseases that still account for an estimated 97 per cent of global health funding (Marrero *et al.*, 2012; Nugent and Feigl, 2010).

The hunt for solutions to the 'grand challenges' of global health is of course laudable and the avalanche of funding from private philanthropic donors such as Gates, Bloomberg and Rockefeller has not only completely changed the face of global health science but also and arguably the contractual role of the state within this science (McGoey, 2014). However, and as Richard Horton contends, because 'the appropriation of human health by medical scientists and the health professions has created a medicine that claims its authority through the ideology of technoevangelism' (Horton, 2014b, 218), the problems that this evangelism purports to solve have been reconfigured in ways that seem to sit uncomfortably with the holistic discourse promulgated by the SDGs (Sachs, 2012). This is an argument that has been elaborated in depth by Vincanne Adams (2013a, 2013b) in her concern that the type of evidence favoured by this form of science has had the effect of transforming people into numbers, entries on a database or points on a graph. And, while technological efforts to find simple, low-cost solutions to major barriers to health continue apace, the need for these innovations to demonstrate evidence of efficacy and cost-effectiveness can have the unintended consequence of problematising those deemed in need of technological intervention: as victims, inefficient, uneducated or underdeveloped. In turn, when global health is framed as a series of technical problems, these then offer up new market niches for bioscientific ingenuity and public–private product development (Crane, 2013, 180).

What is clear is that 'magic bullet approaches are increasingly the norm in global health; that is, the delivery of health technologies (usually new drugs or devices) that target one specific disease regardless of myriad societal, political or economic factors that influence health' (Biehl and Petryna, 2013, 108). In reality and as the recent experience of Ebola has shown, it is these distal social, economic and political factors that help magnify suffering (after all, where healthcare systems functioned, Ebola was quickly contained). Yet these 'social determinants of health' that are so crucial to driving and addressing the NCD burden (Alleyne *et al.*, 2013) remain largely absent in the frameworks and research priorities of global heath, even as their language permeates the emergent SDG agenda. For the two to align, global health will have to undergo a profound 'paradigm shift' (Buse and Hawkes, 2015).

This 'paradigm shift' means asking difficult and politically unpalatable questions. As the stand-alone SDG health goal is pinned to 13 targets, this will significantly expand the terrain of action beyond the far more constrained horizons of the MDGs. Working towards the SDGs will consequently require a new 'global health architecture' that is inter-sectoral and cross-ministerial, that builds local capacity in sustainable ways and that prioritises prevention over treatment (Herrick, 2014; cf. also Battersby, Chapter 11, this volume). It will also necessitate engagement with the NCD risk factors of tobacco, alcohol and poor diet (Buse and Hawkes, 2015; Stuckler and Basu, 2013), which are amenable only to political economic and regulatory action, as opposed to the individual, technocratic 'fixes' so often favoured by global health science. These are political just as much as they are biomedical or public health issues, especially as preventing further rises in the NCD burden will necessitate tackling 'corporate vectors of disease' (Moodie *et al.*, 2013). It is here that we wish to return to Fassin and his assertion that, rather than a politics of health, what we need is a 'politics of life'. When the necessary 'paradigm shift' is cast in this way, 'global health is less about new problems (or solutions) than about new problematisations . . . that is, new ways of describing and interpreting the world – and therefore of transforming it' (Fassin, 2012, 113). This invokes Osborne's (1997, 174) suggestion that problematisations are 'not modes of constructing problems, but active ways of positing them and experiencing them'. And, as we know, global health has arguably 'more often been defined and illustrated than problematized' (Fassin, 2012, 96); what we now need is a commitment to 'making intelligible what often remains obscured, reformulating problems to allow alternative solutions, resisting individualistic and technical models to highlight the social mechanisms and political issues of global health' (Fassin, 2012, 115). In doing so, it may then be possible to counter the biomedical tendency to 'project coldness and abstraction, faceless publics [and] anonymous populations' to develop a concept of health that 'emphasises the connectedness of each of us to each other, one that understands how our future depends upon extraordinary cooperation between us' (Horton, 2014b, 218). This marks a social scientific search for antidotes to those global health problematisations that work to 'diminish complexity' to produce 'a field of delimitation' (Osborne, 1997, 175) over which science, technology and policy can rationally act. Here, then, critical studies of global health must push to reanimate the kinds of complexities that will so evidently need to be worked *with* if the SDGs have a hope of succeeding. This is the task of a truly interdisciplinary global health, within which geographers clearly have the conceptual tools to stake a significant claim.

Themes and contributions

This book is the result of giving geographers the challenge of rethinking their research and praxis in ways that speak to contemporary and historical global health debates, agendas, politics and practices. More than this, though, by bringing together geographers actively engaged in issues that have been identified as some of global health's new 'existential challenges' (Garrett, 2013), this collection goes beyond what already exists in global health scholarship to enlarge the field beyond medical anthropology and international relations' self-imposed social scientific boundaries. This is important, if only to ensure that global health does not become overly self-referential in its search for an interdisciplinary coherence. This collection thus has expansionist aspirations in the sense of opening up our horizons to what may *also* be global health. Using the themes already explored here, the chapters sit alone and come together with metonymical significance to enable and implore us to enlarge the current canon of global health research and writing to consider the salience of geographical perspectives and agendas. To return then to the opening words of this chapter, this collection hopes to shift global health from being something that is both 'everywhere and nowhere' to instead being 'somewhere'. In *locating* global health – socially, politically, economically, pragmatically – this collection aims to forge new conversations, new lines of inquiry and, in so doing, cement global health as a crucial domain of geographical inquiry.

Part I Global health Imaginaries

In 'HIV, AIDS and the global imaginary', Gerry Kearns explores the sexual and racial imaginaries that informed the way in which epidemiologists first conceptualised and organised data about the global AIDS epidemic. Analysing early epidemiological writings on the AIDS epidemic, he shows how AIDS in black African populations was construed as endemic and heterosexual, in contrast to AIDS in North America and Europe which was viewed as a white homosexual epidemic. Kearns further shows how this distinction was informed by colonial imaginaries of racial continents and chimed with contemporary racist readings of AIDS as African and Africa as a diseased continent and a development basket case. He also examines how this early racialised global imaginary was challenged by African elites and intellectuals like Thabo Mbeki, who articulated an alternative post-colonial imaginary of AIDS as a disease of poverty that can be tackled through African traditional medicine, with all the human costs that we know. David Reubi, in 'Temporal and spatial imaginaries of global health: tobacco, non-communicable diseases and modernity' very much builds on Kearns' contribution.

Examining the work of epidemiologists on the global smoking epidemic, he argues that epidemiological models of the epidemic are informed by postwar modernisation theories and imagine the world as separate geographical regions characterised by different smoking rates, cancer incidence and development levels, and organised along an unilinear axis of progress. As Reubi further points out, these spatialities and temporalities of difference stand in stark contrast to the spatio-temporal logics of sameness that often dominate the global health field. Indeed, influenced by theories of globalisation and ideas of time–space compression, many global health experts tend to see the world as a global village where disease patterns and biomedical solutions are the same for everyone.

In her contribution entitled 'Exemplary or exceptional? The production and dismantling of global health in Botswana', Betsey Brada comes back to and further unpacks the spatio-temporal imaginaries of development and modernisation discussed by Reubi. Her ethnographic study of a large public hospital in Botswana explores the conflicting understandings of global health among African and visiting American clinicians and medical students. She shows the growing popularity of placements in clinics in low- and middle-income countries among American medical students, and the financial importance of being able to offer these placements for American medical schools and their African partners. She also shows the often ambivalent ways in which American students and their clinical supervisors view Botswana and the hospital: from a quintessential locus of global health and African healthcare with diseases of the past and decaying infrastructures, to a place that was almost too sophisticated and wealthy to offer a truly global health African experience. With Sarah Atkinson's chapter, 'Mixing and fixing: managing and imagining the body in a global world', we move from American doctors' imaginations of Africa and global health to imaginaries of the global trade in human organ and other body parts in literary fiction and cinema. In particular, Atkinson explores the different notions of scarcity found in creative writings and films, from stories of illegal immigration and coerced harvesting of body parts, to tales of donations whereby donors continue to live through the recipients of their gifts. She also examines the various concepts of inter-corporality found in novels and cinematographic work, paying particular attention to the ways in which medical tourism and global forms of organ transplant may be read as an incorporation and suppression of the racialised other.

Part II Global health, power and politics

Susan Craddock's contribution – 'Making ties through making drugs: partnerships for tuberculosis drug and vaccine development' – offers an original take on the above-mentioned critique that current global health interventions are overly biomedical or technical to the detrminant of the social, economic and political. Drawing on qualitiave research on a number of international public–private partnerships aiming to develop new vaccines and drugs against tuberculosis, she argues that even biomedical or technical initiatives like these partnerships have social and economic benefits. Specifically, Craddock shows how these partnerships and their drug and vaccine development projects create complex 'social economies' in the low- and middle-income settings in which they work, building clinical and laboratory infrastructures, providing training and employment for local drivers, cleaners, investigators, recruiters and technicians as well as offering health education and engagement programmes to the wider community. As with Craddock's contribution, Jamie Lorimer's chapter, 'Living well with parasitic worms: a more-than-human geography of global health', seeks to trouble and complicate the accepted geographical imaginaries that prevail in the global health field. Indeed, drawing upon insights from the animal studies literature, Lorimer explores the paradox of making concurrent attempts to pathologise both the presence and absence of the hookworm, a parasitic worm that inhabits the intestines of human beings and some vertebrate animals. As he reminds us, campaigns to eradicate hookworms in poor countries of the Global South have, of course, a long history, from imperial programmes to tackle what colonial administrators described as the germ of laziness, to the Rockefeller Foundation's efforts to modernise the American deep south. More recently, however, there has been a movement in the other direction, with attempts by small groups of scientists and citizens in the Global North to re-worm the world. As Lorimer shows, these individuals see the absence of worms in the human biome as the reason for the late twentieth-century epidemic in NCDs and autoimmune diseases.

Like Lorimer, Uli Beisel's contribution 'Resistant bodies, malaria and the question of immunity' seeks to challenge the imaginaries of eradication that shape global health experts' understandings of the relationship between humans and (parasitic) animals. Focusing on contemporary global health efforts to eradicate malaria, Beisel argues that metaphors of entanglements may be better suited than metaphors of war and separation when trying to make sense of our relationship with mosquitoes. Drawing upon the science and technology studies literature on human–animal relationships and upon new understandings of immunology as flexible, complex and non-linear interactions, she explores failed efforts to produce a malaria vaccine, growing resistance to artemisinin among Cambodian mosquitoes and African stories of acquired immunity to malaria to argue that the relationship between human beings and mosquitoes is best conceived of as a multi-species entanglement driven by symmetrical strategies of survival.

With Nele Jensen's chapter 'A genealogy of evidence at the WHO', we leave imaginaries of eradication and animal–human binaries and return to epidemiology and the politics of numbers in global health. Jensen explores the history of Chris Murray's Global Burden of Disease (GBD) project at the WHO at the turn of the century. In Murray's own version of this history, the GBD is an attempt to rationalise global health governance and a natural evolution of the mottoes and practices of evidence-based medicine into the realm of health policy. Jensen disrupts this naturalistic account by outlining the messy political, conceptual and material developments – from documents and Gro Harlem Brundtland reform of the WHO to the elimination of rival forms of evidence-making – that made the GBD project possible at all. She also argues that, rather than the GBD rationalising a pre-existing field of global health, it is the global metrics calculated by

Murray and his team that have made the realm of global health visible, thinkable and amenable to intervention.

Part III When solutions make problems

In 'More than one world, more than one health: re-configuring inter-species health', Stephen Hinchliffe brings us back to both the human–animal and the medical–social binaries already addressed in earlier contributions to this volume, albeit from a different angle. The focus of his chapter is the One World, One Health movement – an attempt at overcoming disciplinary and institutional barriers between public health, animal health and agriculture in an effort to address more efficiently re-emerging infectious diseases. Hinchliffe argues that, because this movement is principally concerned with pathogens and their trans-mission, it fails to take into account the socioeconomic dimensions of infections and, therefore, offers only partial protection against them. He demonstrates this through a series of ethnographic vignettes about animal livestock and zoonotic influenza in the British food industry, showing how a One World, One Health approach cannot account for drivers of infections like precarious working condi-tions and genetically engineered disease-free animals with low immunity. Like Hinchliffe, the aim of Paul Jackson and Caitlin Henry's chapter – 'The needs of the "other" global health: the case of Remote Area Medical' – is to problematise specific aspects of the dominant global health imaginaries. Drawing upon their work with Remote Area Medical (RAM), a North American-based charity providing medical assistance, they start by questioning the assumption that global health is necessarily in the Global South. Indeed, while RAM began by providing medical relief in the Caribbean, East Africa and South Asia, it now carries out the majority of its work in poor North American rural settings, thereby shifting the meaning of the 'remote' in RAM from physical distance to socioeconomic disparity. Pointing to the critical role played by volunteers in the work of RAM, Jackson and Henry also critique the exaggerated emphasis placed on entrepren-eurship and medical techniques in contemporary global health.

In 'Eat your greens, buy some chips: contesting articulations of food and food security in children's lives', Jane Battersby offers a thorough critique of both global and South African nutrition policies today. She begins by outlining the problems inherent to these policies, from the failure to recognise that food security is not just malnutrition but also bad nutrition leading to obesity, to the dangers of allowing the private sector like the food industry and supermarkets to influence health policies to their advantage. Drawing upon ethnographic data with school-children in Cape Town, Battersby furthermore shows the difficulties of ensuring they have access to good nutrition, from them missing breakfast because of their long journey to school, to the unhealthy food options sold by shops and street vendors around the school. Like Battersby's contribution, the final chapter in this edited collection, Clare Herrick's 'Structural violence, capabilities and the exper-iential politics of alcohol regulation' is also located in South Africa and is set against the context of global health's limited engagement with NCDs and their risk factors. Exploring the example of alcohol consumption in Cape Town's poor communities, the chapter uses the framework of structural violence and Sen's capabilities approach to trace the ways in which alcohol consumption and its effects have so often been cast in the language of deviance which, in turn, obscures the ways in which upstream factors contribute to the genesis of harms. Here, the 'problem' of drinkers and their environments becomes central to alcohol's policy framing, guiding policy prescriptions that too often act as another form of structural violence, undermining individual capabilities and engendering the life conditions that perpetuate drinking as a form of coping. This is just one example of the type of 'pathogenic social spiral' (Nguyen and Peschard, 2003, 464) to which geographers and a geography of global health must be critically and reflexively attuned.

References

Adams, P.J. (2013a) Addiction industry studies: understanding how proconsumption influences block effective interventions. *American Journal of Public Health*, 103, 4, e35–e38.

Adams, V. (2013b) Evidence-based global public health: subjects, profits, erasures. In Biehl, J. and Petryna, A. (eds) *When People Come First: Critical Studies in Global Public Health*. Princeton, NJ: Princeton University Press. pp. 54–90.

Adams, V. (ed.) (2016) *Metrics: What Counts in Global Health.* Durham, NC: Duke University Press.

Adams, V., Burke, N.J. and Whitmarsh, I. (2013) Slow research: thoughts for a movement in global health. *Medical Anthropology*, 33, 3, 179–197.

Alleyne, G., Binagwaho, A., Haines, A., Jahan, S., Nugent, R., Rojhani, A. and Stuckler, D. (2013) Embedding non-communicable diseases in the post-2015 development agenda. *The Lancet*, 381, 9866, 566–574.

Anderson, B. (1983) *Imagined Communities: Reflections on the Origin and Spread of Nationalism.* London: Verso.

Anderson, W. (2014a) Making global health history: the postcolonial worldliness of biomedicine. *Social History of Medicine*, 27, 2, 372–384.

Anderson, W. (2014b) Treating the Sick Continent. Available at: somatosphere.net (accessed 1 January 2016).

Beaglehole, R. and Bonita, R. (2010) What is global health? *Global Health Action*, 3.

Berlinguer, G. (1999) Healthand equity as a primary global goal. *Development*, 42, 2, 17–21.

Biehl, J. and Petryna, A. (2013) *When People Come First: Critical Studies in Global Health*. Princeton, NJ: Princeton University Press.

Biehl, J. and Petryna, A. (2014) Peopling global health. *Saúde e Sociedade*, 23, 376–389.

Biehl, J., Petryna, A., Gertner, A. and Picon, P.D. (2009) Judicialisation of the right to health in Brazil. *The Lancet*, 373, 9682, 2182–2184.

Birn, A.E. (2005) Gates's grandest challenge: transcending technology as public health ideology. *The Lancet,* 366, S14–S19.

Bourgois, P. (2003) Crack and the political economy of social suffering. *Addiction Research and Theory*, 11, 1, 31–37.

Brada, B. (2011) 'Not here': making the spaces and subjects of 'global health' in Botswana. *Culture, Medicine, and Psychiatry*, 35, 2, 285–312.

Brown, T. (2011) 'Vulnerability is universal': considering the place of 'security' and 'vulnerability' within contemporary global health discourse. *Social Science & Medicine*, 72, 3, 319–326.

Brown, T. (2014) Geographies of global health. In *The Wiley Blackwell Encyclopedia of Health, Illness, Behavior, and Society*. New York: John Wiley & Sons.

Brown, T. and Moon, G. (2012) Geography and global health, *The Geographical Journal*, 178, 1, 13–17.

Brown, T., Craddock, S. and Ingram, A. (2012) Critical interventions in global health: governmentality, risk, and assemblage. *Annals of the Association of American Geographers*, 102, 5, 1182–1189.

Brown, T.M., Cueto, M. and Fee, E. (2006) The World Health Organisation and the transition from 'international' to 'global' public health. *American Journal of Public Health*, 96, 1, 62–72.

Buse, K. and Hawkes, S. (2015) Health in the sustainable development goals: ready for a paradigm shift? *Globalization and Health*, 11, 1, 13.

Clark, J. (2014) Medicalization of global health 1: has the global health agenda become too medicalized?, *Global Health Action*, 7.

Collier, S. (2011) *Post-Soviet Social: Neoliberalism, Social Modernity, Biopolitics.* Princeton, NJ: Princeton University Press.

Craddock, S. (2000) Disease, social identity, and risk: rethinking the geography of AIDS. *Transactions of the Institute of British Geographers*, 25, 2, 153–168.

Craddock, S. (2012) Drug partnerships and global practices. *Health & Place*, 18, 3, 481–489.

Crane, J. (2011) Scrambling for Africa? Universities and global health. *The Lancet*, 377, 9775, 1388–1390.

Crane, J.T. (2013) *Scrambling for Africa: AIDS, Expertise, and the Rise of American Global Health Science*. New York: Cornell University Press.

Cummins, S., Diez Roux, A. and Macintyre, S. (2007) Understanding and representing place in health research: a relational approach. *Social Science and Medicine*, 65, 1825–1838.

Davies, S., Elbe, S., Howell, A. and McInnes, C. (2014) Global health in international relations: Editors' introduction. *Review of International Studies*, 40, 5, 825–834.

Davis, M. (2005) *The Monster at our Door: The Global Threat of Avian Flu*. New York: The New Press.

De Cock, K.M. and El-Sadr, W.M. (2015) A tale of two viruses: HIV, Ebola and health systems. *AIDS*, 29, 9, 989–991.

Elbe, S. (2010) *Security and Global Health*. Cambridge: Polity Press.

Elbe, S. (2014) The pharmaceuticalisation of security: molecular biomedicine, antiviral stockpiles and global health security. *Review of International Studies*, 40, 5, 919–938.

Epstein, S. (1998) *Impure Science: AIDS, Activism and the Politics of Knowledge*. London: Taylor and Francis.

Epstein, S. (2004) Bodily differences and collective identities: the politics of gender and race in biomedical research in the United States. *Body and Society*, 10, 2–3, 183–203.

Farmer, P. (2004) An anthropology of structural violence. *Current Anthropology*, 45, 3, 305–325.

Farmer, P., Kleinman, A., Kim, J. and Basilico, M. (2013) *Reimaging Global Health: An Introduction*. Berkeley: University of California Press.

Farmer, P.E., Nizeye, B., Stulac, S. and Keshavjee, S. (2006) Structural violence and clinical medicine. *PLoS Med*, 3, 10, e449.

Fassin, D. (2007) Humanitarianism as a politics of life. *Public Culture,* 19, 3, 499–520.

Fassin, D. (2012) That obscure object of global health. In Inhorn, M. and Wentzell, E. (eds) *Medical Anthropology at the Intersections: Histories, Activisms and Futures.* Durham, NC: Duke University Press. pp. 95–115.

Ferguson, J. (2015) *Give a Man a Fish: Reflection on the New Politics of Redistribution.* Durham, NC: Duke University Press.

Forman, L. (2008) Rights and wrongs: what utility for the right to health in reforming trade rules on medicine. *Health and Human Rights,* 10, 2, 37–52.

Gandy, M. (2005) Deadly alliances: death, disease, and the global politics of public health. *PLoS Med,* 2, 1, e4. doi:10.1371/journal.pmed.0020004.

Garrett, L. (2013) *Existential Challenges to Global Health.* New York: New York University Center on International Cooperation.

Gregory, D. (1994) *Geographical Imaginations.* Oxford: Blackwell.

Herrick, C. (2014) (Global) health geography and the post-2015 development agenda. *The Geographical Journal,* 180, 2, 185–190.

Herrick, C. (2016a) Geographical contingencies, contingent geographies and global health. *Annals of the Association of American Geographers,* 106, 3, 672–687.

Herrick, C. (2016b) The post-2015 landscape: vested interests, corporate social responsibility and public health advocacy. *Sociology of Health and Illness.* 38, 7, 1026–1042.

Horton, R. (2013) Offline: Is global health neocolonialist? *The Lancet, 382,* 9906, 1690.

Horton, R. (2014a) Offline: the case against global health. *The Lancet, 383,* 9930, 1705.

Horton, R. (2014b) Offline: reimagining the meaning of health. *The Lancet,* 384, 9939, 218.

Horton, R., Beaglehole, R., Bonita, R., Raeburn, J., McKee, M. and Wall, S. (2014) From public to planetary health: a manifesto. *The Lancet,* 383, 9920, 847.

Ingram, A. (2005) The new geopolitics of disease: between global health and global security. *Geopolitics,* 10, 3, 522–545.

Ingram, A. (2009) The geopolitics of disease. *Geography Compass,* 3, 6, 2084–2097.

Ingram, A. (2013) After the exception: HIV/AIDS beyond salvation and scarcity. *Antipode,* 45, 2, 436–454.

Janes, C.R. and Corbett, K.K. (2009) Anthropology and global health. *Annual Review of Anthropology,* 38, 1, 167–183.

Jasanoff, S. and Sang-Hyun, K. (2015) *Dreamscapes of Modernity: Sociotechnical Imaginaries and the Fabrication of Power.* Chicago, IL: Chicago University Press.

Kearns, G. and Reid-Henry, S. (2009) Vital geographies: life, luck, and the human condition. *Annals of the Association of American Geographers,* 99, 3, 554–574.

Keck, F. (2010) *Un Monde Grippé.* Paris: Flammarion.

Keshavjee, M.S. (2014) *Blind Spot: How Neoliberalism Infiltrated Global Health.* Berkeley: University of California Press.

Kharas, H. and Zhang, C. (2014) New agenda, new narrative: what happens after 2015? *SAIS Review of International Affairs,* 34, 2, 25–35.

Kieny, M.P. and Dovlo, D. (2015) Beyond Ebola: a new agenda for resilient health systems. *The Lancet,* 385, 9963, 91–92.

Kleinman, A. (2010) Four social theories for global health. *The Lancet,* 375, 9725, 1518–1519.

Koplan, J.P., Bond, T.C., Merson, M.H., Reddy, K.S., Rodriguez, M.H., Sewankambo, N.K. and Wasserheit, J.N. (2009) Towards a common definition of global health. *The Lancet,* 373, 9679, 1993–1995.

Lakoff, A. (2010) Two regimes of global health. *Humanity: An International Journal of Human Rights,* Humanitarianism and Development, 1, 1, 59–79.

Livingston, J. (2012) *Improvising Medicine: An African Oncology Ward in an Emerging Cancer Epidemic*. Durham, NC: Duke University Press.

Longhurst, R. (1997) (Dis)embodied geographies. *Progress in Human Geography*, 21, 4, 486–501.

MacPhail, T. (2014) Global Health Doesn't Exist. *Limn* 5.

MacPhail, T. (2015) Data, data everywhere. *Public Culture*, 27, 276, 213–219.

Marrero, S.L., Bloom, D.E. and Adashi, E.Y. (2012) Noncommunicable diseases: a global health crisis in a new world order. *JAMA*, 307, 19, 2037–2038.

Martin, K., Mullan, Z. and Horton, R. (2015) The neglected foundation of global health. *The Lancet Global Health*, 3, Supplement 1, 0, S1–S2.

Matheson, A., Walson, J., Pfeiffer, J. and Holmes, K. (2014) *Sustainability and the Growth of University Global Health Programs*. Washington, DC: Center for Strategic and International Studies.

McGoey, L. (2012) Philanthrocapitalism and its critics. *Poetics*, 40, 2, 185–199.

McGoey, L. (2014) The philanthropic state: market–state hybrids in the philanthrocapitalist turn. *Third World Quarterly*, 35, 1, 109–125.

McGoey, L. (2015) *No Such Thing as a Free Gift: The Gates Foundation and the Price of Philanthropy*. London: Verso.

McInnes, C. and Lee, K. (2012) *Global Health and International Relations*. Cambridge: Polity Press.

Meyers, T. and Hunt, N.R. (2014) The other global South. *The Lancet*, 384, 9958, 1921–1922.

Mold, A. and Reubi, D. (eds) (2013) *Assembling Health Rights in Global Context: Genealogies and Anthropologies*. London: Routledge.

Moodie, R., Stuckler, D., Monteiro, C., Sheron, N., Neal, B., Thamarangsi, T., Lincoln, P. and Casswell, S. (2013) Profits and pandemics: prevention of harmful effects of tobacco, alcohol, and ultra-processed food and drink industries. *The Lancet*, 381, 9867, 670–679.

Nguyen, V-K. and Peschard, K. (2003) Anthropology, inequality, and disease: a review. *Annual Review of Anthropology*, 32, 447–474.

Nugent, R. and Feigl, A. (2010) Where Have All the Donors Gone? Scarce Donor Funding for Non-Communicable Diseases. *Working Paper 228*. Center for Global Development website. Available at: http://www.cgdev.org/content/publications/detail/1424546 (accessed 1 August 2013).

Osborne, T. (1997) Of health and statecraft. In Petersen, A. and Bunton, R. (eds) *Foucault, Health and Medicine*. London: Routledge, pp. 173–188.

Panter-Brick, C. (2014) Health, risk, and resilience: interdisciplinary concepts and applications. *Annual Review of Anthropology*, 43, 431–448.

Panter-Brick, C., Eggerman, M. and Tomlinson, M. (2014) How might global health master deadly sins and strive for greater virtues? *Global Health Action*, 7.

Petryna, A. (2009) *When Experiments Travel: Clinical Trials and the Global Search for Human Subjects*. Princeton, NJ: Princeton University Press.

Pfeiffer, J. and Nichter, M. (2008) What can critical medical anthropology contribute to global health? *Medical Anthropology Quarterly*, 22, 4, 410–415.

Pigg, S.L. (2013) On sitting and doing: ethnography as action in global health. *Social Science & Medicine*, 99, 127–134.

Rayner, G. and Lang, T. (2012) *Ecological Public Health: Reshaping the Conditions for Good Health*. London: Routledge.

Redfield, P. (2013) *Life in Crisis: The Ethical Journey of Doctors Without Borders*. Berkeley: California University Press.

Reubi, D. (2011) The promise of human rights for global health: a programmed deception. *Social Science and Medicine,* 73, 5, 625–628.

Reubi, D. (2013) Health economists, tobacco control and international development: on the economisation of global health beyond neoliberal structural adjustment policies. *BioSocieties,* 8, 205–228.

Reubi, D. (2016a) Modernisation, smoking and chronic disease: of temporality and spatiality in global health. *Health & Place,* 39, 188–195.

Reubi, D. (2016b) Of neoliberalism and global health: human capital, market failure and sin/social taxes. *Critical Public Health,* doi: 10.1080/09581596.2016.1196288.

Reubi, D. and Berridge, V. (2016) The internationalisation of tobacco control, 1950–2010. *Medical History,* 60, 4.

Rose, N. (2001) The politics of life itself. *Theory Culture & Society,* 18, 6, 1–30.

Rowden, R. (2009) *The Deadly Ideas of Neoliberalism: How the IMF Has Underminded Public Health and the Fight Against AIDS.* New York: Zed Books.

Rushton, S. (2015) The politics of researching global health politics: comment on 'Knowledge, moral claims and the exercise of power in global health'. *International Journal of Health Policy and Management,* 4, 5, 311–314.

Rushton, S. and Williams, O. (eds) (2011) *Partnerships and Foundations in Global Health Governance.* Basingstoke: Palgrave-Macmillan.

Sachs, J.D. (2012) From Millennium Development Goals to Sustainable Development Goals. *The Lancet,* 379, 9832, 2206–2211.

Said, E.W. (1977) Orientalism. *The Georgia Review,* 31, 1, 162–206.

Schrecker, T., Chapman, A., Labonte, R. and de Vogli, R. (2010) Advancing equity on the global market place: how human rights can help. *Social Science and Medicine,* 71, 1520–1526.

Shiffman, J. (2014) Knowledge, moral claims and the exercise of power in global health. *International Journal of Health Policy and Management,* 3, 6, 297–299.

Smith, E. (2009) Imaginaries of development: The Rockefeller Foundation and rice research. *Science as Culture,* 18, 4, 461–482.

Sparke, M. and Anguelov, D. (2012) H1N1, globalization and the epidemiology of inequality. *Health & Place,* 18, 4, 726–736.

Sridhar, D. and Batniji, R. (2008) Misfinancing global health: a case for transparency in disbursements and decision making. *The Lancet,* 372, 9644, 1185–1191.

Storeng, K.T. (2014) The GAVI Alliance and the 'Gates approach' to health system strengthening. *Global Public Health,* 9, 8, 865–879.

Storeng, K.T. and Behague, D. (2013) Evidence-based advocacy and the reconfiguration of rights language in safe motherhood discourse. In Mold, A. and Reubi, D. (eds) *Assembling Health Rights in Global Context: Genealogies and Anthropologies.* London: Routledge, pp. 149–168.

Storeng, K.T. and Mishra, A. (2014) Politics and practices of global health: critical ethnographies of health systems. *Global Public Health,* 9, 8, 858–864.

Stuckler, D. and Basu, S. (2013) Malignant neglect: the failure to address the need to prevent premature non-communicable disease morbidity and mortality. *PLoS Med,* 10, 6, e1001466.

Stuckler, D., King, L. and Basu, S. (2008) International Monetary Fund programs and tuberculosis outcomes in post-communist countries. *PLoS Medicine,* 5, 7, 1079–1089.

Thomas, C. and Weber, M. (2004) The politics of global health governance: whatever happeneed to 'Health for All By the Year 2000'? *Global Governance,* 10, 2, 187–205.

Venkatapuram, S. (2012) Health, vital goals and central human capabilities. *Bioethics*, 27, 5, 271–279.

Weir, L. and Mykhalovskiy, E. (2010) *Global Public Health Vigilance: Creating a World on Alert*. New York: Routledge.

Wendland, C.L. (2012) Moral maps and medical imaginaries: clinical tourism at Malawi's College of Medicine. *American Anthropologist*, 114, 1, 108–122.

Whatmore, S. (2006) Materialist returns: practising cultural geography in and for a more-than-human world. *Cultural Geographies*, 13, 4, 600–609.

Yach, D. and Bettcher, D. (2000) Globalisation of the tobacco industry influence and new global responses. *Tobacco Control*, 9, 206–216.

Yamey, G., Shretta, R. and Binka, F.N. (2014) The 2030 sustainable development goal for health. British Medical Journal, 349, g5295.

Part I
Global health imaginaries

1   HIV, AIDS and the global imaginary

Gerry Kearns

HIV, AIDS and the global imaginary

The syndrome that later received the name AIDS was first announced by a communication published in the USA by the Centres for Disease Control (CDC): 'In the period October 1980–May 1981, 5 young men, all active homosexuals, were treated for biopsy-confirmed *Pneumocystis carinii* pneumonia [PCP]' (CDC, 1981). Looking principally at the epidemiological discussion of AIDS within the USA, I have noted the persistent homosexualisation of the condition and examined the spatial metaphors through which this prejudice was sustained (Kearns, 2016). In this chapter, I want instead to examine how AIDS has been conceptualised as an issue of global health. I will describe the geographical imaginary of the first attempts to conceptualise AIDS as an issue of global health. I will outline some of the consequences of this global imaginary for AIDS policies, both in the USA and in South Africa.

When David Stoddart (1986, 154) wrote about geography as a form of scientific prediction based on observations of spatial proximity, he claimed to be describing the geographical method of exploration. Yet exploration was not really like extending a jigsaw puzzle, piece by adjacent piece, but, rather, some concept of the overall picture, a global imaginary, helped explorers interpret the new data that they produced. I use the term 'imaginary' in the sense intended by Jean-Paul Sartre when he wrote of imaginary objects that manifest in the 'synthetic acts of consciousness [where] there appear at times certain structures that we call imaging consciousness' (Sartre, 2004[1940], 7). The imaginary object helps us make sense of our perceptions and in this work of imagination there is a normative invest-ment. Webber remarks that, for Sartre, 'the patterns of salience and significance in our surroundings that motivate our actions result partly from the ways we imagine the world could be' (Webber, 2004, xxvi). Louis Althusser made a similar point when he suggested that 'Ideology represents the imaginary relationship of individuals to their real conditions of existence' (Althusser, 1971[1970], 162). A global imaginary, then, may be an understanding of how the world is and works, and it can organise our apperception of new data about the world.

In a thrilling survey of what they call 'the myth of continents', Lewis and Wigen (1997) explicate the Eurocentrism of the continental. The global imaginary of continents set up various oppositions between Europe and a series of others. Time and again, the discourse of continents legitimated European colonialism by presenting Africa as primitive (Mudimbé, 1988), Asia as enervated (Said, 1978) and America as degenerate (Pagden, 1982). Continental thinking is over-determined both by environmentalism and by racism: other places were understood as somehow less suitable than Europe as an ecumene for progressive civilisation (Glacken, 1967) and peoples indigenous to places outside Europe were thought to be incapable of sustained progress, even if they may once have been (Carew, 1988a, 1988b). This continental imaginary and its associated racism were central to the early epidemiological concepts of the global impact of AIDS.

Mapping global AIDS

Very soon after the first cases among, and early deaths from opportunistic infections of, young gay men, physicians in the USA reported cases among people other than gay men. Within one month of its first report on PCP among young gay men, the CDC announced cases among heterosexual injecting drug users (Shilts, 1987, 83) and, in January 1982, when it published a summary of the new epidemic detailing 158 cases either of PCP or of another opportunistic infection, Kaposi's Sarcoma (KS), the CDC identified 12 cases among men thought to be exclusively heterosexual (CDC, 1982a, 251). The epidemic in the USA was known to be diverse almost from its inception, and yet the earliest attempts to make sense of the epidemic at a global scale projected the space of the USA as sustaining a homosexual epidemic (Kearns, 2016). This was not simply a broad generalisation, since separate epidemics were hypothesised and were assigned to distinct global spaces.

In one of a clutch of articles in which they announced their geographical model of AIDS, researchers from the Special Program on AIDS of the World Health Organisation (WHO), together with colleagues from Belgium, Canada, Tanzania, and from the World Bank, announced that:

> The available data on reported AIDS cases and HIV-1 seroprevalence provide a reasonable description of the current global patterns of infection and severe or fatal disease due to HIV-1 infection. Three distinct epidemiologic patterns of infection and disease can be distinguished.
>
> (Piot *et al.*, 1988, 574)

Epidemiological reasoning is often spatial, inferring process from patterns of prevalence, tracks of transmission or clustering of cases. The WHO epidemiologists identified three groups of countries based, they argued, on the pattern of AIDS (Piot *et al.*, 1988, 577; see Figure 1.1). Pattern I countries had an epidemic where '[h]omosexual/bisexual men and intravenous drug abusers [were] the major affected groups' (Piot *et al.*, 1988, 576). Since the 'mid-1970s or early 1980s' AIDS had been established in the Pattern I countries of 'Western Europe, North America, some areas in South America, Australia, [and] New Zealand'

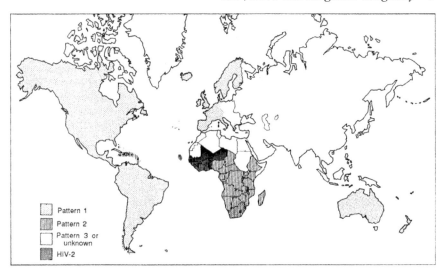

Figure 1.1 Patterns of HIV-1 infection in the world.
Source: Piot *et al.* (1988).

(Piot *et al.*, 1988, 576). The Pattern 2 countries of 'Africa, Caribbean, [and] some areas in South America' had, from the '[e]arly to late 1970s', an epidemic that was '[p]redominantly heterosexual' (Piot *et al.*, 1988, 576). In the rest of the world ('Asia, the Pacific Region (minus Australia and New Zealand), the Middle East, Eastern Europe, and some rural areas of South America'), the epidemic had started a little later, the '[e]arly to mid-1980s', and there was a '[v]ery low prevalance of HIV' (Piot *et al.*, 1988, 576). There are a number of problems with this identification of distinct epidemics in different places, and in particular with the continental basis of the classification of epidemics.

In the first place, the data were so patchy that generalising to the level of individual continents was a heroic undertaking. The epidemiologists at the WHO knew that their data were incomplete, particularly, they believed, in the case of the countries of Africa:

> Reporting of AIDS cases from Africa has in general been delayed and incomplete. The reasons for this include the limited access of large segments of the population to health care facilities where the diagnosis of AIDS can be established, the low efficiency of surveillance systems, the general lack of facilities for the diagnosis of AIDS, and the reluctance of some governments to officially acknowledge the existence of AIDS until 1987.
>
> (Piot *et al.*, 1988, 573–574)

A great deal of effort was expended in cajoling countries into admitting the presence of AIDS within their borders. Once a single AIDS case had been conceded, the WHO could follow up by asking for, and recommending the form of, a national AIDS prevention and treatment strategy. As of early December 1987, the WHO had received notification of AIDS in 129 of the 161 countries submitting mortality reports. Thus, if similar countries were grouped together, the documented experience of some might serve as proxy for the profile of vulnerability unacknowledged in others. In this first decade of the epidemic, global health data served advocacy rather than planning (Ghys *et al.*, 2006). Projecting a global pandemic engaged the attention of multilateral agencies, justifying expenditure and intervention by the WHO, and later the World Bank and other agencies of the United Nations (UN).

Interpolation and exceptions

To project a global epidemic, it would help if the map had no gaps. The maps produced by the epidemiologists were based, although with significant exceptions, on countries grouped into continents. Thus, Asia was typified as having the Type III epidemic with low prevalence and an epidemic starting in the mid-1980s. Yet, in 1988, there had been no cases at all reported from Afghanistan, Bangladesh, Bhutan, Brunei, Dar-es-Salaam, Burma, Kampuchea, North Korea, Laos, Maldives, Mongolia or Vietnam, and only three each from China, Indonesia and Sri Lanka (Panos, 1989a). The map in the *Science* article of 1988 is less confident than the text, indicating only that for Asia, North Africa and Eastern Europe there was 'Pattern 3 or unknown' (Piot *et al.*, 1988, 577), but in another article of the same year, the same region is given as 'Pattern III' without qualification (Chin and Mann, 1988, s250). All of Western Europe was shown as having a Pattern 1 epidemic, with predominantly homosexual transmission and an epidemic starting in the period from the mid-1970s to the early 1980s. Cumulative data reported for September 1989 showed that in several of the countries of Western Europe more than two-thirds of the AIDS cases reported had indeed been for people identifying as homosexual (ranging from 81 per cent in the United Kingdom down to 67 per cent in Denmark, with the Netherlands, Finland, Iceland, Sweden, Norway, West Germany and Belgium falling in descending order between the two). However, in Austria, Portugal, Ireland, Malta, Spain and Italy, this group was not the majority of the epidemic, making up only 16 per cent of the epidemic in Italy and 18 per cent in Spain (Panos, 1989b). Identifying the epidemic as primarily about sexuality (homosexual in Pattern I countries, heterosexual in Pattern II) hid the vulnerability of injecting drug users (by September 1989, 66 per cent of cumulative AIDS cases in Italy, and 62 per cent in Spain; Panos, 1989b).

In an article of 1990, Chin gave HIV infection rates by gender for each continent. It can only have been interpolation that produced for Europe and Australasia precisely the same estimated rates; one in 200 for males and one in 1400 for females (Chin, 1990, s280). It might appear at first blush that this is no more than the developmental logic that Reubi (2015) finds in the global epidemiological understanding of tobacco addiction. However, I will suggest that this interpolation was based on racialised common sense about continents. A global imaginary of racial continents gave the general pattern; and the racial basis of this reasoning is further indicated by the distribution of exceptions. The Americas, north, south and central, were shown as Pattern I, apart from a part of the Caribbean that included Haiti (Piot *et al.*, 1988, 577). Paul Farmer (1992) has remarked upon Haiti's status as the first black republic in the western hemisphere (1804) and as thereby raising the ire of contemporary white slave-owning societies, most notably the USA. Its status as a sort of speck of Africa in the backyard of the USA is a measure of the persistent stigma attaching to this small country (Potter, 2009). In 1988, there were several countries in the Caribbean which had yet to report even as many as ten cases of AIDS and the only countries reporting substantial numbers of cases were Haiti and Puerto Rico; coincidentally the places with perhaps the most intense interaction with the USA (Panos, 1989a). At this time, the 5715 AIDS cases in the Caribbean (Panos, 1989a) were swamped by those of the USA (102,621 cases by August 1989; Panos, 1989b). Over its vast territory the cumulative case prevalence in the USA was 407 cases reported per million people living in 1989, compared to 298 per million in Haiti, but 574 in Puerto Rico and 1345 in the Bahamas. To single out the Caribbean epidemic while treating as a single unit the contiguous land mass of the Americas, north and south, follows a suggestive racial historical geography.

The same logic extends to the preliminary mapping of Africa. Once more there was a very broad-brush geography: North Africa as Pattern III and the rest of Africa Pattern II. But, again, there is a significant exception: South Africa. In an article of 1988 this was the only country in the world shown as having a complex epidemic, a mix of Pattern I and Pattern II. We might ask why this one place was shown as having a mixed epidemic: both a heterosexual and a homosexual epidemic. This conclusion was certainly not dictated by the data. In fact, in terms of cases reported, the AIDS epidemic in South Africa looked very like the so-called Pattern 1 countries. As of 19 April 1988: 'A total of 98 cases had been notified and broken down into risk categories . . . – the majority of cases (81%) falling into the male homosexual/bisexual category' (Schoub *et al.*, 1988, 153). In fact, 81 per cent was equal to the comparable figure for the United Kingdom, the European country with the highest proportion of its cases reported for men identified as homosexual.

On the face of it, it seems odd to have introduced an exception for South Africa, highlighted as the only mixed epidemic in Africa, indeed anywhere in the world. The 98 cases in South Africa from an African total of 19,141 reported by 31 October 1988 (Chinn and Mann, 1988, s249) hardly constituted a significant epidemiological exception at the time. On purely numerical grounds, it would have been more accurate to say that the USA, rather than South Africa, was a mix of Pattern 1 and Pattern 2. It is tempting to conclude that South Africa was characterised as a combination of two patterns because, like oil and water, its black and white people were understood as separate populations, and with a majority black population but a minority white government at the time the characterisation as South Africa as black and hence as likely to have a Pattern 2 epidemic was as questionable as the characterisation of the country as white and thus to be included with the other white countries as having a Pattern 1 epidemic.

African AIDS

The racialisation of epidemiological reasoning is clear in the way that being African was constructed as itself predisposing people to contracting AIDS. An early communication in *The Lancet* about AIDS among people of African origin began by listing the known risk groups for AIDS, remarking that the condition had been found in 'homosexual or bisexual men, in drug addicts, in haemophiliacs, and in Haitian immigrants'; but, the authors remarked: 'To our knowledge there is no report of AIDS and opportunistic infections in previously healthy Black Africans with no history of homosexuality or drug abuse' (Clumeck *et al.*, 1983). Absent identification as homosexual, or as injecting drug users, or haemophiliacs, then, the description of AIDS among black Africans hospitalised in Belgium 'suggests that Black Africans, immigrants or not, may be another group predisposed to AIDS' (Clumeck *et al.*, 1983). Jan Zita Grover (1987) carefully unpicked the dangers of focusing upon risk groups rather than risk behaviours and here we can see very clearly that the risk group language stigmatised identities or, in this case, the occupants of a whole continent, or, rather, the black inhabitants of that continent.

This had consequences for the ways in which AIDS was thought about in some African countries producing, for example, a strongly racialised understanding of AIDS in South Africa. Schoub and co-workers described the AIDS cases among 79 homosexual men as 'a Western AIDS pattern occurring mainly in the white population', whereas the cases of '[seven] black patients' represented 'the beginnings of heterosexually acquired African AIDS' (Schoub *et al.*, 1988, 153). The white men were described as Western, but the black people were African. This is the global imaginary of early AIDS epidemiology, wherein racialised continents structured understandings about the development and expectations about the future trajectory of the epidemic. This imaginary drew upon long-standing notions of darkest Africa (Jarosz, 1992) but in developing an idea of African AIDS, epidemiologists gave a new twist to the idea of Africa as a place where nature was just too strong for local culture, reinforcing a fatalistic view of Africa as naturally a development basket case (Dada, 1990; Patton, 1990). AIDS became an index of an African fatality that clung both to the land and to its black people. Much the same may be said of the association of AIDS with Haiti, in effect, 'the stigmatization of an entire nation' (Pape and Johnson, 1993, s345):

> Stigma stains the imaginary and informs our understanding of Haiti. . . . Perhaps stigma is paired with AIDS even more frequently than the ubiquitous phrase 'the poorest country in the Western Hemisphere' is yoked to Haiti. As Elizabeth Abbott has argued, 'AIDS stamped Haiti's international image as political repression and intense poverty never had.'
> (Jean-Charles, 2011, 63, quoting Abbott, 1988, 255)

Alongside the treatment of being African/black as a risk factor, much of the early epidemiology also proposed that African AIDS was different, and that African

AIDS included the AIDS among black Haitians. One early article, reporting on Uganda, suggested that there was infection with HIV (at the time called HTLV-III and LAV) but that the clinical expression in Uganda suggested the presence of a distinctive disease:

> The first patients were seen in 1982 and new ones are being seen with increasing frequency. Most patients present with fever, an itchy maculopapular rash, general malaise, prolonged diarrhoea, occasional respiratory symptoms, and oral candidiasis, but the most dominant feature is extreme wasting and weight loss. Hence the syndrome is known locally as slim disease.
>
> (Serwadda *et al.*, 1985, 849)

In Uganda they observed that '[s]lim disease occurs predominantly in the heterosexually promiscuous population' (Serwadda *et al.*, 1985, 849). In the Rakai district, bordering Tanzania, HTLV-III was endemic with 10 per cent of adults tested showing seropositivity. In this region the border was crossed repeatedly by traders, and, from 1980, by Tanzanian soldiers. Of 15 traders tested, ten were positive: 'These traders admitted to both heterosexual and homosexual casual contacts. Tanzanian soldiers ... have had frequent heterosexual contact with the local population' (Serwadda *et al.*, 1985, 852). Many of the early cases of AIDS among African people were reported by epidemiologists in Europe, particularly Belgium and France which saw African patients who had either travelled to Europe for treatment or who fell ill while in Europe, as with: 'A previously healthy, married 23-year-old black woman [who] left Zaire for Belgium in June 1981. Neither she nor her husband were drug abusers. Eight days after arriving in Belgium she was hospitalized with fever, weakness, subclavicular adenopathy, and splenomegaly' (Offenstadt *et al.*, 1983). She died in March 1982 after clinical tests had already established the collapse of her immune system in the manner diagnostic of AIDS.

Epidemiologists who had been working on AIDS among black African men treated in Belgium noted the epidemiological and clinical distinctiveness of African AIDS: the sex ratio of patients was more even, and the opportunistic infections among cases from Africa were 'quite similar to those reported among AIDS patients in Haiti, but [were] slightly different from those in the USA' (Colebunders *et al.*, 1985, 10). Reporting on AIDS in the tropics, one early work by Belgian epidemiologists distinguished between an epidemic spread ('un envoi épidémique'; Taelman and Piot, 1984, 331) of the disease in the USA on the one hand, and a disease that could be considered endemic in central Africa and in Haiti such that one might speak of these regions as hearths or at least focii of the disease: '[L]es médecins haïtiens identifient un foyer de SIDA en Haïti confirmant ainsi l'endémicité du SIDA dans ce pays' (ibid.). This distinction in epidemiological pattern separated the Western from the African/Haitian diseases, suggesting that the rapid spread in the first was subsequent to the earlier undetected establishment of the second. Yet, neither of the works cited on AIDS in Haiti offered such a speculation.

One of the studies did indeed suggest that AIDS in Haiti, and among Haitians in the USA, had a distinctive clinical expression, principally 'diarrhoea, fever, weight loss, and *Candida* oesophagitis' (Malebranche *et al.*, 1983, 876), but the authors made no comment on the endemicity of AIDS in Haiti and did not propose that there was a different type of AIDS in Haiti. On the contrary, they suggested that the gastro-intestinal conditions they observed were unlikely to be 'directly related to the putative causal agent of AIDS' but were probably 'related to infectious complications of the underlying immune disorder' (Malebranche *et al.*, 1983, 877). In other words, the mix of opportunistic infections varied with context, climatic or social, but AIDS was fundamentally the same disease. The other study from Haiti cited by Taelman and Piot, rather than identifying differences between Haiti and the USA, in fact underlined the similarities both in the nature of the disease and in the moment of its appearance:

> The first cases of Kaposi's sarcoma and opportunistic infections in homosexual men in the United States were documented in early 1978. We do not believe that AIDS was present in Haiti before 1978. This contention is supported by the clinical experience of the practicing pathologists and dermatologists in Haiti and by our inability to identify earlier cases through examination of autopsy and biopsy records. It also seems likely that Haitians would have presented to U.S. hospitals sooner if AIDS had been occurring in Haiti before 1978.
>
> (Pape *et al.*, 1983, 949)

In drawing a distinction between epidemic AIDS in the USA and endemic AIDS in Haiti, or in Africa, the epidemiologists were over-reaching the evidence. There was a similar bias towards distinguishing African/Haitian AIDS from US AIDS even in the discussion of the sickness among Haitian immigrants inside the USA. The first report from the CDC covered 34 cases, of which 30 were male, and in this respect very like the majority of cases in the USA at that time. However, the CDC reported that '[n]one of the 23 Haitian males questioned reported homosexual activity, and only one gave a history of IV drug abuse' (CDC, 1982b, 360). Rather than questioning the reliability of this testimony, the CDC made Haitians a distinct risk group alongside homosexuals, intravenous drug users and haemophiliacs. This construction of Haitian/African AIDS had serious consequences, and not only for Haiti where the collapse of tourism was immediate: '[T]he Haitian Bureau of Tourism estimated that tourism declined from 75,000 visitors in the winter of 1981–82 to under 10,000 the following year' (Farmer, 1992, 146).

Postcolonial AIDS

The epidemiological construction of a distinctively African AIDS was readily identified as racist by many cultural critics (Austin, 1990; Bass, 1998; Dada, 1990; O'Malley, 1992; Patton, 1990; Treichler, 1989; Watney, 1989). A Canadian journalist, Renée Sabatier (1988), covering the epidemic from a third-world perspective, identified both the risks of the AIDS epidemic for developing countries and also documented the racism and prejudice that informed many AIDS policies. In 2001, contemplating the provision of expensive combination antiretroviral (ARV) therapy in Africa, the head of the United States Agency for International Development was in despair. Africans, he said, 'don't know what watches and clocks are', and thus could not be expected to stick to a treatment regime that required time discipline in the ingesting of medicines (Attaran, 2007). AIDS was fated for Africa, both natural and untreatable. In fact, when effective therapies were provided, compliance among African people was found to be better than in North America itself (Attaran, 2007).

My argument thus far has been that the geographical imaginary that shaped perceptions and representations of AIDS in epidemiology found it too easy to organise the world around racialised continents. I have suggested that there was a policy intention behind interpolation, with data being stretched to allow the concept of a global epidemic, presenting AIDS as a crisis to which every state must needs respond. I have also claimed that the treatment of certain spaces as exceptions to the continental geography of AIDS underlined the essentially racial basis of this geography. I have further proposed that in distinguishing African from Western AIDS, epidemiologists often went further than the data dictated and certainly drew inferences that were resisted by some scientists from the countries that were designated as Pattern II, the African AIDS.

Alongside the racialised categories of some global epidemiological models, there was certainly also explicitly racist commentary in other quarters. The scientific work was sometimes the occasion or excuse for sensationalist and offensive commentary in the mass media (Lupton, 1994). The link between science and tabloid journalism was a commonsense global imaginary of the West. It has two main parts. The first is that epidemic disease is naturally localised in certain deviant groups who are thereby a risk to the 'general population' (Grover, 1987). The second is that epidemic disease comes from outside the West. Of course, this builds on a long history from the Asiatic cholera of the 1830s (Morris, 1976) to the Asiatic flu of 1889 to 1890, 'the first named flu pandemic' (Ryan, 2008, 16). In both respects, Western common sense is animated by disgust in precisely the way Nussbaum (2004, 14) indicates: 'its thought-content is typically unreasonable, embodying magical ideas of contamination, and impossible aspirations to purity, immortality, and nonanimality.' The black body was implicated both socially and spatially in this geopolitics of disgust, as the diseased 'other' both inside and outside the West.

This directly and indirectly endangered black lives. With the disease incorporated into the general white disgust at black bodies, it became very difficult for people of colour to acknowledge their own vulnerability. Respectable black opinion distanced itself from the sorts of bodies stigmatised by racist commentary, bodies that injected drugs or had sexual relations outside heterosexual marriage (Cohen, 1999). Needle-exchange schemes were represented as attempts to promote drug use among African-Americans and on those grounds rejected, as when New York City's first African-American mayor closed down one such programme (Anderson, 1991). In a study of sex education and HIV prevention in the USA, Patton (1996) noted that the representation of African-American males as deviant, as early and hyper-sexualised, produced defeatism, invalidating programmes that may otherwise have addressed their needs. In broad terms, African-Americans were ill-served by what Geary (2014, 18) describes as 'the discourse of queers'; that is, by their treatment as deviants.

Similar difficulties attended the reception of African AIDS discourse in the African countries themselves. In reaction to the stigmatising of Africa as the source of AIDS, and in the mid-1980s, the introduction by Western countries of testing for students and other visitors from certain African countries, commentators in Africa challenged the Western science and the Western policies. At a time when there were more AIDS cases reported from many Western than from African countries, Ochieng (1987), for example, suggested that if the West were truly concerned to limit the spread of the disease it would screen its own residents before allowing them to travel abroad, rather than imposing restrictions upon visitors from Africa. In a comprehensive review of all the grounds for scepticism, Chirimuuta and Chirimuuta (1987, 3) asked: 'How is it possible that this predominantly American disease has been attributed to the African continent?' Their reply was unequivocal: '[T]he medical "experts", the media and the public at large are affected by the insidious and unrecognised disease of racism' (p. 136).

There was justified scepticism about claims that AIDS was widespread and of long standing in Africa, and that AIDS in Africa and among people of African descent was very different from Western AIDS. There was also justified anger that, in concluding so quickly that AIDS was best understood as an African disease, Western scientists and commentators were repeating the stereotypes current during the colonial era; that Africa was naturally disease-ridden, and that only Western technology could mitigate the impress of an unfavourable African disease-ecology. However, in reacting against the colonialist construction of diseased Africa, African politicians and scientists ran the risk of viewing AIDS only as a Western projection lacking any other substance. As more African people became infected with the HIV virus, and later died from the opportunistic infections, denying the reality of AIDS became ever more dangerous, reaching its apogee in the arguments of Thabo Mbeki when, as president of South Africa, he took direct control of his country's anti-HIV programmes. This new discourse on AIDS was an alternative global imaginary and, in retaining as an explicit rejection the earlier colonialist discourses on diseased Africa, it deserves to be called postcolonial.

Mbeki's postcolonial concept of AIDS challenged the Type I/Type II global imaginary. Mbeki repudiated what he called the 'African exceptionalism' that presented African people as 'a peculiar species of humanity' (Mbeki, 1998a). This exceptionalism, he argued, was colonialist:

> To perpetuate their imperial domination over the peoples of Africa, the colonisers sought to enslave the African mind and to destroy the African soul.

They sought to oblige us to accept that as Africans we had contributed nothing to human civilization; except as beasts of burden. . . . In the end, they wanted us to despise ourselves, convinced that, if we were not sub-human, we were, at least, not equal to the colonial master and mistress.

(Mbeki, 1998b)

To repudiate the neo-colonial hold of such ideologies, African peoples must, he suggested, cultivate a profound autonomy:

[S]trengthening the genuine independence of African countries and continent in their relations with the major powers and enhancing their role in the determination of the global system of governance in all fields, including politics, the economy, security, information and intellectual property, the environment and science and technology.

(Mbeki, 1999)

Autonomy would redress 'the perception that as a continent we are condemned forever to depend on the merciful charity which those who are kind are ready to put into our begging bowls', and, in 'a genuine liberation', would put 'an end to the tragic sight of the emaciated child who dies because of hunger or is ravaged by curable diseases because their malnourished bodies do not have the strength to resist any illness' (Mbeki, 1998a). As Gevisser (2007) has shown, this vision of an African renaissance informed most aspects of Mbeki's presidency (1999–2008), including its AIDS policies.

When the International AIDS Conference came to Durban in 2000, Mbeki, as president of South Africa, welcomed its delegates in a speech that reached back, beyond the introduction of successful anti-retroviral therapies in 1996, to the arguments of the WHO in 1995, and quoted the opening of the report:

The world's most ruthless killer and the greatest cause of suffering on earth is listed in the latest edition of WHO's International Classification of Diseases, an A to Z of all ailments known to medical science, under the code Z59.5. It stands for extreme poverty.

(WHO, 1995, 1)

This code is part of Chapter 21 of the *International Statistical Classification of Diseases and Related Health Problems* (10th revision). This section concerns 'Factors influencing health status and contact with health services', and supplements but does not replace the classification of diseases. The WHO classification identifies the 'underlying cause of death', the 'precipitating cause' that is preventable:

The most effective public health objective is to prevent the precipitating cause from operating. For this purpose the underlying cause has been defined as '(a) the disease or injury which initiated the morbid events leading directly to death, or (b) the circumstances of the accident or violence which produced the fatal injury.'

(WHO, 2004, 23)

The WHO specifically counsels that the codes in Chapter 21 should 'not be used . . . for primary mortality coding' and that they are to be understood as recording 'some circumstance or problem . . . which is not in itself a current illness or injury' (WHO, 2008, 1091). Metaphorically, one might see poverty as a cause of death and, in the wake of the bacteriological revolution, epidemiologists continued to speak of the 'predisposing causes' of sickness, with the disease organism conceptualised as the seed and the weak body or insalubrious environment understood to be its receptive soil (Warboys, 2000, 206). However, Mbeki presented HIV disease (B20–B24 in the ICD classification) and Extreme Poverty as alternative causes of death and in contemplating 'the collapse of immune systems among millions of [African] people' he concluded that with a crisis of this magnitude, 'we could not blame everything on a single virus' (Mbeki, 2001[2000], 29).

In this, of course, Mbeki was drawing upon a scepticism about Western medicine stemming in part from the work of Ivan Illich (1974). It was also reinforced by a New Public Health movement that emphasised the social determinants of health and the necessity for preventive rather than curative approaches to sickness (Ashton and Seymour, 1988). This culminated in the WHO's adoption of a positive conception of health with its Ottawa Charter for Health Promotion in 1986 where health was described as not only the absence of disease but as a state of 'complete physical, mental and social well-being' (WHO, 2009, 1). Mbeki held to an extreme version of this perspective, seeing Western medicine as both iatrogenic and as a conspiracy to defraud non-Western countries.

Against the Western medicine AZT (Azidothymidine), Mbeki, even before becoming president, had championed an African drug (Virodene), engineering the removal of the people at the Medicines Control Council who considered the African drug inefficacious (Myburgh, 2009). In this respect, Mbeki drew upon the views of what Youde (2007) calls a 'counter-epistemic community', a group of scientists intensely sceptical of viral explanations of AIDS and suspicious of the motives of other scientists promoting expensive treatments (AZT) for a condition that they had themselves defined (HIV disease). Together with others, including Peter Mokaba, a close adviser who subsequently died of AIDS, he wrote a long and rambling report on AIDS for the national executive committee of the African National Congress (Kenyon, 2008). After reviewing the history of colonial public health policies, and the racist epidemiological writings identified by Chirimuuta and Chirimuuta, the 'dissertation' (Anon., 2002, 102) argued that HIV was only one of the threats to African immune systems; poverty and nutrition were more important. Furthermore, it asserted that 'anti-retroviral drugs can neither cure AIDS nor destroy the HI virus' (Anon., 2002, 7).

Acting on this belief, Mbeki pressured his minister of health, Manto Tshabalala-Msimang, to promote African treatments, including garlic, beetroot and lemon juice, for boosting immune systems (Sidley, 2000). His administration also advocated the trial of African pharmaceuticals rather than ARVs. As Nicoli Nattrass (2012) has argued, there were serious consequences to all this. In the first place, at a time when AZT was making inroads into mother-to-child in utero transmission, South African mothers were denied this medication. Nattrass estimated that 300,000 lives could have been saved if such a prophylactic measure had been instituted. The international pressure on Mbeki was formidable. Ironically, this very proud African was seen by colleagues as having brought shame upon Africa, and, moreover, as denying South Africa access to discounted drugs. In December 2007, he was replaced as head of the ANC by Jacob Zuma whom in 2005 he had dismissed from the post of deputy president following a corruption scandal over arms sales. In September 2008 Zuma got the earlier conviction overturned and a court decided that Mbeki had brought the case against Zuma on petty political grounds (Shange, 2016). The National Executive Committee of the ANC censured Mbeki who immediately resigned as president (Lindow, 2008). Mbeki's postcolonial reading of AIDS was directly responsible for his losing both status and office.

A new global imaginary

With time, the first global imaginary of Type I/Type II countries was modified. Soon after the first maps (see Figure 1.1), the mixture of types was broadened out from South Africa, and in 1989 it was suggested that 'Latin America is in evolution from Pattern I to Pattern II epidemiology and is now classified separately as Pattern I/II' (Sato *et al.*, 1989, s304). By 1992, many questioned the utility of including Asia, Eastern Europe, North Africa and the Middle East as a Type III pattern, characterised only by late onset. Jonathan Mann and co-workers concluded in 1992 that: 'As useful as the patterns were for developing initial understanding of differentiation within the global epidemic, the WHO nomenclature of 1987 rapidly grew out of date and needed replacement' (Mann *et al.*, 1992, 17).

Not only this increasing complexity but also a different conception of disease ecology provoked a new global imaginary. The new conceptualisation of AIDS owed most to Mann's own work. In 1984, Mann was appointed by the CDC to lead a research team investigating heterosexual AIDS in Zaire. The team he joined was emphasising the 'different and important pattern [in central Africa] compared with that of AIDS in other areas' (Piot *et al.*, 1984, 68) and Mann was a co-author of the article in *Science* from which Figure 1.1 was taken (Piot *et al.*, 1988). In 1986, Mann went to the WHO and set up the WHO's Global Programme for AIDS. In his 1987 briefing on AIDS to the UN General Assembly, Mann distinguished three epidemics. The first was of the HIV virus and this would be followed after some years by cases of AIDS as the immune systems of the HIV-infected persons declined to the point where opportunistic infections would manifest. Alongside the epidemics of HIV and later of AIDS, Mann identified a 'third epidemic, of social, cultural, economic and political reaction to AIDS, [which] is also worldwide and is as central to the global AIDS challenge as the disease itself' (Mann, 1987, 1). This third epidemic would be intensified by '[f]ear and ignorance' (p. 3).

Mann was developing some of the ideas of the New Public Health that Mbeki had also been inspired by. In stressing the social and political determinants of health, Mann was also drawing upon the success of the capabilities approach as a new paradigm in global development thinking (Nussbaum, 2011). Mann interpreted the idea that human rights were essential to human flourishing as also suggesting that human rights were vital for organic integrity and longevity. This suggested, he argued, that female education was as vital to health as others find it essential to economic growth (Klasen, 2002). His new geography highlighted the global differences in the Human Development Index (Wahlberg, 2007) and related these to contrasting trajectories in the HIV/AIDS pandemic.

In this context, Mann elaborated a broad vision of the relations between health and human rights, suggesting that the promotion of human rights advanced health and that abridging those rights endangered health (Mann *et al.,* 1994). This human rights agenda structured the new global imaginary of Geographic Areas of Affinity (GAA) that Mann developed as an alternative to the Type I/Type II patterns for describing the global pandemic (Mann *et al.*, 1992). Countering HIV infection by promoting good education, by limiting AIDS sicknesses, by removing the stigma that prevented people from seeking treatment, and by countering social fragmentation, by including HIV-positive people as full and equal members of society, effective human rights should be, argued Mann, at the heart of national and global AIDS policies. For this reason, the GAA were defined not only on the basis of epidemiology but also as incorporating societal factors such as the Human Development Index, the Human Freedom Index, an indicator of gender equality, and a measure of the underlying rate of urbanisation. This new global imaginary was not fully accepted at the WHO, and in particular by Director General Hiroshi Nakajima. Frustrated by a leadership that conceded too much to AIDS policies setting collective protection against individual rights, Mann resigned in 1990 (Hilts, 1990).

This is an alternative global imaginary to the racialised conception of the Type I/Type II, and while it shares some features with Mbeki's postcolonial inversion of racialised geographies, it articulates something quite different. It does not treat colonialism and its legacies as a central feature of the epidemic. It asserts an inverse correlation between female empowerment and HIV vulnerability which is troubled by the evidence that intense repression of extramarital sexuality in some Islamic theocracies, or coercive imprisonment of gay men in Cuba, do indeed reduce some forms of risky behaviour, but with consequences for civil liberties that should be contested on their own terms. In other words, Mann's epidemiological imaginary is also ideological and empirically vulnerable but the full elaboration of those dimensions will require a further and longer paper.

The political salience of global disease imaginaries could not be more clear than in the fates of Thabo Mbeki and of Jonathan Mann. How we understand disease shapes how we configure global geopolitics, and, just as clearly, how we understand global interdependence affects the way we imagine our vulnerability to disease. Mbeki responded in a postcolonial register to the racialised readings in early AIDS epidemiology, and Mann responded in a liberal manner to the burden of disease stigma likewise created by those racialised readings. Medical Geography is always also Geopolitics.

References

Abbott, E., 1988. *Haiti: The Duvaliers and Their Legacy*. New York: McGraw Hill.

Althusser, L., 1971[1970]. 'Ideology and ideological state apparatuses', trans. B. Brewster, in L. Althusser, *Lenin and Philosophy and Other Essays*. New York: Monthly Review Press, pp. 127–186.

Anderson, W., 1991. 'The New York needle trial: The politics of public health in the Age of AIDS.' *American Journal of Public Health* 81(11): 1506–1517.

Anon., 2002. 'Castro Hlongwane, Caravans, Cats, Geese, Foot and Mouth and Statistics: HIV/Aids and the Struggle for the Humanisation of the African.'

Ashton, J. and Seymour, H., 1988. *The New Public Health: The Liverpool Experience*. Milton Keynes: Open University Press.

Attaran, A., 2007. 'Adherence to HAART: Africans take medicines more faithfully than North Americans.' *PLoS Med.* 4(2): e83; doi: 10.1371/journal.pmed.0040083.

Austin, S.B., 1990. 'Aids and Africa: United States media and racist fantasy.' *Cultural Critique* 14: 129–141.

Bass, J.D., 1998. 'Hearts of darkness and hot zones: The ideologeme of imperial contagion in recent accounts of viral outbreaks.' *Quarterly Journal of Speech* 84(4): 430–337.

Carew, J., 1988a. 'Columbus and the origins of racism in the Americas: Part one.' *Race and Class* 29(4): 1–19.

Carew, J., 1988b. 'Columbus and the origins of racism in the Americas: Part two.' *Race and Class* 30(1): 33–57.

CDC [Gottlieb, M.S. *et al.*], 1981. '*Pneumocystis* Pneumonia – Los Angeles.' *Morbidity and Mortality Weekly Report* 30(21) (5 June): 250–252.

CDC [Curran, J.W. *et al.*], 1982a. 'Task Force on Kaposi's Sarcoma and Opportunistic Infections: Epidemiologic aspects of the current outbreak of Kaposi's sarcoma and opportunistic infections.' *New England Journal of Medicine* 306(4) (28 January): 248–252.

CDC, 1982b. 'Opportunistic infections and Kaposi's sarcoma among Haitians in the United States.' *Morbidity and Mortality Weekly Report* 31(26) (9 July): 353–354, 360–361.

Chin, J., 1990. 'Global estimates of AIDS cases and HIV infections' *AIDS* 4(suppl. 1): S277–S283.

Chin, J. and Mann, J.M., 1988. 'The global patterns and prevalence of AIDS and HIV infection.' *AIDS* 2(suppl. 1): s247–s252.

Chirimuuta, R.C. and Chirimuuta, R., 1987. *AIDS, Africa and Racism*. Burton-on-Trent: Chirimuuta.

Clumeck, N., Mascart-Lemone, F., de Maubeuge, J., Brenez, D. and Marcelis, L., 1983. 'Acquired immune deficiency syndrome in black Africans.' *Lancet* 321(8325) (19 March): 642.

Cohen, C.J., 1999. *The Boundaries of Blackness: AIDS and the Breakdown of Black Politics*. Chicago, IL: University of Chicago Press,

Colebunders, R., Taelman, H. and Piot, P., 1985. 'Acquired immunodeficiency syndrome (AIDS) in Africa: A review.' *Tropical Doctor* 15: 9–12.

Dada, M., 1990. 'Race and the AIDS agenda', in T. Boffin and S. Gupta (eds), *Ecstatic Antibodies: Resisting the AIDS Mythology*. London: Rivers Oram Press, pp. 85–95.

Farmer, P.E., 1992. *AIDS and Accusation: Haiti and the Geography of Blame.* Berkeley, CA: University of California Press.

Geary, A.M., 2014. *Antiblack Racism and the AIDS Epidemic.* New York: Palgrave Macmillan.

Gevisser, M., 2007. *Thabo Mbeki: The Dream Deferred.* Johannesburg: Jonathan Ball.

Ghys, P.D., Walker, N. and Garnett, G.P., 2006. 'Improving analysis of the size and dynamics of AIDS epidemics.' *Sexually Transmitted Infections* 82(Supplement 3): 1–2.

Glacken, C.J., 1967. *Traces on the Rhodian Shore: Nature and Culture in Western Thought from Ancient Times to the End of the Eighteenth Century.* Berkeley, CA: University of California Press.

Grover, J.Z., 1987. 'AIDS: Keywords.' *October* 43: 17–30.

Hilts, P.J., 1990. 'Leader in U.N.'s battle on AIDS resigns in dispute over strategy.' *New York Times*, 17 March; Available at http://www.nytimes.com/1990/03/17/us/leader-in-un-s-battle-on-aids-resigns-in-dispute-over-strategy.html (accessed 12 March 2016).

Illich, I., 1974. *Medical Nemesis: The Expropriation of Health.* Edinburgh: Edinburgh University Press.

Jarosz, L., 1992. 'Constructing the Dark Continent: Metaphor as geographic representation of Africa.' *Geografiska Annaler* 74B: 105–115.

Jean-Charles, R.M., 2011. 'The sway of stigma: The politics and poetics of AIDS representation in "Le president a-t-il SIDA" and "Spirit of Haiti".' *Small Axe* 15(3): 62–79.

Kearns, G., 2016. 'Queering epidemiology', in G. Brown and K. Brown (eds), *Ashgate Companion to Geographies of Sex and Sexualities.* Burlington, VT: Ashgate, pp. 263–273.

Kenyon, C., 2008. 'Cognitive dissonance as an explanation of the genesis, evolution and persistence of Thabo Mbeki's HIV denialism.' *African Journal of AIDS Research* 7(1): 29–35.

Klasen, S., 2002. 'Low schooling for girls, slower growth for all? Cross-country evidence on the effect of gender inequality in education on economic development.' *World Bank Economic Review* 16(3): 345–373.

Lewis, M.W. and Wigen, K.E., 1997. *The Myth of Continents: A Critique of Metageography.* Berkeley: University of California Press.

Lindow, M., 2008. 'Why South Africa's Mbeki resigned.' *Time*, 20 September; available at http://content.time.com/time/world/article/0,8599,1843112,00.html (accessed 12 March 2016).

Lupton, D., 1994. *Moral Threats and Dangerous Desires: AIDS in the News Media.* London: Routledge.

Malebranche, R., Guérin, J.M., Laroche, A.C., Elie, R., Spira, T., Drotman, P., Arnoux, E., Pierre, G.D., Péan-Guichard, C., Morisset, P.H., Mandeville, R., Seemayer, T. and Dupuy, J-M., 1983. 'Acquired Immunodeficiency Syndrome with severe gastrointestinal manifestations in Haiti.' *Lancet* 322(8355) (15 October): 873–878.

Mann, J.M., 1987. 'Statement at an informal briefing on AIDS to the 42nd session of the United Nations General Assembly on Tuesday 2th October 1987.' *WHO/SPA>/ INF/87.12*; available at http://apps.who.int/iris/bitstream/10665/61546/1/WHO_SPA _INF_87.12.pdf (accessed 12 March 1987).

Mann, J.M., Tarantola, D.J.M. and Netter, T.W., 1992. *AIDS in the World.* Cambridge, MA: Harvard University Press.

Mann, J.M., Gostin, L., Gruskin, S., Brennan, T., Lazzarini, Z. and Fineberg, H.V., 1994. 'Health and human rights.' *Health and Human Rights* 1(1): 6–23.

Mbeki, T., 1998a. *The African Renaissance, South Africa and the World*. Tokyo: United Nations University; available at http://archive.unu.edu/unupress/mbeki.html (accessed 12 March 2016).

Mbeki, T., 1998b. *The African Renaissance*. Pretoria: Department of International Relations and Cooperation; available at http://www.dfa.gov.za/docs/speeches/1998/mbek0813.htm (accessed 12 March 2016).

Mbeki, T., 2002[1999]. Speech by the President of South Africa, Thabo Mbeki, at the launch of the African Renaissance Institute, Pretoria, 11 October 1999. Durban: African Union Summit; available at http://www.au2002.gov.za/docs/speeches/mbeki991011.htm (accessed 12 March 2016).

Mbeki, T., 2001[2000]. 'Speech by the President of South Africa, Thabo Mbeki, at the opening session of the 13th International AIDS Conference: Durban, 9 July 2000.' *Jornal brasileiro de Doenças Sexualmente Transmissíveis* 13(1): 17–19.

Morris, R.J., 1976. *Cholera 1832: The Social Response to an Epidemic*. London: Croom Helm.

Mudimbé, V.Y., 1988. *The Invention of Africa: Gnosis, Philosophy, and the Order of Knowledge*. London: James Currey.

Myburgh, J., 2009. 'In the beginning there was Virodene', in K. Cullinan and A. Thom (eds), *The Virus, Vitamins and Vegetables: The South African HIV/AIDS Mystery*. Auckland Park, South Africa: Jacana, pp. 1–15.

Nattrass, N., 2012. *The AIDS Conspiracy: Science Fights Back*. New York: Columbia University Press.

Nussbaum, M.C., 2004. *Hiding from Humanity: Disgust, Shame and the Law*. Princeton, NJ: Princeton University Press.

Nussbaum, M.C., 2011. *Creating Capabilities: The Human Development Approach*. Cambridge, MA: Belknap Press.

Ochieng, P., 1987. 'Africa not to blame for AIDS.' *New African* 232: 25.

Offenstadt, G., Pinta, P., Hericord, P., Jagueux, M., Jean, F., Amstutz, P., Valade, S. and Lesavre, P., 1983. 'Multiple opportunistic infection due to AIDS in a previously healthy black woman from Zaire.' *New England Journal of Medicine* 308(13): 775.

O'Malley, J., 1992. 'The representation of AIDS in Third World development', in J. Miller (ed.), *Fluid Exchanges: Artists and Critics in the AIDS Crisis*. Toronto: University of Toronto Press, pp. 169–176.

Pagden, A., 1982. *The Fall of Natural Man: The American Indian and the Origins of Comparative Ethnology*. Cambridge: Cambridge University Press.

Panos, 1989a. 'Datafile.' *WorldAIDS* 3 (May): 15–20.

Panos, 1989b. 'Datafile.' *WorldAIDS* 6 (November): 6–8.

Pape, J.W. and Johnson Jr., W.D., 1993. 'AIDS in Haiti, 1982–1992.' *Clinical Infectious Diseases* 17(Supplement 2): s341–s345.

Pape, J.W., Liataud, B., Thomas, F., Mathurin, J-R., St Amand, M-M.A., Boncy, M., Pean, V., Pamphile, M., Laroche, A.C. and Johnson, W.D., 1983. 'Characteristics of the Acquired Immunodeficiency Syndrome (AIDS) in Haiti.' *New England Journal of Medicine* 309(16): 945–950.

Patton, C., 1990. 'Inventing "Africa AIDS" ', in C. Patton, *Inventing AIDS*. London: Routledge, pp. 77–97.

Patton, C., 1996. *Fatal Advice: How Safe-Sex Education Went Wrong*. Durham, NC: Duke University Press.

Piot, P., Plummer, F.A., Mhalu, F.S., Lamboray, J-L., Chin, J. and Mann, J.M., 1988. 'AIDS: An international perspective.' *Science* NS 239(4840) (5 February): 573–579.

Piot, P., Taelman, H., Minlangu, K.B., Mbendi, N., Ndangi, K., Kalambayi, K., Bridts, C., Quinn, T.C., Feinsod, F.M., Wobin, O., Mazebo, P., Stevens, W., Mitchell, S. and McCormick, J.B., 1984. 'Acquired Immunodeficiency Syndrome in a heterosexual population in Zaire.' *Lancet* 324(8394) (14 July): 65–69.

Potter, A.E., 2009. 'Voodoo, zombies, and mermaids: U.S. newspaper coverage of Haiti.' *Geographical Review* 99(2): 208–230.

Reubi, D., 2015. 'Modernisation, smoking and chronic disease: Of temporality and spatiality in global health.' *Health & Place*; doi: 10.1016/j.healthplace.2015.04.004.

Ryan, J.R., 2008. 'Past pandemics and their outcome', in J.R. Ryan (ed.), *Pandemic Influenza: Emergency Planning and Community Preparedness*. Boca Raton, FL: CRC Press, pp. 1–22.

Sabatier, R., 1988. *Blaming Others: Prejudice, Race and Worldwide AIDS*. London: Panos.

Said, E.W., 1978. *Orientalism*. New York: Vintage Books.

Sartre, J-P., 2004 [1940]. *The Imaginary: A Phenomenological Psychology of the Imagination*, trans. J. Webber. London: Routledge.

Sato, P., Chin, J. and Mann, J.M., 1989. 'Review of AIDS and HIV infection: Global epidemiology and statistics.' *AIDS* 3(suppl. 1): s301–s307.

Schoub, B.D., Smith, A.N., Lyons, S.F., Johnson, S., Martin, D.J., McGillivray, G., Padayachee, G.N., Naidoo, S., Fisher, E.L. and Hurwitz, H.S., 1988. 'Epidemiological considerations of the present status and future growth of the acquired immunodeficiency syndrome epidemic in South Africa.' *SAMJ. South African Medical Journal* 74(20 August): 153–157.

Serwadda, D., Sewankambo, N.K., Carswell, J.W., Bayley, A.C., Tedder, R.S., Weiss, R.A., Mugerwa, R.D., Lwegaba, A., Kirya, G.B., Downing, R.G., Clayden, S.A. and Dalgleish, A.G., 1985. 'Slim disease: A new disease in Uganda and its association with HTLV-III infection.' *Lancet* 326(8460) (19 October): 849–852.

Shange, N., 2016. 'Mbeki said Zuma would be taken care of should he resign – lawyer.' *News24*, 17 January; available at http://www.news24.com/SouthAfrica/News/mbeki-said-zuma-would-be-taken-care-of-should-he-resign-lawyer-20160117 (accessed 12 March 2016).

Shilts, R., 1987. *And the Band Played On: Politics, People and the AIDS Epidemic*. New York: St Martin's Press.

Sidley, P., 2000. 'Clouding the AIDS issue.' *British Medical Journal* 320(7240): 1016–1016.

In Stoddart, DR 1986. *On Geography and its History*. Oxford: Blackwell.

Taelman, H. and Piot, P. 1984. 'Le SIDA en région tropicale: Les foyers haïtien et africain.' *Annales de la Société Belge de Médecine Tropicale* 64: 331–334.

Treichler, P., 1989. 'AIDS and HIV infection in the Third World: A First-World chronicle', in B. Kruger and P. Mariani (eds), *Remaking History*. Seattle, WA: Bay Press, pp. 31–86.

Wahlberg, A., 2007. 'Measuring progress: Calculating the life of nations.' *Distinktion: Journal of Social Theory* 8(1): 65–82.

Warboys, S., 2000. *Spreading Germs: Disease Theories and Medical Practice in Britain, 1865–1900*. Cambridge: Cambridge University Press.

Watney, S., 1994[1989]. 'Missionary positions: AIDS, "Africa" and race', in S. Watney, *Practices of Freedom: Selected Writings on HIV/AIDS*. London: Rivers Oram Press, pp. 109–127.

Webber, J., 2004. 'Philosophical introduction', in J-P. Sartre, *The Imaginary: A Phenomenological Psychology of the Imagination*, trans J. Webber. London: Routledge, pp. xiii–xxvi.

WHO [World Health Organization], 1995. *The World Health Report 1995: Bridging the Gaps*. Geneva: World Health Organization.

WHO, 2004. ICD-10. *International Statistical Classification of Diseases and Related Health Problems* (10th revision), Volume 2, 2nd edn. Geneva: World Health Organization.

WHO, 2008. ICD-10. *International Statistical Classification of Diseases and Related Health Problems* (10th revision), Volume 1, 2008 edn. Geneva: World Health Organization.

WHO, 2009. *Milestones in Health Promotion: Statements from Global Conferences*. Geneva: World Health Organization.

Youde, J.R., 2007. *AIDS, South Africa and the Politics of Knowledge*. Burlington, VT: Ashgate.

2 Temporal and spatial imaginaries of global health

Tobacco, non-communicable diseases and modernity

David Reubi

Introduction

Influenced by the theories on globalisation that became so pervasive following the end of the Cold War, many of those who have written on global health assume that the last decades of the twentieth century have been marked by an accelerated compression of time and space (e.g. Beaglehole and McMichael, 1999; Walt, 2000). For them, the world has become a global village characterised by political, economic and social integration as well as temporal simultaneity. This, they contend, is the consequence of trade liberalisation policies and technological innovations like air travel and the Internet, which have brought about growing flows of people, knowledge, capital and goods around the world. Applying these ideas to public health and biomedicine, these commentators explain that the world we now live in is characterised by a convergence of disease patterns, biomedical knowledge and public health strategies. Often these arguments have been made in relation to infectious diseases, as with the idea that air travel has allowed for the rapid spread of microbes around the global (e.g. Garrett, 1995; Youde, 2012). More importantly for us, similar ideas have also been articulated about non-communicable diseases (NCDs) and their risk factors and, specifically, the smoking epidemic and the chronic diseases to which it contributes (e.g. Yach and Bettcher, 1999; Lee, 2003). So, for example, many commentators have argued that smoking and lung cancer are a global epidemic caused by trade liberalisation and multinational tobacco companies. Likewise, others have argued that 'global advocacy' in the field of tobacco control was made possible by the Internet, which allowed activists from around the world to 'interact simultaneously' (e.g. Yach and Bettcher, 2000; Lee and Collin, 2005).

There is little doubt that these temporalities and spaces of globalisation shape many theories, practices and materialities in today's global health and chronic disease complex (McGoey *et al.*, 2011); but, as an emerging body of research suggests, there are other, often-conflicting spatio-temporal logics at work within this complex (e.g. Tousignant, 2013; Beisel, 2014; cf. also Lakoff and Collier, 2008; Fassin, 2012; Anderson, 2014). This chapter contributes to this research by arguing that there exists, within the contemporary field of global tobacco control, what I term temporalities and spaces of modernisation that have been extremely influential, and stand in stark contrast to the spatial and temporal logics of globalisation. To do so, I examine a statistical model of the global smoking epidemic that has shaped the way tobacco control advocates have thought for the past 20 years and which was elaborated by epidemiologist Alan Lopez and his colleagues at the World Health Organisation (WHO) in the early 1990s. Specifically, drawing upon extensive archival and ethnographic research on the international tobacco control movement,[1] I unpack how this model links the different temporal phases of the epidemic with particular disease patterns, public health policies, geographical regions and levels of development. I also show how many of its assumptions can be traced back to postwar modernisation and development theories. I conclude by exploring what this may mean for our understanding of global health. However, before doing so, I examine the temporalities and spaces of globalisation that may be found in much of the literature on global health.

Temporalities and spatialities of globalisation

In *The Condition of Postmodernity*, geographer David Harvey argued that the world was experiencing a 'time–space compression':

> As space appears to shrink to a 'global village' of telecommunications . . . and as time horizons shorten to the point where the present is all there is . . . so we have to learn to cope with an overwhelming sense of *compression* of our spatial and temporal worlds.
>
> (Harvey, 1989, p. 240)

Harvey further observed that this time–space compression, which had been ongoing since at least the mid-nineteenth century, had recently accelerated because of radical changes in the nature of capitalism and revolutions transport and communication technologies. While particularly influential, Harvey was certainly not alone in articulating these ideas. Indeed, the last decades of the twentieth century saw a growing number of publications and debates on this topic, so much so that ideas about time–space compression and globalisation more generally had gained widespread acceptance by the late 1990s (May and Thrift, 2001; Scholte, 2005).

It is therefore no surprise that these ideas have been so influential among many of those writing about global health over the past 15 years (e.g. Walt, 2000; Lee and Collin, 2005).[2] Borrowing from the work of Marshall McLuhan, David Harvey, Anthony Giddens and others, these writers imagine that the post-Cold War period has been marked by 'a process of increasing economic, political and social interdependence and global integration' (Yach and Bettcher, 1998, p. 735). 'Time and space', they feel, is 'collapsing' (Yach and Bettcher, 2000, p. 206). The world is becoming a 'global village' (Lee and Collin, 2005, p. 15) with 'a sense of transworld simultaneity and instantaneity' (Lee, 2003, p. 105) and a 'shared cosmopolitan culture' (Yach and Bettcher, 2000, p. 206). Following the literature on globalisation, these writers view this 'process of closer integration' as being the result of two key factors (Walt, 2000, p. 1). The first is 'neoliberalism' and, specifically, 'trade liberalisation' (Lee, 2003, p. 65; Harman, 2012, p. 5). The second is the 'revolution in communications and transportation technologies' from the Internet to the aeroplane (Daulaire, 1999, p. 22). These factors, they believe, enable the ever growing 'flows of information, goods, capital and people across political and geographical boundaries' that bring about a global convergence of social, political and economic life (ibid.).

What is innovative in these writings on global health is the way in which they perceive public health and biomedicine through the lens of globalisation and time–space compression (Brown *et al.*, 2006; Fassin, 2012). Thus, for these writers, the world is 'a global health village' characterised by a convergence of disease patterns, biomedical expertise and public health interventions (Yach and Bettcher, 2000, p. 736). Often, these arguments are made in relation to infectious diseases (e.g. Garrett, 1995; Weinberg, 2005; Youde, 2012). Many of these writers argue, for example, that the development of air travel has led to 'the microbial unification of the world' by allowing for the rapid spread of pathogenic micro-organisms (Berlinguer, 1999, p. 18). Another illustration is the way in which the development of new Internet-based, epidemiological surveillance systems allow public health authorities across the globe to know about and guard against pandemics 'in real time' as they unfold (e.g. Weir and Mykhalovskiy, 2010; Caduff, 2014).

Importantly for us, many commentators writing on global health have applied ideas about globalisation and time–space compression to their analysis of NCDs and their risk factors. Some of them have written about the relationship between trade liberalisation in the food industry and the rise of unhealthy diets and NCDs like diabetes (e.g. Smith, 2003; Chopra, 2005). Others have explored the impact of globalisation on the alcohol industry and the chronic disease burden (e.g. Gilmore, 2009; Collin *et al.*, 2014). But most of these commentators have focused on smoking (e.g. Yach and Bettcher, 1999; Lee, 2003; Collin, 2005). The reasons for this are mainly historical: smoking was the first NCD risk factor to be addressed in global health with the adoption of the *WHO Framework Convention on Tobacco Control (FCTC)* in the early 2000s and which now serves as a model for tackling other key NCD risk factors (Yach *et al.*, 2003; WHO, 2003; Casswell and Thamarangsi, 2009). For these commentators, smoking is perceived as a 'global epidemic' defined by worldwide mortality and morbidity figures. One author, for example, argues that 'the global tobacco epidemic' killed an 'estimated four million people' per year around the world (Collin, 2003). 'Transnational tobacco companies', they suggest, are the main driver of this epidemic (Collin, 2005, p. 114). Taking advantage of recent trade liberalisation efforts, these companies are expanding their markets around the globe through sophisticated advertising and marketing campaigns purporting to spread a 'shared [smoking] culture' articulated around 'global [cigarette] brands' and the notion of 'the global smoker' (Yach and Bettcher, 1999; Collin, 2003). These different commentators also draw upon ideas about globalisation and time–space compression to rethink the public health strategies deployed to stop the smoking epidemic. To illustrate, some argue that in order to 'impact tobacco consumption throughout the world' one needs 'global norms and legal instruments' such as the *FCTC* (Yach and Bettcher, 1998, p. 740; Harman, 2012, p. 38). Similarly, others comment that new communication technologies like the Internet have 'profoundly improved' the 'prospects for global advocacy' by allowing experts and activists everywhere to 'interact simultaneously' (Yach and Bettcher, 1998, 2000).

Contextualising the Lopez model

There is no doubt that these temporalities and spatialities of globalisation play an important role within today's global health field, but they are certainly not the only concepts of time and space to shape this field. The temporal and spatial forms associated with an influential epidemiological model of the smoking epidemic elaborated by Alan Lopez and others good examples of such alternative concepts of time and space.[3] However, before we look at these forms in more detail, it is important that we discuss the context in which the model was developed. Lopez's model – which outlines how the smoking epidemic develops in a population over time by charting changes in prevalence, mortality, public attitudes and policies – was designed in the early 1990s by three WHO experts: Lopez, an Australian demographer who worked as chief epidemiologist for the Geneva-based organisation's *Tobacco or Health Programme (THP)*; Neil Collishaw, a sociologist and long-term anti-smoking advocate from Canada also based at the *THP*; and Tapani Piha, a specialist in community medicine from Finland who worked on tobacco control for the WHO's Regional Office for Europe (WHO Europe). The three men outlined their epidemiological model in an article entitled 'A Descriptive Model of the Cigarette Epidemic in Developed Countries', which appeared in 1994 in *Tobacco Control* – the leading journal in the field of international tobacco control (Lopez *et al.*, 1994).

The Lopez model was part of growing international efforts to address the smoking epidemic at the time (Reubi and Berridge, 2016). The internationalisation of tobacco control has a long history stretching back to the 1960s and the organisation of the World Conferences on Tobacco or Health every few years, but it is really from the 1980s onward that international efforts in the field really picked up. One important initiative, though probably not as influential as the International Union against Cancer's *Smoking and Cancer Programme*, was the *THP* where Lopez and Collishaw devised their model. As the WHO's first permanent programme on tobacco control, the *THP* was an understaffed and underfunded operation that, among others, developed standardisation protocols for smoking prevalence surveys and carried out capacity-building workshops in the developing world (Chollat-Traquet, 1990). Another, similar initiative, albeit a more regional one, was the *Action Plan for a Tobacco-Free Europe* launched by WHO Europe and for which Piha was a consultant (WHO Europe, 1993). An important aspect of international tobacco control efforts during this period was the problematisation of smoking in what was then called 'the Third World' (Reubi, 2013). Up until the 1980s, experts believed that chronic diseases and contributing risk factors such as smoking were exclusive to the rich, industrialised nations of the North and that the developing world was all about infectious diseases, malnutrition and poverty. The publication of the WHO report on *Smoking Control in Developing Countries* in 1983 marked a shift in thinking (WHO, 1983). Increasingly, there was a recognition that the smoking epidemic was spreading to the Third World. This, it was imagined, was the result of raising disposable incomes associated with successful economic development and modernisation as well as the tobacco industry's efforts to create new markets throughout Latin America, Asia and Africa. It was to prevent developing countries from facing the additional burden of smoking-related diseases that international initiatives like the *THP* sought to build tobacco control capacity in the Third World.

The Lopez model was also part of late twentieth-century efforts by epidemiologists to formulate credible, global estimates for smoking prevalence and smoking-attributable mortality. At the time, there were a lot of doubts about the reliability of the numbers on smoking produced by the WHO. As an expert involved in international tobacco control efforts during this period remembered:

> We always questioned smoking statistics in those days. Especially those from the WHO, which we thought must simply be wrong.

These doubts were not limited to the data about smoking prevalence and smoking-attributable mortality but extended to the global mortality estimates for most diseases and risk factors published by the WHO (Smith, 2013). The reasons for these doubts were multiple. First, in many countries – indeed, most developing countries – there were no nationwide surveys on smoking habits and no national death registers from which to draw data on tobacco-related mortality (Mackay and Crofton, 1996). Second, the epidemiological models to estimate smoking prevalence and smoking-attributable mortality when data were missing were often very crude (WHO, 1990). Third, there were many instances of double-counting within WHO, with all departments attributing deaths to the diseases for which they were responsible to increase their funding (Smith, 2013). The increasing numbers of epidemiological investigations conducted around that time were often framed as a solution to these problems of reliability. Alan Lopez himself was closely associated with two of these investigations, which directly fed into and shaped the model of the smoking epidemic he developed with Collishaw and Piha. The first was a research project led by Oxford epidemiologist Richard Peto which computed more reliable, global figures for smoking-attributable mortality using a novel estimation technique (Peto and Lopez, 1990; Peto *et al.*, 1994). The second investigation was the Global Burden of Disease project led by Christopher Murray at Harvard which sought to establish global estimates of mortality and disability to allow for more rational policy-making (Murray and Lopez, 1996).

The Lopez model has been and continues to be hugely influential in the field of global tobacco control. The article in *Tobacco Control* where the model was outlined in 1994 has been cited more than 850 times according to Google Scholar.

Unsurprisingly, most experts and activists in the field know and regularly refer to it. As two high-profile tobacco control experts observed:

> The Lopez model has been incredibly influential. . . . It is still used as a frame of reference today even though it was published 20 years ago.

> [The Lopez model] is still as valid today as it was twenty years ago. I still very much use it my work. For all its potential problems, it generally fits what is going on.

The importance of the model in shaping the thinking of tobacco control advocates around the globe was also recently recognised by the editors of the leading journal in the field: *Tobacco Control*. The journal's 20-year anniversary issue, which sought to review 'the major achievements' in the field, contained one article by Peto, Lopez and others in which they revisited and, aside from a change to smoking and smoking-attributable mortality rates for women, confirmed the overall validity of their 1994 'landmark model' in the light of new epidemiological data (Malone and Warner, 2012, pp. 72–73; Thun *et al.*, 2012). The model was also very influential for advocacy and policy-making. Indeed, both tobacco control experts and historians agree that, together with the new epidemiological estimates provided by Peto and his colleagues, it played a decisive role in the adoption of the *FCTC* in the early 2000s (Reynolds and Tansey, 2012). More recently, experts mandated by the Bill and Melinda Gates Foundation used the Lopez model to show the surprisingly large number of lives that could be saved through the prevention of the upcoming smoking epidemic in sub-Saharan Africa, thereby legitimising philanthropy's efforts to develop a tobacco control movement across the subcontinent (Blecher and Ross, 2014).

Of time and space in the Lopez model

To unpack the notions of time and space that underpin the Lopez model, one needs to examine the way in which the model imagines the smoking epidemic. As already mentioned, the model outlines how the epidemic develops in the population of a country over a 100-year time period. The model is based on statistical data from a few Western countries and, in particular, the USA and the UK, which were among the first to experience the epidemic and where there has been the necessary epidemiological infrastructure to record smoking prevalence and smoking-related mortality (Berridge, 2007; Brandt, 2007). Many of the assumptions around which the Lopez model is built, such as the 100-year period over which the epidemic is represented, derive from the particularities of this data. The model identifies four successive, 25-year-long phases – which Lopez and his colleagues term Stage I, Stage II, Stage III and Stage IV – through which the epidemic unfolds. For all four stages, the epidemic is characterised along three explicit variables. The first is smoking prevalence, understood as 'the percentage of the adult population who smoke regularly' (Lopez *et al.*, 1994, p. 243). The second is smoking-related mortality, defined as the 'numbers of deaths' caused by smoking 'through a variety of diseases, principally several sites of cancer, major vascular diseases and chronic lung diseases' (ibid.). Given the difference in smoking patterns among men and women in the USA and the UK, the model further breaks down these first two variables by male and female. The third variable, which unlike the first two is not numerical, is public attitudes towards smoking and the state of tobacco control policies.

Lopez and his colleagues offer both a narrative and a graphic account of the four stages of the epidemic using these three variables (cf. Figure 2.1). Stage I describes the beginning of the smoking epidemic: male prevalence starts rising reaching 15 per cent, while female prevalence remains low 'because of socio-cultural factors' which discourage women from smoking; 'death and disease due to smoking are not yet evident'; and 'smoking becomes socially acceptable and tobacco control strategies remain underdeveloped, with priority being given to reducing malnutrition and the burden of infectious diseases' (Lopez et al., 1994, p. 244). Stage II sees the epidemic develop further: male prevalence continues to grow rapidly, peaking at 60 per cent; female prevalence increases dramatically to reach over 30 per cent; smoking-related deaths among men start rising, typically mirroring the rise in smoking prevalence with a 20-year time-lag because of the late onset of lung cancer, chronic obstructive pulmonary disease and some cardio-vascular diseases; and tobacco control policies remain weak, with 'a lack of public and political support, in part because of the risks of tobacco use may still not be widely understood' (ibid.).

Stage III seems to represents a turning point in the epidemic: 'male prevalence begins to decline' to around 40 per cent, while female prevalence plateaus at 40 per cent before decreasing; smoking-related mortality among men rises dramatically, accounting for 30 per cent of all deaths by the close of the period; smoking-attributable mortality among women also starts to grow; at the same time, public attitudes towards smoking change, with 'knowledge about the health hazards of tobacco [now] generally widespread' and smoking becoming a 'socially abnormal behaviour' leading to the implementation of tobacco control policies (Lopez et al., 1994, pp. 244–245). Stage IV represents the tail end of the epidemic: 'smoking prevalence for both sexes continues to decline'; smoking-related mortality among men begins to slowly decrease, while mortality among women is still increasing, reaching 20 per cent by the end of the stage; and public attitudes towards smoking harden and anti-smoking policies become more comprehensive (ibid., p. 245).

Crucially for the argument made here, there is a fourth, unspoken variable along which Lopez and his colleagues characterise the smoking epidemic: the level of economic development of the country in which the epidemic is unfolding. Indeed, they implicitly posit that the more developed a country is, the more it will have progressed through the stages of the smoking epidemic. Moreover, they tacitly associate the level of development and stages of the epidemic with different geographical regions. This is evident in the way Lopez and his colleagues relate particular stages of the epidemic to particular countries. Thus, they explain that 'many developing countries, primary in sub-Saharan Africa, are currently in Stage I', which is characterised by growing smoking prevalence rates among men and no tobacco control policies

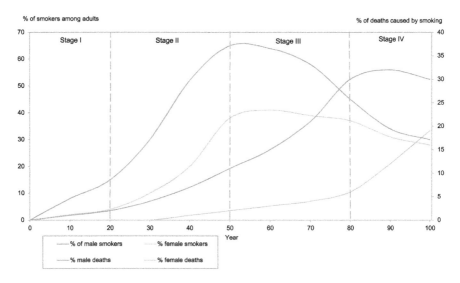

Figure 2.1 The Lopez model of the smoking epidemic.
Source: Adapted from Lopez *et al.* (1994, p. 246).

owing to the prioritisation of malnutrition and infectious diseases by governments and health experts (Lopez *et al.*, 1994, p. 246). Similarly, they assert that countries that are further along in their economic development 'such as China, Japan and other countries of Asia, Latin America and North Africa' are in Stage II, which is typified by dramatic increases in smoking prevalence, a lack of awareness about the dangers of tobacco and weak tobacco control policies (ibid.). In contrast, they argue that most of the rich, industrialised 'countries of Western Europe, along with Australia, Canada and the US, are nearing the end of Stage III or [have passed] into Stage IV', which are marked by a decline in smoking prevalence, public opposition to smoking and comprehensive tobacco control policies (Lopez *et al.*, 1994, pp. 245–246).

By linking smoking with development and geography, Lopez and his colleagues were tapping into ideas about tobacco in the developing world that had become common among public health experts after the early 1980s, when smoking was being identified as a problem for the Third World (Reubi, 2013). One such idea was the notion that developed and developing countries were at opposite ends of the smoking epidemic (e.g. WHO, 1983; Peto *et al.*, 1994). In the former, it was believed, the epidemic was subsiding, while in the latter, the epidemic was only just beginning. As a prominent tobacco control expert argued:

> The difference between developed and developing countries is one of timing. . . . A lot of what is going on right now in the developing world is not dissimilar to what went on in the developed world, many, many decades ago.

Closely related to this first idea was the view that 'smoke-and-health consciousness in [developing] societies lags behind that of the developed world by two or three decades' (Warner, 1984, p. 37). As one academic with an extensive experience of the global tobacco control field noted:

> In many developing countries, you do not see any support for tobacco control at any level – no governmental policies, no governmental agencies, no anti-smoking movement, no research. There is just not much of anything.

Another important idea about smoking and development that dominated the global tobacco control field after the 1980s was the notion that the two major causes of the tobacco epidemic in the Third World were: (1) the successful economic development of countries in the Global South, which meant that their citizens were getting richer and had more spending power for discretionary items like cigarettes; and (2) the tobacco industry's expansion into the developing world to take advantage of this new spending power and compensate their declining sales of cigarettes in the North (e.g. WHO, 1983; Stebbins, 1990; Warner, 2000). Unsurprisingly perhaps, many international tobacco control advocates bemoaned the relationship between successful economic development and increasing smoking rates, describing it as 'defective modernization' and an illustration of 'the Third World modernizing all too quickly' (Warner, 1984, p. 37; Stebbins, 1990, p. 228).

The Lopez model did not only reiterate these pre-existing ideas about smoking and development; it elaborated them further. To start with, the model made it clear that not all developing countries were the same in terms of smoking patterns, public attitudes to smoking and tobacco control policies. As mentioned above, it tacitly assumed that countries that were more developed were at a more advanced stage of the tobacco epidemic. And it correlated these differences in smoking and development to particular geographical regions, with Asian and Latin American nations associated with higher levels of development, greater smoking prevalence and superior tobacco control programmes than African societies. As one international activist observed:

> The model shows that you cannot lump all developing countries together . . . there are Asian and Latin American countries that one might still refer to as developing countries where there is heavy smoking by males, very low smoking by females . . . there are African countries where smoking is still relatively novel, where smoking is still very much on the rise and very much at the beginning of the epidemic.

Furthermore, the Lopez model also bestowed scientific legitimacy upon many of these pre-existing ideas about development and smoking with scientific legitimacy. It did so by translating these ideas into numbers and graphs, and by having them published in an internationally recognised academic journal (Latour, 1990; Porter, 1995). This was important for global tobacco control activists, who had come to view scientific truth as a marker of their moral integrity and an advantage they had over the tobacco industry (Larsen, 2008).

It is important to note that the Lopez model's relationship with developed countries is not the same as with developing countries. For the former, the model is 'historical in nature' in the sense that they are currently in Stage IV after having effectively gone through the previous three stages (Lopez *et al.*, 1994, p. 245). In contrast, for the latter the model is more dynamic. Indeed, while these countries are currently located in Stage I or Stage II, their future is still indeterminate to a certain extent. One prospect is to do as developed societies have done before and go through the next two or three stages of the epidemic as described in the Lopez model. That means letting the epidemic follow its course before tackling it in Stage III and Stage IV. But, as Lopez and his colleagues point out, developing countries 'can prevent history repeating itself' and chose for themselves a better, healthier future (ibid.). This necessitates them taking 'strong public health measures to arrest the growth of tobacco consumption' at 'earlier stages of the epidemic' and, specifically, 'during Stage I or Stage II' (Lopez *et al.*, 1990, pp. 245–246). This, of course, was possible because of the extensive knowledge about smoking and how to tackle it accumulated by experts in the Global North. As Lopez and his colleagues explained, developing countries 'have the advantage of knowing the serious health consequences of smoking' and have at their disposal an array of already existing 'effective prevention interventions' to address the problem (Lopez *et al.*, 1990, p. 245).

Intriguingly, Lopez and his colleagues use the case of Singapore – the poster child of successful economic development and modernisation – to illustrate their point (Reubi, 2010). As they explain, in the 1970s, the Southeast Asian Republic was both at the start of its development effort and 'in the early part of Stage II of the cigarette epidemic', with smoking prevalence at about 42 per cent among men and 10 per cent among women and weak tobacco control policies (Lopez *et al.*, 1994, p. 246). Twenty years later, in the 1990s, at a time when Singapore was close to becoming a developed nation, it should, if it had let the epidemic run its course unchecked, have been entering Stage III, with smoking prevalence at 60 per cent among men and 40 per cent among women and still weak anti-smoking policies. Instead, it had, in the 1970s, adopted comprehensive tobacco control measures borrowed from Europe and North America, which had brought smoking prevalence rates down to 33 per cent among men and 3 per cent among women – figures that were more akin to the end of Stage IV than the start of Stage III. In other words, at the same time that the Asian city state was going through an accelerated process of modernisation, it had also managed to progress through Stages II and III of the smoking epidemic at about two to three times the 'normal' speed.

Temporalities and spaces of modernisation

Many of the spatio-temporal notions that underpin the work of Lopez and his colleagues can be traced back to the modernisation and development theories that dominated the field of international politics after the Second World War (Escobar, 1995; Ekbladh, 2011). As Wahlberg (2007) shows, these theories are built around a distinctive conception of human progress centred on nation-states and stages of development. For proponents of these theories, all states and their populations go through the same sequence of stages as they progress from underdevelopment to development. Modelled on the history of the rich, industrialised nations of North America and Europe, these stages are characterised by particular social, political, economic, demographic and epidemiological conditions. As Wahlberg (2007) further shows, there were many examples of this way of conceptualising and grading progress in the development literature. An influential one was the model outlined by Walt Rostow in *The Stages of Economic Growth*. At one end of the development continuum was 'traditional society', which, Rostow believed, was characterised by 'pre-Newtonian science and technology', 'family and clan connexions', 'fatalism' and a reliance on 'agriculture' (Rostow, 1960, pp. 4–5). At the other end was 'the age of high mass-consumption' typified by high 'income', an 'urban' population 'working in offices' and 'durable consumer goods' such as 'automobiles' (ibid., pp. 10–11). In between these two poles, Rostow talked about 'take-off' and 'drive to maturity', which he associated with the 'building of an effective centralised national state', the emergence of 'banks and institutions for mobilising capital', a 'new type of enterprising men', 'new industries' and an embrace of 'modern science' (ibid., pp. 6–10).

Another influential example of this way of conceptualising progress was Abdel Omran's paper on 'The Epidemiological Transition'. The distinctive aspect of Omran's work was the addition of demographic and epidemiological dimensions to the stages of development outlined by Rostow. Thus, according to Omran (1971, pp. 533–534), traditional society, which he termed 'the Age of Pestilence and Famine', was not only defined by the social, political and economic traits outlined by Rostow but also by high fertility, low life expectancy, infectious diseases and malnutrition. Likewise, Omran posited that Rostow's age of mass consumption, which he called 'the Age of Degenerative and Man-Made Disease', was not only characterised by a central state, industrialisation and science, but also by low fertility, high life expectancy, ageing populations and chronic disease (ibid.). Most of these ideas developed by Rostow and Omran could be found in what was probably the most influential postwar conceptualisation of human progress: the categories of 'Industrialised Countries' (First World), 'Centrally Planned Economies' (Second World) and 'Middle and Low Income Countries' (Third World) outlined by the World Bank in its first *World Development Report* (World Bank, 1978, p. ix). Indeed, the Bank associated development not only with 'economic growth', industrialisation, 'improvements in transportation, communications and electric power', a 'dynamic entrepreneurial class' and 'technological sophistication', but also with 'a rapid expansion of education systems, growing literacy, improvements in nutrition and health conditions', 'greater urbanisation' and 'reduced fertility' (ibid., pp. 1–7).

These stages of development allowed experts in the field to judge the progress and development of nations by situating them in both time and space. Unsurprisingly, North American and European countries were deemed to be in the later stages of development and associated with progress and modernity. To illustrate, Rostow linked his age of high mass consumption with 'the United States', 'Western Europe and Japan' (Rostow, 1960, p. 11). In contrast, the poor, developing nations of the Global South were thought to be in the earlier stages of development and viewed as traditional and backward. In its 1978 report, for example, the Bank identified most countries in sub-Saharan Africa as Low Income while it described the majority of nations in Southeast Asia and Latin America as Middle Income (World Bank, 1978). The location of a country in time and space, however, was not immutable. Specifically, modernisation theorists believed that Third World countries could improve their levels of development and move to a more advanced stage, thus reducing the spatio-temporal gap that separated them from North America and Europe (Ekbladh, 2011). Such efforts at accelerated development were made possible by technical and financial assistance from developed countries and generally involved the establishment of a strong, centralised state together with the creation of the physical infrastructure and human resources necessary for rapid industrialisation (Reubi, 2010).

The parallels between modernisation theories and the Lopez model are readily apparent. To start with, both are articulated around the idea that all countries go through the same successive stages – stages of development for modernisation theories; stages of the smoking epidemic for the Lopez model. Furthermore, in both cases, these stages are modelled on the history of Europe and America, assuming thereby that all developing countries should follow the same path as the rich, industrialised nations of the Global North. This assumption has, in the case of modernisation theories, been extensively criticised for foreclosing alternative paths of development (Escobar, 1995). It has also been problematic for the Lopez model, with, for example, women in most developing countries not taking up smoking as the model predicted (Thun *et al.*, 2012). Another parallel between modernisation theories and the Lopez model is that they both characterise each of the stages a country goes through by an amalgam of economic, political, social, demographic and epidemiological features. Similarly, in both cases, the sequence of stages is used to position a country in time and space, making it possible to group it with some nations and differentiate it from others. Finally, both modernisation theories and the Lopez model assume that a country in the early stages of development or the smoking epidemic can, by drawing on the knowledge accumulated by experts in North America and Europe, choose to progress faster through the remaining, successive stages.

Conclusion

I have sought to draw attention to some of the temporal and spatial logics at work in the field of global health and chronic disease. As I have showed, many commentators writing on global health have been strongly influenced by globalisation theories and notions of time–space compression. The world, they believe, is becoming a 'global village' characterised by temporal simultaneity and a convergence of political, economic and social life. This process of convergence, they also believe, is the result of the ever growing global flows of information, capital and goods across political and geographical boundaries made possible by trade liberalisation and revolutions in communication and transportation. Applying these ideas to health, they argue that the world is increasingly characterised by a global convergence of disease patterns, biomedical knowledge and public health strategies. To validate their claims, these commentators point to a range of recent developments in global health. Some relate to infectious diseases such as the rapid spread of microbes associated with air travel and Internet-based epidemiological surveillance systems that allow public health authorities to tackle epidemics 'in real time'. But many others relate to chronic diseases and the smoking epidemic in particular, including: the worldwide dissemination of unhealthy behaviours like smoking brought about by trade liberalisation and multinational tobacco corporations; transnational anti-smoking advocacy networks made possible by Internet-based communication technologies; and the adoption of global public health norms like those of the *FCTC*.

There is little doubt that temporalities and spatialities of globalisation shape many of the institutions, theories and practices that make up the contemporary field of global health and chronic disease. But, as I have argued in this chapter, they are not the only notions of time and space at work within this field. Rather, they work alongside many other, often contradictory spatio-temporal logics. The temporalities and spatialities underpinning the Lopez model explored in this chapter are a case in point. Unlike the temporalities and spatialities of sameness described in much of the literature on global health, the Lopez model is articulated around temporalities and spatialities of difference. This, of course, is not the difference celebrated by postmodern thinkers (e.g. Lyotard, 2004; Bauman, 2005), but the difference of modernisation theories built around nation states, sequential stages and progress. Indeed, the Lopez model, in stark contrast to the 'one world, one time, one health' mantra of globalisation, divides the world into nation states and orders them along epidemiological, geographical and development lines.

More generally perhaps, this chapter also speaks and contributes to the growing body of critical studies in global health (e.g. Fassin, 2012; Biehl and Petryna, 2013; Anderson, 2014). According to these scholars, the field of global health is characterised by 'tensions and contradictions' as well as by 'failures and resistances' (Fassin, 2012, pp. 107 and 113). They encourage us to recognise this 'uneven terrain' and think of 'the globalisation of health . . . as a heterogeneous and contested historical phenomenon' (Fassin, 2012, p. 99; Anderson, 2014, p. 372). This article very much follows this lead, depicting how different, even contradictory, spatio-temporal logics, each with their own strengths and weaknesses, work alongside each other within the global health field. Furthermore, it shows the importance of knowledge and expert discourses such as globalisation and modernisation theories in the making of the notions and practices that are part of and inform contemporary global health, something also repeatedly emphasised in critical studies of global health (e.g. Lakoff and Collier, 2008; Reubi, 2013; Gaudillière, 2014).

Acknowledgements

An earlier version of this chapter was published in *Health & Place*, Volume 39, pp. 188–195. I would like to thank the public health activists and experts interviewed for this research. I would also like to thank Simon Rushton for his insightful observations, which helped to markedly improve this chapter. Earlier versions were presented at the Cancer Cultures Conference at the Anthropology Department at University College London, the Royal Geographical Society's Annual Conference and the British International Studies Association's Annual Conference. I would like to thank the participants for their helpful and constructive comments. Last but not least, I am very grateful to the Wellcome Trust for their generous financial support through a Small Medical Humanities Research Grant and a Society and Ethics Research Fellowship.

Notes

1 This research was articulated around three main data-collection strategies: (1) articles were gathered from a literature search on global tobacco control in major online databases and the British Library catalogue; (2) documents were obtained from organisations active in global tobacco control such as the WHO and the Framework Convention Alliance; and (3) over 100 semi-structured interviews were conducted with tobacco control experts and advocates in accordance with standard ethical principles and procedures (cf. Latour, 1993; Prainsack and Wahlberg, 2013). This corpus of texts and interviews was examined to identify the notions of temporality and spatiality around which the advocates and experts that make up the global tobacco control movement conceptualise, narrate and experience the smoking epidemic. Although these advocates and experts often come from different socio-economic and geographical backgrounds, it is important to note that their styles of thinking and reasoning are remarkably similar and consistent over time (Fleck, 1979; Hass, 1992; Hacking, 2002).

2 While the literature on globalisation and health has been very influential within the field of global health, it has existed alongside two other bodies of work. The first is the research on cost-effectiveness and the global burden of disease carried out by epidemiologists and economists like Dean Jamison, Christopher Murray and Alan Lopez. Concerned with health planning and financing in low- and middle-income countries, this work does not engage with theories of globalisation and is, like the Lopez model, markedly influenced by modernisation theories (e.g. Jamison *et al.*, 1993; Murray and Lopez, 1996). The second is the anthropological and geographical research that is deeply sceptical of the global and celebrates the local, emphasising resistance to, mistranslation and re-appropriation of biomedical and public health discourses by community leaders, doctors and patients in particular places (e.g. Kelly and Beisel, 2011; Livingstone, 2012; Lawhon and Herrick, 2013).

3 As science and technology studies have suggested (e.g. Evans, 1999; Morgan and Morrison, 1999; Sismondo, 1999), scientific models like the epidemiological model devised by Lopez and his colleagues are best understood as heterogeneous assemblages of scientific theory, mathematical techniques, moral values, social categories, graphic representations, empirical data and narratives. At once representations, predictions and tools for intervention, they are critical in the production of contemporary scientific and political truths.

References

Anderson, W., 2014. Making Global Health History: The Postcolonial Worldliness of Biomedicine. *Social History of Medicine* 27(2): 372–384.

Bauman, Z., 2005. *Liquid Life*. Polity Press, Cambridge.

Beaglehole, R. and McMichael, A., 1999. The Future of Public Health in a Changing Global Context. *Development* 42(2): 12–16.

Beisel, U., 2014. On Gloves, Rubber and the Spatio-Temporal Logics of Global Health. Available at somatosphere.net (accessed 13 October 2014).

Berlinguer, G., 1999. Health and Equity as a Primary Global Goal. *Development* 42(2): 17–21.

Berridge, V., 2007. *Marketing Health Smoking and the Discourse of Public Health in Britain, 1945–2000*. Oxford University Press, Oxford.

Biehl, J. and Petryna, A., eds, 2013. *When People Come First: Critical Studies in Global Health*. Princeton University Press, Princeton, NJ.

Blecher, E. and Ross, H., 2014. *Tobacco Use in Africa: Tobacco Control Through Prevention*. American Cancer Society, Atlanta.

Brandt, A., 2007. *The Cigarette Century*. Basic Books, New York.

Brown, T.M., Cueto, M. and Fee, E., 2006. The World Health Organization and the Transition from 'International' to 'Global' Public Health. *American Journal of Public Health* 96(1): 62–72.

Caduff, C., 2014. Sick Weather Ahead. *Cambridge Anthropology* 32(1): 32–46.

Casswell, S. and Thamarangsi, T., 2009. Reducing Harm from Alcohol: Call to Action. *The Lancet* 373: 2247–2257.

Chollat-Traquet, C., 1990. WHO Tobacco or Health Programme. In Durston, B. and Jamrozik, K., eds, *Tobacco and Health 1990*. Health Department, Perth, Western Australia, pp. 314–316.

Chopra, M., 2005. The Impact of Globalization on Food. In Lee, K. and Collin, J., eds, *Global Change and Health*. Open University Press, Maidenhead, pp. 42–52.

Collin, J., 2003. Think Global, Smoke Local. In Lee, K., ed., *Health Impacts of Globalization*. Palgrave Macmillan, Basingstoke, pp. 61–85.

Collin, J., 2005. The Global Economy and the Tobacco Pandemic. In Lee, K. and Collin, J., eds, *Global Change and Health*. Open University Press, Maidenhead, pp. 111–125.

Collin, J., Johnson, E. and Hill, S., 2014. Government Support for Alcohol Industry: Promoting Exports, Jeopardising Global Health? *British Medical Journal* 348: g3648.

Daulaire, N., 1999. Globalization and Health. *Development* 42(2): 22–24.

Ekbladh, D., 2011. *The Great American Mission*. Princeton University Press, Princeton, NJ.

Escobar, A., 1995. *Encountering Development*. Princeton University Press, Princeton, NJ.

Evans, R., 1999. Economic Models and Policy Advice. *Science in Context* 12(2): 351–376.

Fassin, D., 2012. The Obscure Object of Global Health. In Inhorn, M. and Wentzell, E., eds, *Medical Anthropology at the Intersections*. Duke University Press, Durham, NC, pp. 95–115.

Fleck, L., 1979. *Genesis and Development of a Scientific Fact*. University of Chicago Press, Chicago, IL.

Garrett, L., 1995. *The Coming Plague*. Penguin, New York.

Gaudillière, J-P., 2014. De la santé publique internationale à la santé globale. In Pestre, D., ed., *Le gouvernement des technosciences*. Editions La Découverte, Paris, pp. 65–96.

Gilmore, A., 2009. Action Needed to Tackle a Global Drink Problem. *The Lancet* 373(9682): 2174–2176.

Hacking, I., 2002. *Historical Ontology*. Harvard University Press, Cambridge, MA.

Harman, S., 2012. *Global Health Governance*. Routledge, Abingdon, Oxon.

Harvey, D., 1989. *The Condition of Postmodernity*. Blackwell, Cambridge.

Hass, P., 1992. Epistemic Communities and International Policy Coordination. *International Organization* 46(1): 1–35.

Jamison, D.T., Mosley, W.H., Measham, A.R. and Bobadilla, J.L., eds, 1993. *Disease Control Priorities in Developing Countries*. Oxford University Press, Oxford.

Kelly, A. and Beisel, U., 2011. Neglected Malarias: the Frontlines and Back Alleys of Global Health. *Biosocieties* 6(1): 71–87.

Lakoff, A. and Collier, S., eds, 2008. *Biosecurity Interventions: Global Health and Security in Question*. Columbia University Press, New York.

Larsen, L.T., 2008. The Political Impact of Science. *Science and Public Policy* 35(10): 757–769.

Latour, B., 1990. Drawing Things Together. In Lynch, M. and Woolgar, S., eds, *Representation in Scientific Practice*. MIT Press, Cambridge, pp. 19–68.

Latour, B., 1993. *The Pasteurization of France*. Harvard University Press, Cambridge, MA.

Lawhon, M. and Herrick, C., 2013. Alcohol Control in the News: The Politics of Media Representations of Alcohol Policy in South Africa. *Journal of Health, Politics, Policy and Law* 38(5): 989–1025.

Lee, K., 2003. *Globalization and Health*. Palgrave Macmillan, Basingstoke.

Lee, K. and Collin, J., eds, 2005. *Global Change and Health*. Open University Press, Maidenhead.

Livingstone, J., 2012. *Improvising Medicine: an African Oncology Ward in an Emerging Cancer Epidemic*. Duke University Press, Durham, NC.

Lopez, A., Collishaw, N. and Piha, T., 1994. A Descriptive Model of the Cigarette Epidemic in Developed Countries. *Tobacco Control* 3(3): 242–247.

Lyotard, J-F., 2004. *The Postmodern Condition*. Manchester University Press, Manchester.

Mackay, J. and Crofton, J., 1996. Tobacco and the Developing World. *British Medical Bulletin* 52(1): 206–222.

Malone, R.E. and Warner, K.E., 2012. Tobacco Control at Twenty. *Tobacco Control* 21(2): 74–76.

May, J. and Thrift, N., 2001. *TimeSpace: Geographies of Temporality*. Routledge, London.

McGoey, L., Reiss, J. and Wahlberg, A., 2011. The Global Health Complex. *BioSocieties* 6: 1–9.

Morgan, M. and Morrison, M., eds, 1999. *Models as Mediators*. Cambridge University Press, Cambridge.

Murray, C.J.L. and Lopez, A.D., eds, 1996. *The Global Burden of Disease*. Harvard University Press, Cambridge, MA.

Omran, A., 1971. The Epidemiologic Transition. *Milbank Memorial Fund Quarterly* 49(4/1): 509–538.

Peto, R. and Lopez, A.D., 1990. The Future Worldwide Health Effects of Current Smoking Patterns. In Durston, B. and Jamrozik, K., eds, *Tobacco and Health 1990*. Health Department, Perth, Western Australia.

Peto, R., Lopez, A.D., Boreham, J., Thun, M. and Heath, C., 1994. *Mortality from Smoking in Developed Countries, 1950–2000*. Oxford University Press, Oxford.

Porter, T., 1995. *Trust in Numbers.* Princeton University Press, Princeton, NJ.

Prainsack, B. and Wahlberg, A., 2013. Situated Bio-Regulation: Ethnographic Sensibility at the Interface of STS, Policy Studies and the Social Studies of Medicine. *Biosocieties* 8: 336–359.

Reubi, D., 2010. The Will to Modernize. *International Political Sociology* 4: 142–158.

Reubi, D., 2013. Health Economists, Tobacco Control and International Development. *Biosocieties* 8(2): 205–228.

Reubi, D., & Berridge, V. (2016). The Internationalisation of Tobacco Control, 1950–2010. Medical History, 60(4). 10.1017/mdh.2016.97.

Reynolds, L.A. and Tansey, T., eds, 2012. WHO Framework Convention on Tobacco Control. *Wellcome Witnesses to Twentieth Century Medicine*, Vol. 43. Queen Mary University of London, London.

Rostow, W.W., 1960. *The Stages of Economic Growth.* Cambridge University Press, Cambridge.

Scholte, J.A., 2005. *Globalization: A Critical Introduction.* Palgrave Macmillan, Basingstoke.

Sismondo, S., 1999. Models, Simulations and their Objects. *Science in Context* 12(2): 247–260.

Smith, J.N., 2013. The New Book of Life. Available at www.jeremynsmith.com (accessed 15 September 2014).

Smith, R., 2003. The Impact of Globalization on Nutrition Patterns. In Lee, K., ed., *Health Impacts of Globalization.* Palgrave Macmillan, Basingstoke, pp. 86–104.

Stebbins, K.R., 1990. Transnational Tobacco Companies and Health in Underdeveloped Countries. *Social Science and Medicine* 30(2): 227–235.

Thun, M., Peto, R., Boreham, J. and Lopez, A.D., 2012. Stages of the Cigarette Epidemic on Entering its Second Century. *Tobacco Control* 21(2): 96–101.

Tousignant, N., 2013. Broken Tempos. *Social Studies of Science* 43(5): 729–753.

Wahlberg, A., 2007. Measuring Progress. *Distinktion* 14: 65–82.

Walt, G., 2000. Globalization and Health. Paper presented at Medact Meeting, 13 May, London.

Warner, K.E., 1984. Toward a Global Strategy to Combat Smoking. *Journal of Public Health Policy* 5(1): 28–39.

Warner, K.E., 2000. The Economics of Tobacco. *Tobacco Control* 9: 78–89.

Weinberg, J., 2005. The Impact of Globalization on Emerging Infectious Disease. In Lee, K. and Collin, J., eds, *Global Change and Health.* Open University Press, Maidenhead, pp. 53–62.

Weir, L. and Mykhalovskiy, E., 2010. *Global Public Health Vigilance.* Routledge, New York.

WHO, 1983. *Smoking Control Strategies in Developing Countries.* WHO, Geneva.

WHO, 1988. *Smokeless Tobacco Control.* WHO, Geneva.

WHO, 1990. *Report of a WHO Consultation on Statistical Aspects of Tobacco-Related Mortality.* WHO, Geneva.

WHO, 2003. *WHO Framework Convention on Tobacco Control.* WHO, Geneva.

WHO Europe, 1993. *Action Plan for a Tobacco-Free Europe.* WHO Europe, Copenhagen.

World Bank, 1978. *World Development Report, 1978.* World Bank, Washington, DC.

Yach, D. and Bettcher, D., 1998. The Globalization of Public Health. *American Journal of Public Health* 88(5): 735–741.

Yach, D. and Bettcher, D., 1999. Globalization of Tobacco Marketing, Research and Industry Influence. *Development* 42(2): 25–30.

Yach, D. and Bettcher, D., 2000. Globalisation of the Tobacco Industry Influence and New Global Responses. *Tobacco Control* 9: 206–216.

Yach, D., Hawkes, C., Epping-Jordan, J. and Galbraith, S., 2003. The WHO's Framework Convention on Tobacco Control: Implications for Global Epidemics of Food-Related Deaths and Disease. *Journal of Public Health Policy* 24(3–4): 274–290.

Youde, J., 2012. *Global Health Governance*. Polity Press, Cambridge.

3 Exemplary or exceptional?

The production and dismantling of global health in Botswana

Betsey Behr Brada

Introduction

As the editors of this volume have observed, global health must be understood as something emergent, contextual and contingent. Rather than asking *where* it is, we must instead investigate the conditions under which global health seems self-evident. Drawing upon ethnographic observations of interactions among the staff of a large hospital in southern Africa and visiting American (i.e. US) clinicians and trainees, this chapter sheds light on the production and dismantling of global health as a pedagogic object.

The rise to prominence of global health as a key pedagogical object in contemporary US medical training over the past two decades cannot be overstated. With the increasing politicisation of the distribution and quality of healthcare in the USA, more and more medical students and medical educators have found their moral compasses pointing overseas. With the meteoric rise in status among medical students of leaders such as Paul Farmer and organisations such as Partners in Health and Médecins Sans Frontières/Doctors without Borders and the development of new US-driven aid programmes such as the President's Emergency Plan for AIDS Relief (PEPFAR), 'global health' has emerged as a primary site of moral professional practice for young Americans, something seemingly less available in the USA. While directors of American global health training programmes at both undergraduate and professional levels describe themselves as responding to this intense student interest, American medical educators also increasingly regard global health as an indispensable component of contemporary training (Drain *et al.*, 2007; Fauci. 2007; Panosian and Coates, 2006).

In this context, short-term rotations, or clinical electives, consisting of six to eight weeks of clinical practice in a so-called 'resource-poor' setting have become enormously popular across medical schools and specialisations (Evert *et al.*, 2007; Grudzen and Legome, 2007; Haq *et al.*, 2000; Houpt *et al.*, 2007; Nelson *et al.*, 2008; Thompson *et al.*, 2003). These programmes are highly valued for offering contemporary medical students a pedagogical experience that is at once technical and moral. On the one hand, their importance is shaped by complaints about laws and technologies that keep American trainees distant from patients' bodies. American medical trainees visiting Botswana complained that their encounters with patients in the USA were governed by laboratory tests and other diagnostic technologies, leaving students feeling as though decisions had been made for them. American medical educators found these encounters similarly frustrating: medical practice requires a 'feel' that technologies could not provide, they told me, but students had few opportunities for the 'hands-on' practice elementary to shaping a competent medical practitioner.

On the other hand, for American educators and students alike, the most important facet of short-term global health rotations went beyond the acquisition of technical skill or manual dexterity. They were prized instead for their capacity to cultivate a student's moral orientation. Both educators and students feared the dehumanising effects of contemporary medical training and practice. One educator explained it this way: A 'humanitarian impulse', he said, drew many students to medicine but was lost in the course of medical training. By trading the truncated and heavily technicised interactions of the USA for the seeming immediacy of a hospital in southeastern Botswana where they palpated bodies and performed blood draws and lumbar punctures, American students could reconnect to this sentiment. From this point of view, Referral Hospital offered a context wherein students could provide hands-on care for a needy and underserved population, honing their technical skills while rekindling a sense of empathy by interacting with patients grateful for the ministrations of even unlicensed trainees. Even just a few weeks in southern Africa seemed to hold the power to morally transform students in ways that America's quotidian racism, poverty and inequality did not seem to offer.

Global health rotations, such as the one that is the focus of this chapter, promised students the chance to recalibrate their relationship to their objects of work – that is, patients and patients' bodies – and, in so doing, transform themselves into humane novice practitioners (Shaywitz and Ausiello, 2002). The assumption that travel holds the capacity to precipitate such moral transformations, Claire Wendland reminds us, is not limited to contemporary medicine: short stints in Paris offered early nineteenth-century American medical trainees a platform from which 'to advocate for medical reforms that some characterized as returns to Hippocratic tradition' (Wendland, 2012: 116). Biomedicine as a discipline faces an intractable problem: teaching students the techniques of deeply invasive and dehumanising bodily encounters while also cultivating a proper affective orientation towards the practice of medicine (Becker *et al.*, 1961; Bosk, 2002; Fox and Lief, 1963; Good, 1995). Global health rotations are only the most recent response to this challenge (Fox, 1999; Wendland 2012), yet they serve as a key site for the cultivation of a caring and empathetic disposition among contemporary novice practitioners.

Despite its promises, in everyday practice global health is not nearly as self-evident as its popularity and traction as a constituent element of US-based medical training would suggest. Scholars have drawn attention to the unequal abilities of different actors to classify themselves and their activities and institutions as participatory in 'global health' (Brada, 2011; Crane, 2010, 2013; Wendland, 2012). This inequality is reflected both in the terms by which transnational engagements are framed and the day-to-day activities that constitute them. Even as 'collaboration' and 'partnership' have emerged as the primary terms by which powerful Northern institutions characterise their interventions in the Global South, scholars have pointed to the ways in which these projects themselves both generate and rely on the very inequalities they propose to address (Crane, 2013: 7; Kenworthy, 2014), and that the inequalities that suffuse global health treatment and research projects become unacknowledged public secrets (Geissler, 2013). Key to these dynamics is the mutual constitution of spaces and the subjects imagined to legitimately inhabit them, and the policing of these spaces and identities in order to maintain these distinctions (Brada, 2016; Prince, 2014; Sullivan, 2011, 2012; Whyte *et al.*, 2013).

If the *where* of global health is uncertain and in need of maintenance, so too is the *when*. As David Reubi (2015) argues, even as proponents of global health programming assert the converge, similarity and simultaneity of disease patterns, they also retain a modernist conceptualisation of linear development wherein nations progress through sequential stages and wherein a national population's responses to an epidemic may be modelled and predicted in advance. Even as the ideas of HIV as a global epidemic and the universal applicability of biomedicine regardless of context underpinned American interventions in Botswana, Referral Hospital also seemed to promise a glimpse into American medicine's imagined past: therapies long since abandoned, drugs not yet rendered ineffective due to resistance. The idea of Botswana as a place where medicine was out of date offered even American trainees a superior standing relative to local practitioners. Of course, the modernist tendency to view Africa as an iteration of Europe's past is well documented (Fabian, 1983; Ferguson, 1999). Yet at times Referral Hospital's grounding in this teleology unravelled: Referral Hospital seemed too advanced, Botswana's epidemic too well managed to illustrate the general features of 'Africa' and serve as a quintessential site of global health. These uneven tempos (cf. Toussignant, 2013), the shifting position of Referral Hospital relative to other temporal frames, offered local practitioners opportunities to imagine a moment when Botswana might disentangle itself from global engagements and the trajectories they entail.

In what follows, I argue that the hospital's self-evidence as a site of global health depends on claims regarding the kinds of subjects and objects seen to inhabit it, claims that had to be maintained and could, in some circumstances, be undermined. 'Global health' is an argument, a position, rather than a discrete activity defined by institutional, geographical or moral parameters (Brada, 2011). At stake in the stability of these claims was the ability of visiting students to constitute themselves as novice experts who had, in fact, encountered global health, and the related problem for their medical school in establishing itself as an institution capable of offering global health experiences to its students. My data are drawn from ethnographic fieldwork conducted at Referral Hospital, Botswana's largest hospital, between 2006 and 2008. Specifically, my research focused on a partnership between the hospital and a private American medical school, Eastern University Medical School (EUMS). At times, EUMS personnel regarded the hospital – and by extension, Botswana's healthcare system, and the country at large – as representative of an imagined Africa more generally, providing a glimpse of a quintessentially global health context. At other times, however, these visitors saw the hospital and its staff and patients as exceptions to general rules thought to apply to both the African continent at large and to global health. These interactions highlight global health's instability as a pedagogic object: While the hospital's presumed capacity to illustrate the general features of global health and Africa justified the presence of US actors and institutions, its failure to adequately do so was always immanent.

I begin with an examination of Botswana, and its HIV epidemic in particular, as a site of global health. I then demonstrate the ways in which EUMS visitors made global health apparent to one another at Referral Hospital and examine the ways in which Referral Hospital's features were taken as epitomes of larger scale phenomenon: that is, how Referral Hospital stood in for Botswana, and even for the African continent as a whole. I then highlight ways in which visiting Americans inadvertently disrupted the stability of Referral Hospital as a site of global health. I conclude by arguing that the contingency of 'global health' illuminates transnational subjects and engagements that US-driven global health programming tends to occlude, and opens up an opportunity for Batswana practitioners to reflect on and to re-imagine the terms by which they and their hospital engage 'global health'.

Botswana's epidemic as an ambivalent site of global health

As I have argued elsewhere, Botswana is both a highly likely and highly unlikely place in which to do 'global health' (2011). During the period of British colonization from the late nineteenth century to the mid-1960s, the Bechuanaland Protectorate, as it was called, remained an arid site of underdevelopment, its population largely significant to imperial agendas only insofar as they provided a source of labour for South African industry (Livingston, 2005; Morapedi, 1999; Schapera, 1947). Shortly after independence in 1966, however, Batswana discovered extensive diamond deposits, and entered into an arrangement whereby the proceeds of mining were returned to the state (Gulbrandsen, 2012).[1] This arrangement generated one of the fastest growing economies in the world, and led to the rapid development of government-sponsored education, healthcare and infrastructure. Lauded as 'an African success story', a 'miracle' of stable democratic governance, steady economic growth and investment in infrastructure, Botswana has largely managed to avoid debt to international financial institutions and the crippling structural adjustment programmes that have accompanied it, and is frequently regarded as an exception to the rules of poverty, corruption and warfare governing the rest of the continent (Acemoglu *et al.*, 2003; Good, 1992, 2008; Gulbrandsen, 2012; Maipose, 2009; Parsons, 1993; Samatar, 1999; Werbner, 2004).

Despite this astonishing rate of state-sponsored development and the country's reputation for economic prosperity and good governance, by 2001 Botswana had one of the highest HIV prevalence rates in the world. The number of deaths attributed to the virus continued to rise, peaking at more than 15,000 in 2003 alone (UNAIDS, 2013). In addition, like other countries in the region, Botswana's epidemic has wreaked havoc upon professional cadres, striking those who possessed the training and abilities most needed to manage the epidemic. Furthermore, Botswana's relatively robust public health infrastructure, oriented towards decentralised preventative public health services, was unprepared for the burden of hospital-based care and chronic debility to which the epidemic gave rise (Livingston, 2004, 2012). Until very recently, for example, the country lacked the capacity to train physicians within its borders. Nursing training has been available at missionary institutions since the days of the Protectorate and, more recently, at public educational institutions, but the government has historically relied on a mixture of foreign health professionals and foreign-trained Batswana to fill other positions in public hospitals. While plans for a medical school have been under discussion since the mid-1990s, the University of Botswana's Faculty of Medicine graduated its first class only in 2015.

These factors form the context in which then President Festus Mogae publicly declared in 2001 his fear that Botswana faced 'extinction' as a nation, his determination to explore the feasibility of free public treatment with anti-retroviral medications (ARVs), and his appeals for international assistance (Farley, 2001). While international policy circles continued to emphasise prevention and palliative care, Botswana's national leadership launched sub-Saharan Africa's first free public HIV treatment programme and began distributing ARVs. By 2004, more than 20,000 patients were receiving ARVs and the programme continued to expand as the Ministry of Health implemented routine HIV testing in healthcare settings (Ramiah and Reich, 2005). But the ambitious programme taxed Botswana's already overburdened public health sector. US-based private foundations and medical schools, eager to participate in the worldwide expansion of HIV treatment, began developing connections with Botswana in order to support the treatment programme, focusing primarily on training practitioners to manage patients on long-term ARV treatment and developing the infrastructure on which the treatment programme relied.

All of this has added up to something of a conundrum. For one thing, as perplexing as Botswana's epidemic was to outsiders who regarded the country as a model of development in Africa, it was no less so for many Batswana, who did not recognise in themselves the deviant sexualities and general backwardness they associated with the disease (Heald, 2005; MacDonald, 1996). While more than 300,000 of Botswana's approximately two million citizens are living with HIV, descriptions of Botswana as backward, abject and 'AIDS-ridden' (Thomma, 2003) can sit awkwardly against Batswana's pride in their political stability, economic viability and a peaceful postcolonial transition in a region where these are rare, as well as their experience of national leadership vis-à-vis HIV. In addition, Botswana's government was heavily involved in ARV treatment from the very beginning. In contrast to South Africa where political battles have surrounded HIV treatment, forcing the citizenry to wrest a matter of life and death from a recalcitrant state (Comaroff, 2007; Decoteau, 2013), Botswana's ARV programme has served as a means by which the government has shored up its legitimacy (Gulbrandsen, 2012). The stability of diamond prices, too, has arguably lent itself to the persistence of modernist teleologies of development perhaps longer than elsewhere in Africa (Ferguson, 1999, 2006).

Notwithstanding the degree to which Botswana lives up to its reputation for exceptionality, then, even in the midst of the epidemic individual Batswana continue to feel the presence of the state in their everyday lives in the form of schools, roads, clinics, boreholes and, more recently, ARVs. 'Whatever else you can say about [former President] Mogae,' I was told several times, 'he brought us treatment.' In short, while Botswana possesses many features of a quintessential site of 'global health' – a devastating epidemic, an overtaxed public health infrastructure, a population in need of complex forms of medical care – its political and economic stability cut both ways. They contribute to the ease and convenience with which US institutions establish programmes in Botswana while also making it difficult to cast Botswana as a site of a generic 'global health' wherein transnational intervention is the *sine qua non* of healthcare.

'Do all the procedures you can': producing global health

As the government of Botswana began laying plans for the national ARV treatment programme in the early 2000s, infectious disease specialists from EUMS were invited via a series of personal connections to help formulate the policies guiding the treatment programme. These physicians began dropping in on Referral Hospital's adult medical wards, which bore the brunt of the epidemic and its associated infections, such as tuberculosis. EUMS students began finding their way to Gaborone for a few weeks at a time, and by 2004 EUMS had placed a few physicians in Gaborone year-round. This rather haphazard arrangement evolved into a full EUMS firm, or medical team composed of specialists and trainees, that oversaw cases. Despite significant differences between medical systems and curricula, over the next few years EUMS formalised its partnership with Referral Hospital around two objectives. First, EUMS offered to provide training and mentoring for the junior physicians of the ward, known as medical officers (MOs). Many of these MOs were Batswana who had received government sponsorships to study medicine overseas that required them to work in the public sector upon returning home. While they were supervised by specialised physicians, or attendings, there were no formal opportunities for advanced training, such as a residency, available to them in Botswana. To that end, there were always a few infectious disease specialists from EUMS rotating through the ward for a few weeks or months at a time.

Second, EUMS established a six-week rotation for its medical students that promised to expose them to 'global health'. For EUMS educators and administrators, the absence of a local medical school created the possibility that EUMS students could fill an unoccupied niche. This assumption was further grounded in a perceived congruence between students' need for clinical experience and patients' need for care amid presumably inadequate and incompetent local practice, a perception that allowed EUMS personnel to see the relationship as at least mutually beneficial, even benevolent. The school's investment in this aspect of the programme was considerable: EUMS covered the cost of the flight and provided room and board in an expensive set of apartments near the hospital.

As discussed above, both students and educators prized the rotation for its capacity to transform students' subjectivities. But for EUMS students the most immediate value of this niche lay in the opportunity to practise the blood draws, lumbar punctures, and other invasive procedures used in the diagnosis and treatment of HIV as well as other conditions. By restricting the programme to students in their fourth year of training, EUMS ensured they had some basic clinical experience, but their access to patients' bodies in Botswana was far greater than in the USA. 'We'll be great residents', one student explained to me, indicating the degree to which the opportunity to perform invasive procedures on Batswana patients offered them a professional edge over their colleagues back home. 'Do procedures', students leaving Gaborone at the end of their six weeks counselled their incoming classmates. 'Do all the procedures you can.'

Students' access to patients' bodies, then, often served for them as the most obvious sign of 'global health'. This access, and the presumed congruence of needs and deficiencies that grounded it, offered EUMS students a kind of circular reasoning. This must be global health; why else would they, unlicensed trainees, be doing it? To the extent that 'global health' emerged as a coherent object of pedagogy between EUMS instructors and their students, then, it did so through a determined focus on what Referral Hospital lacked in comparison to an imagined US counterpart. These comparisons frequently acquired a temporal dimension. 'Local' drugs, treatment protocols and practitioners were obsolete; visiting Americans, even novices, could provide up-to-date medical care, almost as if by visiting Botswana they travelled into the past (Brada, 2011). Anxious to establish their credibility as novice 'global' practitioners, EUMS students vied with one another to deride 'local' resources, practices and personnel in their instructors' presence. In this context 'global health' better captured the capacity for American medical students to inhabit and lay claim to a specific trajectory of moral and professional formation than it described either the geographical distribution of threats to health or the distribution of medical experts committed to remedying them.

'Not bad for an African hospital'

While individual students valued the rotation for its ability to contribute to their individual skill sets and careers, EUMS had a broader stake in the rotation's existence. Although the school's reputation as an elite institution increasingly hinged upon its ability to incorporate overseas travel into its curricula, EUMS had few other international programmes, and senior administrators placed ever more pressure on the rotation at Referral Hospital to illustrate EUMS' engagement in global health. To that end, EUMS instructors frequently spoke of Referral

Hospital as though it stood in for not just the entire country of Botswana but for the entire African continent. 'Well, here in Africa, you'll see that', instructors might explain to students upon encountering unfamiliar or even, to their eyes, inadequate or out-of-date therapies. Indeed, at times students' criticisms and complaints reached such a pitch that EUMS instructors were forced to remind their students that, its myriad faults notwithstanding, Referral Hospital was 'not bad for an African hospital'.

As a quintessential example of African healthcare, Referral Hospital was called upon to represent the failures and inadequacies of a particularly *African* AIDS epidemic epitomised not just by the absence of treatments but by the absence of practitioners knowledgeable about treatment. This led to some strange and awkward encounters, as when Dr Sam, a retired American infectious disease expert, was invited by EUMS to spend several weeks at Referral Hospital. At his lecture, which EUMS instructors had heavily encouraged both their own students and Referral Hospital's MOs to attend, he began by talking about intestinal parasites, a condition of little concern in Botswana, observing that 'the average Vietnamese person has three worms'. To the consternation of his American hosts, Dr Sam's subsequent observations misconstrued the basic epidemiology of southern Africa as he estimated a much lower HIV prevalence rate and a much higher rate of parasites than was the case.

Through these contrasts, EUMS instructors and students mutually constituted 'global health' as a practice that entailed visiting Americans travelling to and returning from sites that seemed to demand their expertise, a practice from which African experts were largely excluded (cf. Crane, 2010, 2013). Here, 'global health' as an expert stance requires not a mastery of the context in which a medical professional finds him- or herself but the ability to move authoritatively from one context to another and the constitution of these disparate situations as objects of expert intervention, as reflected by Dr Sam's frequent allusions to Vietnamese parasitic infections (Carr, 2010). The specific features of a country seem almost incidental. In addition, visiting 'Africa' seemed to hold out to American experts an opportunity to intervene in an earlier phase of the epidemic, to redeem past mistakes and perhaps capture an elusive glory (cf. Crane, 2013; Reubi, 2015; Toussignant, 2013). For example, Dr Sam recalled with some nostalgia treating AIDS in San Francisco in the early 1980s: the virus had not yet been identified and both diagnosis and treatment posed formidable challenges. Such authoritative movement requires the constitution of a hierarchy of recognisable categories – abject patients, ignorant and helpless local practitioners, visiting experts – and their arrangement in time. But as powerful as these categorisations may seem, they required maintenance and were subject to contestation, re-evaluation and even, as the following section illustrates, inadvertent redefinition in the hands of those recruited to reinforce them.

'Anything this sophisticated': global health dismantled

Using Referral Hospital to showcase global health's quintessential features was not nearly as straightforward as EUMS instructors might have hoped. Students expected to encounter a 'resource-poor setting', but upon arrival many struggled to discern differences in practices, materials and approaches, and even terminology from actual deficiencies. Their efforts to constitute themselves as experts were hampered by their unfamiliarity with the conventions that governed Referral Hospital. While some of these forms of knowledge were local to Botswana's health system, such as the highly regarded audiology services at a smaller hospital in Ramotswa, some 35 km south of Gaborone, others were more 'global': terms such as *FBC* for 'full blood count' are used widely across the Commonwealth of Nations and beyond, but such terms flummoxed EUMS students accustomed to ordering a *CBC* (complete blood count). While an encounter with these conventions might be regarded as the stuff of global health practice itself, EUMS students often met them with frustration: this unfamiliarity threatened their primary goals; that is, it undermined their capacity to intervene rapidly and effectively in patients' bodies, and to demonstrate to their local colleagues what such rapid and effective intervention looked like (cf. Cicourel, 1995; Macdonald, 2002).

Frustrated by an inability to perform proficiently in a new environment, students tended to imagine that their mastery of global health depended on identifying which of its novel characteristics were, in fact, deficiencies. They did not, then, respond positively to discussions that emphasised the sophistication of Referral Hospital and its staff. In June 2007 Dr Paul, a senior infectious disease specialist at a university in the western USA, was invited to Referral Hospital for four weeks by the head of the EUMS' division of infectious disease, with whom he had a long friendship. Dr Paul had worked in North Africa in the early 1980s and his polite and affable manner distinguished him among visiting Americans at Referral Hospital. One bright winter morning, he and I joined a team composed of Dr Adu, a Ghanaian specialist employed by Referral Hospital, Dr Moseki, a Motswana MO, and three EUMS students as they made their way down the long, narrow ward and stopped to examine a patient receiving treatment for cryptococcal meningitis. As Dr Adu discussed the patient's condition with a nurse, Dr Paul discovered that, rather than relying solely on India Ink for diagnosis, Referral Hospital's lab had the capacity to culture cerebrospinal fluid (CSF) collected via lumbar puncture and to test it for cryptococcal antigens. 'I'm surprised to find anything this sophisticated [in sub-Saharan Africa] outside South Africa,' he remarked excitedly to the rest of us. 'In southern Sudan we tested for crypto using India Ink,' he continued. 'This patient would have died.'

Such comparisons presented two problems to EUMS students. First, even if students were able to draw comparisons from one 'global health' space to another (Brada, 2011), as trainees they were generally unable to draw them across time. Reminiscences such as Dr Paul's reminded them of their status as novitiates vis-à-vis global health and conflicted with the idea that Americans temporarily inserted themselves into backward and parochial health systems where they practised an advanced medicine by virtue of being American, regardless of age or experience. But more importantly, Dr Paul's remark cast doubt on the capacity of Referral Hospital to serve as an exemplary space of global health. Instead, his comparison emphasised Referral Hospital's *exceptionality* vis-à-vis global health and its idealized site in an undifferentiated and generically abject 'Africa'. If the legitimacy of their six-week rotation lay in an encounter with abject subjects and the identification and correction of unsophisticated and obsolete practices, then such assessments of the diagnostic technologies and treatments available in southeastern Botswana and the practitioners who wielded them could only undermine that legitimacy.

Likewise, even Dr Sam in his lecture, as he rehearsed an overview of HIV morbidity and mortality in sub-Saharan Africa, conceded that it might not entirely apply to 'this little paradise'. Surprised, perhaps even dismayed, that Botswana was not the 'Africa' he anticipated, Dr Sam also found Referral Hospital to be out of step temporally, inasmuch as its lack of excitement stemmed from its failure to recapitulate the heady (and horrifying) early days of the epidemic in the USA. Local African practitioners, he concluded dubiously, might learn to manage patients on long-term ARV therapy, but the tedium of managing a chronic condition that characterised Botswana's treatment era offered no challenge to an expert such as himself. 'The excitement [of the epidemic] is disappearing', he concluded with obvious disappointment.

A greener pasture

While Dr Paul's and Dr Sam's reactions to the practices they encountered at Referral Hospital dismayed EUMS students, these reactions were received with more ambivalence by the ward's MOs. On the one hand, these junior physicians grumbled about missing labs, drug stock-outs and the other inconveniences that coloured day-to-day practice on the ward, and they could sometimes be found bemoaning the unavailability of the MRI (magnetic resonance imaging) scans they knew from their studies overseas. They drew comparisons of their own from a wide range of experiences: Dr Moseki, for example, had done her medical training in the Caribbean and North America before returning to Botswana. On the other hand, the MOs sometimes bristled when they sensed Botswana was being held up as the epitome of a poor, benighted African country. They resisted the generalisations of 'Africa' offered by visiting speakers such as Dr Sam. One sees cases of leishmaniasis in Mozambique, not Botswana, one MO politely objected; scabies is a pressing problem in *East* Africa, countered another. Wary of painting all EUMS personnel with the same brush, Dr Moseki nevertheless found EUMS students' attitudes consistent enough to speculate that the students were given explicit instructions regarding what they would find at Referral Hospital: 'They come here with the mentality that they're saviours of black people, as if they've been told, "You're going there to save the Africans."'

Here, Dr Moseki found herself in a double-bind. To admit that Referral Hospital had any faults whatsoever seemed to capitulate to the idea that Referral Hospital – and, by extension, Botswana as a whole, including Dr Moseki herself – was nothing more than a token of a type, an instantiation of representations of Africa promulgated in American global health training programmes: poor, diseased, incapable and in need of outside assistance. But even positive assessments of the hospital and of healthcare in Botswana more broadly, such as those voiced by Dr Paul and Dr Sam, sat uneasily with Dr Moseki and her colleagues insofar as they reflected a surprise that Botswana had somehow escaped the abject state in which Africa was presumed to lie. In these instances both Botswana's status as an exemplary site of global health *and* as an exception to it were troubling: taken together, they pointed to the contingency of the spatial and temporal logics informing global health training programmes, such as EUMS's programme at Referral Hospital, and to the power claimed by US institutions in setting the terms by which global health is imagined. Dr Moseki put it this way:

> Pretty soon . . . they [EUMS] are gonna find a greener pasture somewhere in some poor backward African place and that's where they'll go because they need . . . to feel like they're saviours. [And]. . . here [at Referral Hospital], we'll be like, 'You don't really do much', and they'll go.

Here Dr Moseki imagines a moment when Referral Hospital cannot provide the context for EUMS students and practitioners to engage in global health. EUMS personnel themselves, upon encountering unexpected technologies, bureaucratic constraints on their activities, and the banal routine of chronic disease maintenance, also sometimes imagined it, grumbling drily about 'Africa lite'. This uncertainty reveals less about Botswana than it highlights the instability of global health as a pedagogic object, a fantasy that demands a configuration of a technologically deficient healthcare system wherein American saviours act expeditiously towards abject Africans. That this global health is a fantasy is made even more apparent by the difficulty of finding a place for someone like Dr Moseki, a Motswana with clinical experience in the West Indies, the northern plains of the USA and southern Africa, within it.

Conclusion

In an essay on interactions between Malawian medical students and visiting foreigners at Malawi's College of Medicine, Claire Wendland cautions us that 'depicting clinical tourism as invariably extractive, neocolonial, or exploitative would disregard many cases in which students' travels lead to long-lasting connections among Malawians and expatriates that appear to enrich all concerned' (Wendland, 2012: 116). By highlighting the unequal terms by which global health is imagined and institutionalised, my objective in this chapter has not been to place limits on the experiences of individual Batswana and American medical personnel, either trainees or experts, or to suggest that this inequality precludes the mutually enriching engagements Wendland describes. Instead, I have highlighted both the stakes for US medical educators and their trainees in stably locating 'global health' and the inability of one hospital in southeastern Botswana – and arguably, any one hospital – to consistently embody the general features of global health and to represent 'Africa' in a generic sense.

MacDonald, D.S. (1996) Notes on the Socio-Economic and Cultural Factors Influencing the Transmission of HIV in Botswana. *Social Science and Medicine* 42(9): 1325–1333.

Macdonald, M.N. (2002) Pedagogy, Pathology and Ideology: The Production, Transmission and Reproduction of Medical Discourse. *Discourse and Society* 13(4): 337–367.

Maipose, G. (2009) Botswana: The African Success Story. In *The Politics of Aid: African Strategies for Dealing with Donors*, ed. L. Whitfield, pp. 108–130. Oxford: Oxford University Press.

Morapedi, W.G. (1999) Migrant Labour and the Peasantry in the Bechuanaland Protectorate, 1930–1965. *Journal of Southern African Studies* 25(2): 197–214.

Nelson, B.D., C.C. Anne, P.K. Lee, M. Newby, R. Chamberlin and C. Huang (2008) Global Health Training in Pediatric Residency Programs. *Pediatrics* 122(1): 28–33.

Panosian, C. and T.J. Coates (2006) The New Medical ''Missionaries'' – Grooming the Next Generation of Global Health Workers. *New England Journal of Medicine* 354(17): 1771–1773.

Parsons, N. (1993) Botswana: An End to Exceptionality? *Round Table* 325: 73–82.

Prince, R.J. (2014) Navigating 'Global Health' in an East African City. In *Making and Unmaking Public Health in Africa: Ethnographic and Historical Perspectives*, ed. R.J. Prince and R. Marsland, pp. 208–230. Athens: Ohio University Press.

Ramiah, I. and M. Reich (2005) Public–Private Partnerships and Antiretroviral Drugs for HIV/AIDS: Lessons from Botswana. *Health Affairs* 24(2): 545–551.

Reubi, D. (2015) Modernisation, Smoking and Chronic Disease: Of Temporality and Spatiality in Global Health. *Health & Place* 39: 188–195.

Samatar, A.I. (1999) *An African Miracle: State and Class Leadership and Colonial Legacy in Botswana Development*. Portsmouth: Heinemann.

Schapera, I. (1947) *Migrant Labour and Tribal Life, a Study of Conditions in the Bechuanaland Protectorate*. London: Oxford University Press.

Shaywitz, D.A., and D.A. Ausiello (2002) Global Health: A Chance for Western Physicians to Give and Receive. *American Journal of Medicine* 113(4): 354–357.

Sullivan, N. (2011) Mediating Abundance and Scarcity: Implementing an HIV/AIDS Targeted Project Within a Government Hospital in Tanzania. *Medical Anthropology* 30(2): 202–221.

Sullivan, N. (2012) Enacting Spaces of Inequality Placing Global/State Governance Within a Tanzanian Hospital. *Space and Culture* 15(1): 57–67.

Thomma, S. (2003) Bush Pledges U.S. Support in AIDS-Ridden Botswana. Knight Ridder Tribune News Service, 10 July: 1.

Thompson, M.J., M.K. Huntington, D. Hunt, L.E. Pinsky and J.J. Brodie (2003) Educational Effects of International Health Electives on U.S. and Canadian Medical Students and Residents: A Literature Review. *Academic Medicine* 78(3): 342–347.

Toussignant, N. (2013) Broken Tempos: Of Means and Memory in a Senegalese University Laboratory. *Social Studies of Science* 43(5): 729–753.

Wendland, C. (2012) Moral Maps and Medical Imaginaries: Clinical Tourism at Malawi's College of Medicine. *American Anthropologist* 114(1): 108–122.

Werbner, R. (2004) *Reasonable Radicals and Citizenship in Botswana: The Public Anthropology of Kalanga Elites*. Bloomington, IN: Indiana University Press.

Whyte, S.R., M.A. Whyte, L. Meinert and J. Twebaze (2013) Therapeutic Clientship: Belonging in Uganda's Projectified Landscape of Care. In *When People Come First: Critical Studies in Global Health*, ed. J. Biehl and A. Petryna, pp. 140–165. Princeton, NJ: Princeton University Press.

4 Mixing and fixing

Managing and imagining the body in a global world

Sarah Atkinson

Introduction

A defining characteristic of the globalisation of healthcare provision has been the movement of people for health-related purposes involving both health personnel seeking improved terms of employment within a globalising labour market and health service users seeking improved access, quality or costs across a global market for major medical interventions. This emergence of new markets for medical care at a global scale reflects a combination of the increasing ease of travel, the development of biomedical technologies for reproduction and recon-struction of the body and the liberalisation of cross-border trade. As such, these new opportunities for medical travel involve multiple geographies of the body, including concerns of borders and boundaries, ethics and inequalities, resource flows and the nature of care at a global scale. Geographers of health have begun to explore the issues that arise from this rapid growth in medical travel, but to date most have directed research attention to the challenges and opportunities for those countries providing services for medical tourists (Johnston *et al.*, 2015a, 2015b) and to the complexities of how the relations of neoliberalism and the market unfold in different settings (Parry *et al.*, 2015). This chapter engages the practices of medical tourism involving the exchange of body parts through attention to scarcity and inter-corporeality in terms of their real and imagined relations and tensions. Scarcity is a fundamental relation underpinning medical tourism in which not only timely and less costly care is sourced but also scarce and vital bodily material. Inter-corporeality has received far less research attention in terms of how medical intervention through sharing of body parts, fluids or reproductive processes confronts and reworks traditions of nationalised and racialised identities to enable practices that both revalue and re-exploit other bodies. This attention to how various types of borders are dissolved, redrawn and policed as bodies are brought together, often literally, in contemporary and future global health markets comple-ments existing geographical work on global health by exploring how we do and might imagine, confront and negotiate the relations and tensions of scarcity and inter-corporeality arising in this kind of medical tourism. The chapter thus has as its primary focus the lived and imagined ways of framing the relations and tensions of scarcity and inter-corporeality in the case of transplant tourism.

Literary fiction and film are an important source to exploit for those interested in not only the lived experiences but also the imaginaries of scarcity and inter-corporeality in relation to organ donation and procurement. Such creative forms situated in present and future fictional worlds afford nuanced, rich explorations of the multiple and complex ways of imagining, confronting and negotiating scarcity and inter-corporeality. These worlds, and the tales of events and lives within them, are here treated as complementary empirical resources to the narrative accounts of human experience captured through interview-based or ethnographic methodologies. A novel or film gives the space for the characters to tell their stories and display their emotions, situated in particular times, places and relationships, but these stories are also complemented with an authorial commentary, verbal or visual observations, as well as the opportunity to make explicit hidden values or unpredictable reactions. These are approaches that emphasise how, in negotiating our own values and practices, we draw upon multiple options and resources, 'culturally available narratives, stories, scripts, discourses, systems of knowledge or . . . ideologies' (Seale, 2003: 514). Literary fiction and film offer us explorations of negotiating such resources and experiences and as such constitute a data source to be mined following the traditions of early geographical engagements with the humanities (Marston and De Leeuw, 2013). Drawing upon literary fiction and film in this way can open up a field of geohumanities and health within wider moves by the discipline to revisit our relationship with the arts and humanities (Dear *et al.*, 2011; Marston and De Leeuw, 2013).

Geographers working on health and medicine have had some limited direct engagement with this trend: drawing upon literary fiction in relation to how landscapes and places relate to healing and health (Gesler, 2003; Tonnellier and Curtis, 2005; Foley, 2015); engagements with new health practices as a form of spirituality (Philo *et al.*, 2015); participation in the creative arts as contributing to health or well-being (Atkinson and Robson, 2012; Atkinson and Scott, 2015). Literary fiction and film also offer alternative engagements and future imaginings through which to expand our available options and resources and to explore their various implications. In this sense, literary fiction and film not only provide a nuanced mirror to and exploration of existing discourses but exercise their own agency in influencing how we engage, celebrate or caution against alternative modes of practice (Kitzinger, 2010). Literary fiction and film that have broached issues of transplant technologies and trade include, on the one hand, elaborations of existing discourses of scarcity and inter-corporeality and, on the other, science fiction explorations of new and different responses to the challenges of organ procurement and donation. Thus, the chapter, as a side-effect, also makes a secondary contribution to the geographies of global health in the engagement with the geohumanities, new sources of data and new modes of agency in how imaginary worlds reflect and inform our practices at local and global scales (Atkinson, 2016).

Geographies of medical tourism

Movement from one country to another for the purposes of accessing medical care is not a new phenomenon; the elite of low- and middle-income countries have always sought the most recent technologies and higher quality care that are unavailable locally from other countries with better resourced health services, a trend that continues (Snyder *et al.*, 2015a). What is new is the rapid rise in the numbers of those seeking medical intervention in countries other than their own and particularly the rise in the movement of nationals from high-income countries seeking expensive medical interventions at lower costs in middle- and low-income countries. In some cases, patients may be referred from their own healthcare system for treatment in another country through a bilateral agreement between the countries concerned; some seek healthcare from a country other than their own as expatriates currently living there or as tourists taken ill during their vacations and for whom health costs are likely to be covered by insurance. However, the phenomenon of interest is the expansion of a new healthcare sector catering to private patients who intentionally elect to self-refer for medical interventions across international borders and usually cover the costs for such services as an out-of-pocket payment. This is the phenomenon referred to as medical tourism or healthcare export. For example, in Europe, several post-socialist countries report relatively large annual increases (4 to 5%) in the proportion of total health expenditure exported; that is, health services provided to people who are not resident in the nation. These include Hungary, the Czech Republic, Croatia and, most markedly, Slovenia, which showed a 20 per cent increase in health services export each year between 2007 and 2012 (OECD, 2014).This is particularly significant in terms of the potential impact on the National Health Service given that the demand is for more intensive, costly and expert treatments (NaRanong and NaRanong, 2011). For example, the Centers for Disease Control and Prevention (CDC) in the USA estimate that up to 750,000 residents of the USA now travel abroad for care each year, a figure likely to be a conservative estimate, since much of the travel is likely to go undocumented (CDC, 2015); Thailand witnessed a growth in medical tourism over a decade, from almost none to approaching half a million (NaRanong and NaRanong, 2011).

Motivations for travellers include much reduced costs, quicker treatment given long waiting lists at home, availability of the latest technological expertise or access to treatments not permitted in the home country (Petersen and Seear, 2011; Petersen *et al.*, 2014; Snyder *et al.*, 2014). The rise of medical tourism alters the global, regional and local landscapes of healthcare provision and inequalities in access to that provision. The industry has been characterised by the emergence not only of new clinics and hospitals in provider countries but also by a range of associated industries that embed the central medical intervention. Travellers need to be assured of high-quality care and a new industry of facilitation companies serves to meet this demand (Hohm and Snyder, 2015). Some interventions involve a recovery period in a country which is supported through an emerging industry of small-scale recovery 'care homes' offering more personal care and an attractive setting, reflecting the 'tourism' part of the label (Ackerman, 2010). In terms of global health governance, regulating cross-border medical movements and practices is particularly challenging in the absence of standardised international definitions of the relevant components, the historical trajectories and specificities of national regulation of medical practice, and the emergence of an international market for the provision of healthcare in which competition to attract foreign investment may promote deregulation and a globally expressed 'race-to-the-bottom' (Helble, 2011; Schneider, 2015; Whittaker, 2010).

Geographers have begun to engage the phenomenon of medical tourism through two broad approaches or fields of study: as part of health systems and health services research (e.g. Adams *et al.*, 2015a) and as part of research on neoliberal-isation and globalisation (e.g. Greenhough *et al.*, 2015). These are, of course, not discrete categories of research and there is considerable overlap, but they do reflect the primary focus and audiences for the research undertaken. The research group on medical tourism based at Simon Fraser University has produced a substantial body of research since 2010 on a range of healthcare concerns, including the motivations to travel for healthcare (Cameron *et al.*, 2014; Adams *et al.*, 2015b), the potential benefits and pitfalls of developing a medical tourism sector for low- and middle-income countries (Adams *et al.*, 2015a; Johnston *et al.*, 2015a, 2015b), the implications of outward-bound medical tourism for the health systems of low- and middle-income countries (Snyder *et al.*, 2015a), the patterns of health worker migrations related to medical tourism (Crooks *et al.*, 2015; Snyder *et al.*, 2015b), the implications of medical tourism for family physicians in tourists' countries of origin (Snyder *et al.*, 2013) and the ethical, legal and regulatory issues and choices to be negotiated (Adams *et al.*, 2015a). This body of research emphasises the need for attention to the socio-spatial particularities and variations of different medical tourism settings. These studies clearly locate the emerging markets for medical tourism within the context of globalisation but predominantly talk to the community concerned with health systems and associated policy issues (Adams *et al.*, 2015a).

The second body of work takes the processes of globalisation and neoliberal-isation and their varied and situated expressions as the primary focus of their research. This work examines how globalisation and the tenets of neoliberal politics combine with new technologies of communication and biomedicine to reconfigure the provision and access of healthcare, including the rapid increase in the movement of medical patients and professionals, biomedical services and medically relevant body parts (Greenhough *et al.*, 2015; Parry *et al.*, 2015). Research has attended closely to the positionality of those involved in the markets for medical tourism to better understand the differentiated landscapes shaping their choices, decisions and experiences (Parry, 2008). The growth of medical tourism as a market reflects and exemplifies the values of a neoliberal regime: the privileging of individual autonomy as a policy goal; the centrality of consumer choice within a free market economy; the slimming down of state public service provision in favour of privatisation, franchising, contract or outsourcing, including offshore, of elements in service provision; and support for greater flexibility of labour markets and labour provision (Greenhough *et al.*, 2015). However, in the context of a globalising free market for healthcare, the opportunities to realise the claims made for autonomy and choice are unequally distributed and follow existing lines of inequality, including gender, place and culture (England, 2015;

Greenhough *et al.*, 2015; Holliday *et al.*, 2015). This second strand of geographical work on medical tourism is mirrored across the social sciences more widely (see e.g. work in anthropology by Scheper-Hughes, 2002, 2003, and in sociology by Whittaker, 2008), and the dominant analytical discourse has similarly been that seeking medical care through a global market illuminates how the processes of neoliberalisation play out in different settings. Research across the social sciences has thus attended to the different dimensions of unevenness in the dynamics of global medical markets, thereby reaffirming the continued importance of context, history and embodiment.

This unevenness in new markets for medical tourism may also be expressed through variation across different forms of medical intervention. The specific practices of medicine insist on foregrounding the materiality of bodies; when we engage the particular medical technologies that involve the surgical transfer of parts from one body to another in what Waldby termed 'biomedically engineered inter-corporeality' (Waldby, 2002), two further aspects of the unevenness of new markets demand our analytical attention. Waldby (2002) specifically emphasises the ways in which embodied identity is produced through social relations and, drawing on anthropological studies of tissue donations, critiques the overemphasis on the visual in producing embodied identities at the expense of what she calls introceptive data, and perhaps particularly those that become foregrounded in the event of ill-health experiences. Second, the availability of such body matter for certain forms of donation, such as organ transplants, is already significantly behind demand, a shortfall which will only increase in the future given ageing populations and improved medical technologies. Taking these two aspects together, the new possibilities to reinvent and recycle ourselves through replacing or donating body parts, and for fixing bodies through mixing bodies, are accompanied not only by new tensions related to resource flows, inequalities and the nature of care at a global scale, but also by reworking our understandings of sameness and difference in bodily matter. The accommodations made around such tensions are in turn underpinned by emerging new and reworked rhetorics and discourses that enable or block different practices for the procurement of scarce bodily matter through explicit forms of argumentation and implicit or hidden assumptions.

Tensions of scarcity

The forms of discourse which dominate in relation to organ procurement and donation have a distinct pattern in terms of their social and spatial distribution. The dominant analytical discourse related to the global movement of organs for transplant reflects work on medical tourism more widely and continues the emphasis on the workings of globalisation, trade liberalisation and consumer choice. However, this discourse is infused with a far stronger moral resonance than is generally the case in other areas of medical tourism, a moral infusion that is largely condemnatory, a matter for outrage and abhorrence. At its most extreme, the global movements of organs for transplant have been condemned as 'new forms of late modern cannibalism' (Scheper-Hughes, 2002: 1), reflecting the marked tendency for globally scarce organs to move along lines of inequality, from poor to rich, South to North, and to some extent women to men (Scheper-Hughes, 2003). This is a movement that may be illegal and as such invisible, informal or pursued through unethical procedures without consent, or achieved through direct and indirect coercion within a context of structural violence (Galtung, 1969). In marked contrast, the analytical discourse that dominates within high-income countries, or those countries successful in largely upholding regulation, is celebratory through the language of the gift, offering life and hope (Svaenaeus, 2010). Those donating are positioned as generous, even heroic, and recipients as fortunate and saved. These rhetorics of the gift and voluntarism have their roots in the post-Second World War movement for social solidarity and welfare provisions, which in relation to donation was mobilised and theorised as the 'gift relationship' in the influential work of Richard Titmuss (Titmuss, 1970; cf. Fontaine, 2002; Reubi, 2012). The discourse of the generosity or social citizenry of the gift as the basis for donation constitutes the desirable form of organ transplant programmes against which the coerced or commercialised procurement of organs is juxtaposed and against which such self-interest, greed or exploitation appear particularly heinous.

Creative imaginings through film or fiction offer us various entry points in developing a global and critical engagement with these discourses. As a form of knowledge, these media can bring their audiences into close emotional engagement with the realities of living as others, in other bodies, in other social and economic spaces and in other encounters with the processes of globalisation and neoliberalisation. Literature and film enable their audiences to encounter the issues, to confront their own reactions and to reflect on the implications of the rhetoric for different practices. As such, engagement with the creative imaginings of relatively unfamiliar aspects of contemporary societies can illuminate the ways we do and might practice biomedical technologies. Moreover, as the conduit for our reflections on different practices, these creative imaginings have their own agency as strategies themselves for how we encounter and engage other bodies. The exploitative element in the global organ trade has been drawn upon through the genres of the thriller or horror in film. Stephen Frears' thriller *Dirty, Pretty Things* (2002), for example, accompanies the various vulnerabilities to exploitation in the lives of undocumented immigrants in London, including coercion as donors in an illegal organ trade. The protagonists escape, but only by exacting the violence of forced kidney donation back onto the perpetrators of violence. This may make for a sense of satisfaction in cinematic terms through the personal resolution of the problems faced by those characters who have won our sympathies, but only addresses the wider challenges of the underground illegal trade through evoking audience abhorrence.

In a full horror genre, John Stockwell's film *Turistas* (2006) draws upon global inequalities in the organ trade in a different exploration of revenge. The tourists of the title are young, middle-class backpackers from the USA who are kidnapped for the purpose of organ extraction from which one of them dies before they manage to escape. However, in this film, the motivation of the gang extracting the organs is not one of self-interest or financial profit but to redress inequalities in the global flow of organs for transplant. They claim that organs have been stolen from the poor in Brazil for the benefit of rich foreigners and it is time for those countries to pay back. The organs they extract will be taken for donation to the poor in Brazil and as such the violence is enacted in the pursuit of social justice. This inversion of an argument for social justice into an act of violence and coercion serves to undermine any audience sympathies for those fighting for human rights. While exposing some of the issues of a clandestine global trade in organs, both films in different ways effect an important relocation of exploitation, and responsibility for exploitation, away from the wider context of global inequalities and down onto the more localised activities of a criminal sub-class.

Literary explorations of the gift of donation focus on the personal experiential and emotional journeys of those most closely involved. Two novels suggest the emergence of a donation literary genre in that both follow the journeys of several characters connected either to a child who has suddenly and unexpectedly died or to an ill child who benefits from the subsequent act of donation (Snelling, 2008; Wolfson, 2011). The focus on children, a category of person that is both vulnerable and innocent of their ill-health condition, underscores the loss and the benefit by maximising both in terms of the years of life that have been lost and the years of life that are regained in relation to what is considered a normal lifespan. The focus on children thus effectively promotes the gifting of organs to the reader by rendering both loss and benefit wholly unambiguous. At the same time, there is a further benefit in the suggestion that the act of donation, in saving the life of another child, may afford the relatives of the deceased some degree of comfort in the longer term. At the end of Jill Wolfson's book *Cold Hands, Warm Heart* (2011), the mother of the deceased child lays her head against the chest of the recipient child to hear the beating heart of her daughter, the gift that has enabled another young life to be lived.

Part of the underlying difference in these two dominant discourses relates to what may be considered a normal lifespan. While this clearly varies across time and space, the idea itself of 'premature death' is relatively recent, having emerged together with the development of techniques to assess population mortality and longevity rates. As such, the perception of a 'premature death' is 'intimately bound to the spatial and temporal regularities of mortality' (Tyner, 2015: 361). The threat of premature death can be resisted by some better than by others; that is, the resources to prevent premature death can be accessed by some better than by others in the context of scarcity (Kearns and Reid-Henry, 2009). While attention has been given to the illegal trade in organs, the growing market in medical tourism may in reality be the greater challenge to global inequalities in access to organs. Cohen (1999) argued that in the case of the market of live kidney donation in India, the problem for the market was less one of organ scarcity but rather one of recipient scarcity. Those willing to sell were many, given their conditions of poverty and debt; those able to pay the costs of transplantation were fewer. As advances in the technologies of organ transplant enable markets for organs to operate globally, the shortage of local buyers becomes less of an issue.

The current debates on organ procurement now centre on how to increase legal donation by moving beyond the rhetoric of the gift, and two possible policy routes attract the most attention: the opt-out system and the legal sale of organs. A procurement system based on an opt-out register, rather than the more common voluntary opt-in system, has been adopted by only a few countries to date, including Spain and Finland (Lindberg, 2013). Similarly, only one country, Iran, has to date made it legal to sell a kidney, a permission that is actively encouraged through further state incentives to the seller over and above the payment from the buyer. Iran argues that the policy has eradicated its long waiting lists; others argue that the legalised trade does nothing to address the disproportionate sale of kidneys by the same sub-group of the poor and vulnerable that characterise illegal markets (Alesi and Muzi, 2015). While legal systems, such as that of the United Kingdom, formally deny property rights over the human body, such debates broach related areas of contestation over who owns the body and who can exercise consent: opt-out systems effectively position by default the body as belonging to the state after death, albeit with a recognition of personal ownership through a non-consent option; in practice, the medical profession is sensitive to the wishes of the deceased relatives, even to the extent of overruling the deceased's own wishes, at which point ownership over the body is effectively held by the extended kinship group (BBC, 2013; Guardian, 2015); by contrast, arguments for a legalised market for organs reassert private ownership of the body. The Internet also offers routes through which individuals may reassert the private ownership of their body parts by providing virtual spaces in which would-be donors and patients needing an organ, and particularly a kidney, can now meet. This not only moves the act of gifting onto an international scale, but perhaps more importantly permits donors to select the recipients of their body parts. This option to determine the recipient of a donation is implicitly explored in Gabriele Muccino's film *Seven Pounds* (2008), Ben has identified seven strangers to benefit after his suicide, including from his body parts. But first he wants to make sure they are worthy of his gift, invoking a long tradition of judging who is and who is not deserving of charity. Moreover, *Seven Pounds* is an excellent example of how imaginary explorations have their own agency because the film privileges certain motivations for donation over others. Ben initially seeks redemption for his negligent driving which was responsible for seven deaths, but falls in love with one of his beneficiaries and finally sacrifices himself for the sake of a loved and known other. This personalised motive is positioned in the film as superior to a motive of giving back, implicitly undermining the value of donating to society or to humanity. This undermining of a more social commitment, of the giving-over of the body through its excorporations to a social body (Cohen, 2013), aligns with the tenets of a neoliberal project while still adhering to the rhetoric of the heroic gift, and, as such, represents a local accommodation of the distinction between the two dominant analytical discourses of global exploitation and national beatific gifting.

Tensions of Inter-corporeality

Whether cautionary, condemnatory or celebratory, these discourses share two important and related features: first, they focus on the 'donation' (voluntary or coerced) as the critical moment in the transplantation process; and second, the medical act is implicitly presented as a success, the desired route to the recovery of health and of normal living, and the happy end-point to the story. However, social scientists need to pause and interrogate this happy ending and reintroduce the role of biology into our accounts.

Body parts are not as easily interchangeable as explorations of transplants within either neoliberalisation or gifting accounts imply. The body has a fierce system for policing its boundaries through the immune system; the technologies for coinciding with or bypassing the processes of the immune system have been one of the major successes in transplant medicine. The successes of the earliest transplants depended on a very close matching of blood and human leukocyte antigens, and it remains the case that a family member may be the optimal source for an organ. The expansion of modern transplant medicine's potential has come about through the development of pharmacological technologies that can effect a total suppression of the immune system, enabling the introduced organ to pass by the body's rigorous border controls. The immune system and the immunosuppressant drugs, such as cyclosporine, are vital central actants within the processes of transplantation but have received limited attention within social analyses compared with the procurement of organs (for exceptions, see Cohen, 2001; Kierans, 2011). It is the power of the action of these immunosuppressant pharmaceuticals that has widened the pool of potential organ donors for any given recipient and, as such, underpins the possibility of the gift of life from unrelated strangers or the purchase of an organ from those living in poverty in distant countries. Similarly, the organ transplantation process does not end at the point of donation and transfer to the recipient; recipients must continue to take immunosuppressant drugs for the rest of their lives and these drugs not only suppress rejection of the introduced organ, but also rejection of all other noxious entities, leaving transplant recipients particularly vulnerable to other causes of ill-health (Cohen, 2001; Kierans, 2011). This dependency on pharmacological technologies to avoid the rejection of the introduced organ constantly reasserts and reconstitutes a corporeal relation between the recipient and the organ donor in which the presence of the other somewhat paradoxically both enables and threatens life.

Despite the power of immunosuppressant technologies, physicians still match on various biomarkers to maximise the success of transplantation. The relocation of the medical gaze to the molecular scale of bodies is argued to be reworking the forms of biopolitics in the governance of life itself (Rose, 2007). The interactions of molecular and genetic variations with existing socio-political categories of gender and race have generated debate as to whether this relocated gaze may offer an emancipatory discourse in the face of racialised bodies (Reardon, 2012; Skinner, 2006). The possibility to excorporate body parts for the benefit of an unknown other and of incorporating part of the body of an unknown other confronts potential donors and recipients with their own prejudices about different, and particularly racialised, bodies. While Waldby (2002) argued that inter-corporeality in organ exchange may sometimes generate feelings of kinship or profound destabilisations of identity, the growing global market for organs through medical tourism, whether legal or illegal, suggests a detachment or even disregard for the body of the donor.

The exploitation of one set of people by another is not a new phenomenon, but the emergence of a justification for such exploitation through a racialised discourse emerged to resolve a tension between the universal humanism of the enlighten-ment and the inequalities generated by European imperialism and capitalism (Kobayashi, 2004; Skinner, 2006). The construction of 'race' as a category predic-ated on biological difference became naturalised so as to construct the bodies of those colonised as inferior and therefore justifiably subjugated, governed or even enslaved (Kobayashi and Peake, 1994). The mixing of bodies through sexual reproduction within this discourse was often legally prohibited and certainly socially condemned, but genomic projects have demonstrated the high levels that nonetheless occurred and which give witness to the exploitation of women of colour by colonial men (Skinner, 2006). This historic racialisation of bodies in social and political life perpetuates into the present through continued discrimin-ation and resultant inequalities both within and between nation states. The prac-tice of blurring the social and biological continues within organ transplantation through the reworked category of 'ethnicity' in those countries, such as the United Kingdom, where the ethnic classification of persons is used as a proxy for the molecular specificities of tissue matching. In other words, potential donors and recipients are matched by the social proxy of 'ethnicity' rather than by the assess-ment of relevant biological measures (Kierans, 2013).

In medical tourism, the significance of a racialised identity is reflected in how reproductive services are sought through the global market. Whereas new centres for medical tourism that cater for a range of surgical procedures are being inten-tionally developed in postcolonial low- and middle-income countries, white Europeans seeking reproductive donations through the global market predomin-antly prefer services from other European countries (Gunnarson Payne, 2015). In this respect, although the maintenance of a family line through genetic relatedness is sidestepped, the maintenance of the family genealogy through racialised affili-ation remains significant. This is in striking contrast to the practice of those seeking organs to increase their survivability who are willing to accept and incor-porate an organ of a racialised other in concert with the incorporation of immun-osuppressant drugs that may be seen as suppressing the otherness of the transplant organ. To a great extent, the ability to incorporate an organ that originates from a body that is different in molecular terms, whether or not it also differs culturally, ethnically and economically, relies on an understanding of the workings of the body through a mechanical metaphor. Whereas social scientists have challenged biomedicine for seeing bodies only in terms of their component parts and for a binary distinction between body and mind, organ transplantation reasserts these: body parts can function as spare parts, transferable from one setting to another;

identity is independent of the origin of bodily material, although not of overall bodily health. Legal frameworks that insist on the renunciation of ownership of body matter once donated similarly support an understanding of bodily matter as separable from identity (Lock, 2002). The extent to which bodily matter may 'retain some of the values of personhood for many if not most donors and recipients' as argued by Waldby (2002: 240) may vary by type of donation and the particular social role accorded to that issue by society.

There are few accounts of medical tourism for transplantation. Those that exist, as with much of contemporary research, tend to end at the point that an organ has been sourced and the operation undertaken. The biography *Larry's Kidney* (Rose, 2009) follows the journey of US citizen Larry who travels with his cousin, the book's narrator, to source a kidney and a transplantation operation illegally on the global market. The account follows their experiences and emotions in negotiating the health system and culture of a different country and the cousins' relationship with each other in this context. These aspects have been examined through a lens of emotional geographies in terms of confronting otherness (Kingsbury *et al.*, 2012), but not in terms of incorporating otherness, which does not emerge as one of the significant emotional dimensions in the account of Larry's search for a kidney. Receiving and incorporating the organs of a nationally different other seems to involve less of Waldby's 'complex modification of the recipient's embodied identity' (2002: 241) than of the emotional and cross-cultural journey that took Larry to the point of receiving a kidney transplant in the first place. That said, Larry's subsequent experience as a post-transplant patient gets almost no attention and is noted only briefly in an epilogue, indicating his continued ill-health and dependency on immunosuppressants. There has similarly been very little empirical research on post-transplantation experiences that might elaborate the complexities and variations of Waldby's introceptive experiences of transplant incorporations. One of the few studies highlights the continued challenges for organ recipients; as one post-transplantation informant in Mexico states, 'I thought I would be healthy again, and normal, but really I'm just a different kind of patient now' (Crowley-Matoka, 2005: 821).

There is then a bias in the analytical approaches to the global inequalities in organ transplantation that privileges the suffering of donors and underplays that of recipients, and as such generates a further form of inequality, that of an inequality of concern (Kierans, 2011). The discourse of the gift as an altruistic act of beneficence was premised on selective readings of anthropology (Titmuss, 1970; Fontaine, 2002) and is further complemented by anthropological understandings of the gift as part of the social relations of reciprocal exchange, obligation and expectation (Sharp and Randhawa, 2014). The limited ethnographic work that exists with transplant recipients has been framed within the discourse of the gift to disclose the modes of reciprocity that emerge within kin networks and the sense of obligation felt by recipients towards their donor and to the organ itself to follow healthy lifestyle behaviours. Kierans (2011), drawing together anthropological work undertaken in Ireland, Mexico and the Philippines, emphasises the challenges that face the recipients of organ transplantation post-operation, the lack of concern within some healthcare systems and the guilt that recipients feel in the face of expectations by others that they are now restored to health when in reality they are still quite unwell. As Kierans argues in summary, 'Transplantation does extend life, but the lives so extended are radically altered in the process' (2011: 1473).

Tensions of scarcity and inter-corporeality

Improving organ transplantation and improving lives post-transplantation will depend on improving the subtlety of immunosuppressant drug actions or, better still, removing the need for them altogether. The perfect organ match is likely to remain the organ of the identical other, the identical twin or, since most people do not have identical twins, the identical clone. Creative imaginings of future dystopic societies have resolved the tensions of scarcity and inter-corporeality through the production and medical exploitation of a parallel, cloned sub-class to maintain a population's well-being. The narrative of these imaginings hangs on an unequivocal moral position that these practices are to be condemned and the story-line follows how humanity is restored to the exploited bodies. The insights for a critical engagement with contemporary practices of a global market for organ transplantation come not from the condemnation but from the various discourses that are used to justify treating and categorising their supplier population as non-human.

Three examples illustrate this resolution of the tensions of scarcity and inter-corporeality through cloning in future dystopic societies. In the New Earth of the BBC's *Dr Who* (2002), the hospital is run by cat-like nuns who have the knowledge to cure all human ailments. However, the nuns' healing expertise reflects an accelerated rate of knowledge acquisition brought about by experimenting on thousands of human clones which they secretly grow in vaults and infect with diseases. The actions of the sisters are illegal in New Earth but no one is looking too closely at the source of the evident gains. In Michael Bay's *The Island* (2005), customers pay for the growth of customised organs but the scientist-businessman finds it more profitable to produce whole body clones. Similar to New Earth, the exploitation of clones is illegal but again we intuit a society content not to look too closely, a suspicion supported when the non-clone customer is confronted with the reality of his clone double and finds himself unable to act ethically in the face of his potential mortality. By contrast, the society of Kazuo Ishiguro's novel *Never Let Me Go* (2005) openly sanctions cloning to provide a customised organ supply and, as such, requires different and collective strategies to justify the clones' subjugation to organ harvesting. Although the clones are well cared for, especially as they grow up, society's discourses and rhetoric must categorise them as sub-human, even for those most intimately involved with their childhoods. Ishiguro displays the effectiveness of such categorisation: a woman who collects their artwork displays her abhorrence; their headteacher admits that she always had to steel herself to face them.

For us as audience, the location of these scenarios into fictitious futures presents a series of possible, but improbable, undesirable outcomes that we need and indeed will avoid; the audience agrees with the condemnation and reaffirms a need for public debate around new technologies and effective regulation. But treating these examples of exploitation as improbably cautionary tales may over-state both the extent of our condemnation and the power of regulation. Even in the setting in which the clones are most abased, the morality is tinged with a troubling ambiguity. The nuns in *Dr Who* do not act from self-interest; they act from a professional commitment and compassion towards their human patients and justify their actions by arguing that more humane methods of research would have been too slow. This is not a form of argumentation that is unfamiliar to modern audiences; recent scandals of body mining and other misuses of bodily matter have exposed closet and illegal practices by health professionals who claim to be acting for the collective good (BBC, 2010; Dewar and Boddington, 2004).

In *Never Let Me Go*, the language and behaviour of those who care for the cloned children make explicit the ways in which discourse differentiates bodies and underpins the power relations that enable the sustainable exploitation of some bodies by others. Here new rationales are needed; unlike existing discourses that support racism and slavery through biological arguments or bio-logics (Tyner, 2015), discrimination against the corporeal other cannot be grounded in assumed associations and disassociations of genetics, geographical origin and personality deficiencies; differentiation is not based on outward signs of potential group otherness such as colour, dress or religion but on an inward or invisible otherness defined by the personal provenance of bodies. In the future dystopias where two bodies intentionally share the same genetic make-up through the technology of cloning, superiority and dominance are granted on the grounds of which body is authentically human. This human authenticity is granted to the body that was the original first and whose production was resourced through the convention of two parents; identical 'copies' derived through technology and resourced only by one 'parent' do not count as authentically human and, as such, are accorded no claim to human rights.

The possibilities for full human cloning, on which such discrimination would depend, still seem distant. By contrast, discrimination directed to bodies that fail to accord with socially sanctioned body forms or bodily behaviour is very much evident in the present. Lifestyle choices as a basis for discrimination, and bodily exploitation is a theme picked up in Ninni Holmqvist's *The Unit* (2008), a novel which imagines a most plausible future society, a near-future Sweden that has adapted its tradition of a strong collective commitment to the welfare state to encompass a collective response to the demand for scarce organs. At 50, those persons categorised as non-essential must move to the closed 'Unit' of the title from where they will be involved in drug tests and make donations up until their death. The Unit is luxurious, the inhabitants well looked after; the critical aspect here is who counts as essential and who does not, and the Unit is thus populated by those without children, without established partners or not in a valued occupa-tion. This latter may easily be read as not in an economically productive occupa-tion given the disproportionate representation of artists in the Unit. Perhaps more importantly, this hierarchy of value accorded to lifestyle behaviours transforms effortlessly into a hierarchy that is understood as an embodied essentialism. When the main character falls in love and becomes pregnant in the Unit, she cannot be reclassified. As an artist and as a late parent, she is already fatally designated as unsuitable and her child will be adopted by a 'normalised' family.

These future imagined worlds in turn have their own futures hinted at. Both Holmqvist and Ishiguro indicate the fragility of the good care offered to these donor bodies, hinting at a move towards harsher practices. Once bodies are cast as less valued, as amenable to exploitation to save more valued others, then they are already effectively categorised as lesser humans and the discourse that supports an investment in those bodies can be easily transformed into the very different justifications underpinning dehumanising attitudes and practices of abjection.

This chapter has travelled through lived and imagined engagements with the tensions of scarcity and inter-corporeality in the global practices of organ trans-plantation to draw our attention to the importance of the different modes of argu-mentation through which particular practices are justified. In particular, the historical and the potential future blurring of the social and the biological in differentiating bodies as same or different or as more and less valuable takes place within the context of such tensions and the context of increasingly available global markets for medical care. The dominant emphasis in social science analyses on neoliberalism and globalisation privileges the tensions of scarcity in our analyses of medical tourism, but our analyses need to include reflection on how existing modes of differentiation and discrimination might be reworked, renego-tiated or reimagined. Analytical work that can disclose the underlying forms of argumentation that apparently resolve or make invisible the evident tensions of scarcity and inter-corporeality which confront the practices of global transplant tourism is essential work within the processes of ongoing social deliberation about our modes of collective involvement with new and emergent medical tech-nologies. Literature and film afford an alternative and complementary source of nuanced data on the range of possible experiences of those whose lives are directly affected by the accommodations made around the tensions of scarcity and inter-corporeality, and which shape the practices of mixing and fixing bodies in the global market for health and medicine.

References

Ackerman, S. (2010) Plastic paradise: transforming bodies and selves in Costa Rica's cosmetic surgery tourism industry. *Medical Anthropology*, 29: 403–423.

Adams, K., Crooks, V.A., Cohen, G. and Whitmore, R. (2015a) Medical tourism in the tropics. *Global Village*, 13. Available at http://www.aglobalvillage.org/journal/online/medical-tourism-in-the-tropics_krystyna-adams/ (accessed 28 September 2016).

Adams, K., Snyder, J., Crooks, V. and Johnston, R. (2015b) Tourism discourse and medical tourists' motivations to travel. *Tourism Review*, 70: 85–96.

Alesi, F. and Muzi, L. (2015) Kidneys for sale: Iran's trade in organs. Guardian, May. Available at http://www.theguardian.com/society/2015/may/10/kidneys-for-sale-organ-donation-iran (accessed 28 September 2016).

Atkinson, S. (2016) Care, kidneys and clones: the distance of space, time and imagination. In Whitehead, A., Woods, A., Atkinson, S., Macnaughton, J. and Richards, J., eds, *The Edinburgh Companion to the Critical Medical Humanities*, pp. 611–626. Edinburgh: Edinburgh University Press.

Atkinson, S. and Robson, M. (2012) Arts and health as a practice of liminality: managing the spaces of transformation for social and emotional wellbeing with primary school children. *Health & Place* 18: 1348–1355.

Atkinson, S. and Scott, K. (2015) Stable and destabilised states of subjective wellbeing: dance and movement as catalysts of transitions. *Social and Cultural Geography*, 16: 75–94.

Atwood, M. (2011) *Never Let Me Go* by Kazuo Ishiguro. In *M. Atwood In Other Worlds. SF and the Human Imagination*, pp. 168–173. London: Virago.

Bay, M. (2005) *The Island*. USA: Dreamworks.

BBC (2002) New Earth, *Dr Who* Series 2, Episode 1, 15 April. London: BBC.

BBC (2010) Sellafield body parts families given government apology. Available at http://www.bbc.co.uk/news/uk-england-cumbria-11768944, 16 November (accessed 28 September 2016).

BBC (2013) 'Stop Families' from overriding donor consent. Available at http://www.bbc.co.uk/news/health-23260057 (accessed 28 September 2016).

Cameron, K., Crooks, V.A., Chouinard, V., Snyder, J. and Johnston, R. (2014) Motivation, justification, normalization: talk strategies used by Canadian medical tourists regarding their choices to go abroad for hip and knee surgeries. *Social Science and Medicine*, 106: 93–100.

CDC (2015) Medical tourism. Available at http://www.cdc.gov/features/medicaltourism/ (accessed 30 July 2015).

Cohen, L. (1999) Where it hurts: Indian material for an ethics of organ transplantation. *Daedalus*, 128: 135–165.

Cohen, L. (2001) The other kidney: biopolitics beyond recognition. *Body and Society*, 7: 9–29.

Cohen, L. (2013) Given over to demand: excorporation as commitment. *Contemporary South Asia*, 21: 318–322.

Crooks, V.A., Li, N., Snyder, J., Dharamsi, S., Benjaminy, S., Jacob, K.J. and Illes, J. (2015) 'You don't want to lose that trust that you've built with this patient . . .': (dis) trust, medical tourism, and the Canadian family physician–patient relationship. *BMC Family Practice*, 16: 25, Doi 10.1186/s12875-015-0245-6.

Crowley-Matoka, M. (2005) Desperately seeking 'Normal': the promise and perils of living with kidney transplantation. *Social Science and Medicine*, 61: 821–831.

Dear, M., Ketchum, J., Luria, S. and Richardson, D., eds (2011) *GeoHumanities: Art, History, Text at the Edge of Place*. New York: Routledge.

Dewar, S. and Boddington, P. (2004) Returning to the Alder Hey report and its reporting: addressing confusions and improving inquiries. *Journal of Medical Ethics*, 30: 463–469.

England, K. (2015) Nurses across borders: global migration of registered nurses to the US. *Gender, Place and Culture: A Journal of Feminist Geography*, 22: 143–156.

Foley, R. (2015) Indigenous narratives of health: (re)placing folk-medicine within Irish health histories. *Journal of Medical Humanities*, 36: 5–18.

Fontaine, P. (2002) Blood, politics and social science: Richard Titmuss and the Institute of Economic Affairs, 1957–1973. *Isis*, 93: 401–434.

Frears, S. (2002) *Dirty, Pretty Things*. Miramax.

Galtung, J. (1969) Violence, peace, and peace research. *Journal of Peace Research*, 6: 167–191.

Gesler, W.M. (2003) *Healing Places*. Oxford: Rowman & Littlefield.

Greenhough, B., Parry, B., Dyck, I. and Brown, T. (2015) Introduction: the gendered geographies of 'bodies across borders'. *Gender, Place and Culture: A Journal of Feminist Geography*, 22: 83–89.

Guardian (2015) http://www.theguardian.com/australia-news/2015/mar/01/organ-donation-rates-held-back-by-families-refusing-consent-study-finds (accessed 28 September 2016).

Gunnarson Payne, J. (2015) Reproduction in transition: cross-border egg donation, biodesirability and new reproductive subjectivities on the European fertility market. *Gender, Place and Culture: A Journal of Feminist Geography*, 22: 107–122.

Helble, M. (2011) The movement of patients across borders: challenges and opportunities for public health. *Bulletin of the World Health Organization* 89: 68–72.

Hohm, C. and Snyder, J. (2015) 'It was the best decision of my life': a thematic content analysis of former medical tourists' patient testimonials. *BMC Medical Ethics*, 16: 8.

Holliday, R., Bell, D., Hardy, K. and Hunter, E. (2015) Beautiful face, beautiful place: relational geographies and gender in cosmetic surgery tourism websites. *Gender, Place and Culture: A Journal of Feminist Geography*, 22: 90–106.

Holmqvist, N. (2008) *The Unit*, translated from Swedish by Marlaine Delargy. Oxford: One World [2006].

Ishiguro, K. (2005) *Never Let Me Go*. London: Faber and Faber.

Johnston, R., Adams, K., Bishop, L., Crooks, V.A. and Snyder, J. (2015a) 'Best care on the ground' versus 'elitist healthcare': concerns and competing expectations for medical tourism development in Barbados. *International Journal for Equity in Health*, 14: 15, Doi:10.1186/s12939-015-0147-1.

Johnston, R., Crooks, V.A., Snyder, J. and Whitmore, R. (2015b) 'The major forces that need to back medical tourism were ... in alignment: championing development of Barbados' medical tourism sector. *International Journal of Health Services*, 45: 334–352.

Kearns, G. and Reid-Henry, S. (2009) Vital geographies: life, luck and the human condition. *Annals of the Association of American Geographers*, 99: 554–574.

Kierans, C. (2011) Anthropology, organ transplantation and the immune system: resituating commodity and gift exchange. *Social Science and Medicine*, 73: 1469–1476.

Kierans, C. 2013) The emergence of the 'ethnic donor': the cultural production and relocation of organ donation in the UK. *Anthropology and Medicine*, 20: 221–231.

Kierans, C. (2015) Biopolitics and capital: poverty, mobility and the body-in-transplantation in Mexico. *Body and Society*, 21: 42–65.

Kingsbury, P., Crooks, V.A., Snyder, J., Johnston, R. and Adams, K. (2012) Narratives of emotion and anxiety in medical tourism: on *State of the Heart* and *Larry's Kidney*. *Social and Cultural Geography*, 13: 361–378.

Kitzinger, J. (2010) Questioning the sci-fi alibi: a critique of how 'science fiction fears' are used to explain away public concerns about risk. *Journal of Risk Research*, 13: 73–86.

Kobayashi, A. (2004) Critical 'race' approaches in cultural geography. In Duncan, J., Johnson, N.J. and Schein, H., eds, *A Companion to Cultural Geography*, pp. 238–249. Oxford: Blackwell.

Kobayashi, A. and Peake, L. (1994) Unnatural discourse. 'Race' and gender in geography. *Gender, Place and Culture: A Journal of Feminist Geography*, 1: 225–243.

Lindberg, S. (2013) The obligatory gift of organ transplants: the case of the Finnish law on the medical use of human organs, tissues, and cells. *Alternatives: Global, Local, Political*, 38: 245–255.

Lock, M. (2002) *Twice Dead: Organ Transplants and the Reinvention of Death*. Berkeley: University of California Press.

Marston, S. and De Leeuw, S. (2013) Creativity and geography: towards a politicized intervention. *The Geographical Review*, 103: ii–xxvi.

Muccino, G. (2008) *Seven Pounds*. USA: Columbia.

NaRanong, A. and NaRanong, V. (2011) The effects of medical tourism: Thailand's experience. *Bulletin of the World Health Organization*, 89: 336–344.

OECD (2014) *Health at a Glance: Europe, 2014*. OECD Publishing.

Parry, B. (2008) Entangled exchange: reconceptualising the characterisation and practice of bodily commodification. *Geoforum*, 39: 1133–1144.

Parry, B., Greenhough, B., Brown, T. and Dyck, I., eds (2015) *Bodies across Borders: The Global Circulation of Body Parts, Medical Tourists and Professionals*. Farnham: Ashgate.

Petersen, A. and Seear, K. (2011) Technologies of hope: techniques of the online advertising of stem cell treatments. *New Genetics and Society*, 30: 329–346.

Petersen, A., Seear, K. and Munsie, M. (2014) Therapeutic journeys: the hopeful travails of stem cell tourists. *Sociology of Health and Illness*, 36: 670–685.

Philo, C., Cadman, L. and Lea, J. (2015) New energy geographies: a case study of yoga, meditation and healthfulness. *Journal of Medical Humanities*, 36, 35–46.

Reardon, J. (2012) The democratic, anti-racist genome? Technoscience at the limits of liberalism. *Science and Culture*, 21: 25–47.

Reubi, D. (2012) The human capacity to reflect and decide: bioethics and the reconfiguration of the research subject in the British biomedical sciences. *Social Studies of Science*, 42(3): 348–368.

Rose, D.A. (2009) *Larry's Kidney*. New York: Harper Collins.

Rose, N. (2007) *The Politics of Life Itself*. Princeton, NJ: Princeton University Press.

Scheper-Hughes, N. (2002) Bodies for sale – whole or in parts. In Scheper-Hughes, N. and Wacquant, L., eds, *Commodifying Bodies*, pp. 1–8. London: Sage.

Scheper-Hughes, N. (2003) Keeping an eye on the global traffic in human organs. *The Lancet*, 361(9369): 1645–1648.

Schneider, I. (2015) Race to the bottom or race to the top? Governing medical tourism in a globalised world. In Parry, B., Greenhough, B., Brown, T. and Dyck, I., eds. *Bodies across Borders: The Global Circulation of Body Parts, Medical Tourists and Professionals*, pp. 191–210. Farnham: Ashgate.

Seale, C. (2003) Health and media: an overview. *Sociology of Health and Illness*, 25: 513–531.

Sharp, C. and Randhawa, G. (2014) Altruism, gift giving and reciprocity in organ donation: a review of cultural perspectives and challenges of the concepts. *Transplantation Reviews*, 28: 163–168.

Skinner, D. (2006) Racialized futures: biologism and the changing politics of identity. *Social Studies of Science*, 36: 459–488.

Snelling, L. (2008) *One Perfect Day*. New York: FaithWords.

Snyder, J., Crooks, V.A., Johnston, R. and Dharamsi, S. (2013) 'Do your homework . . . and then hope for the best': the challenges that medical tourism poses to Canadian family physician's support of patients' informed decision-making. *BMC Medical Ethics*, 14: 37.

Snyder, J., Adams, K., Crooks, V.A., Whitehurst, D. and Vallee, J. (2014) 'I knew what was going to happen if I did nothing and so I was going to do something': faith, hope, and trust in the decisions of Canadians with multiple sclerosis to seek unproven interventions abroad. *BMC Health Services Research*, 14: 445.

Snyder, J., Byambaa, T., Johnston, R., Crooks, V.A., Janes, C. and Ewan, M. (2015a) Outbound medical tourism from Mongolia: a qualitative examination of proposed domestic health system and policy responses to this trend. *BMC Health Services Research*, 15: 187.

Snyder, J., Crooks, V.A., Johnston, R., Adams, K. and Whitmore, R. (2015b) Medical tourism's impacts on health worker migration in the Caribbean: five examples and their implications for global justice. *Global Health Action*, 8: 27348.

Stockwell, J. (2006) *Turistas (Paradise Lost)*. USA: Fox.

Svaenaeus, F. (2010) The body as gift, resource or commodity? Heidegger and the ethics of organ transplantation. *Bioethical Inquiry*, 7: 163–172.

Titmuss, R.M. (1970) *The Gift Relationship: From Human Blood to Social Policy*. London: Allen and Unwin.

Tonnellier, F. and Curtis, S. (2005) Medicine, landscapes, symbols: '*The country Doctor*' by Honoré de Balzac. *Health & Place*, 11: 313–321.

Tyner, J.A. (2015) Population geography II: Mortality, premature death, and the ordering of life. *Progress in Human Geography*, 39: 360–373.

Waldby, C. (2002) Biomedicine, tissue transfer and intercorporeality. *Feminist Theory*, 3: 239–254.

Whittaker, A. (2008) Pleasure and pain: medical travel in Asia. *Global Public Health: An International Journal for Research, Policy and Practice*, 3: 271–290.

Whittaker, A. (2010) Challenges of medical travel to global regulation: a case study of reproductive travel in Asia. *Global Social Policy*, 10: 396–415.

Wolfson, J. (2011) *Cold Hands, Warm Heart*. London: Walker Books.

Part II

Global health, power and politics

5 Making ties through making drugs

Partnerships for tuberculosis drug and vaccine development

Susan Craddock

Introduction

In the past ten years or so, Product Development Partnerships (PDPs) consisting of non-profit organisations, pharmaceutical companies, philanthropists and universities have formed to develop new vaccines and drugs for tuberculosis and malaria for the first time in decades. Several new drug compounds and vaccine candidates are already moving down the research and development pipeline, causing excitement among researchers, activists and public health practitioners hoping finally to mitigate these diseases in high-burden regions. Yet there are also critiques of PDPs, one being that they focus too narrowly on technological interventions such as drugs, diagnostics, vaccines, and other biomedical tools designed to address specific diseases, to the detriment of broader social and economic measures such as income-generating mechanisms, educational enhancement programmes or nutrition supplement schemes. In so doing, they ignore the conditions in resource-deprived populations producing a range of health problems including but not limited to infectious diseases, even while they might succeed in curing some individuals of specific diseases (Buse and Harmer, 2007; Buse and Walt, 2000). PDPs are also critiqued for diverting limited national health budgets from other, equally trenchant public health issues, and taking their mandate from US, UK or European organisations rather than from the populations targeted for pharmaceutical rollout (Biehl, 2011, 2007). As Vincanne Adams further argues, pharmaceutical research and the scientific methods it relies upon has even caused a shift in the notion of what 'health' even means, in part because research focuses only on those diseases amenable to pharmaceutical potential (Adams, 2010).

These claims all warrant attention, yet what I want to do in this chapter is to complicate the 'either/or' binaries that these critiques establish between pharmaceutical versus socio-economic interventions in global health. I want to do this by suggesting that many interventions encompass within them elements that are both social and technical. This may be easier to see in programmes that are more social and economic in their remit: nutritional supplement programmes, for example, may include new agricultural tools and techniques, and income-generating programmes may include new technologies for running small businesses. Yet even 'technical' interventions such as those championed by PDPs can include social and economic facets. The approaches which four PDPs I highlight in this chapter have to pharmaceutical research, development and dissemination in many ways disrupt these binaries by evidencing social and economic benefits that can accrue precisely *through* the process of pharmaceutical development. This is not to argue against the need for other economic, structural and social interventions into the entrenched poverty and disease nexus, but rather to argue that these binaries do not always exist as such, or are not uniformly displayed across geographies and interventions. This leads to the second point, which is that it is ultimately more productive to move away from the categorisation of interventions and towards a more specific examination of the politics and procedures governing particular interventions. In the case of PDPs, it is constructive to examine areas for improving upon, rather than dismissing, their approaches to pharmaceutical production, and the scientific, governmental and community exchanges they mobilise.

Those PDPs I focus on in this chapter – namely TB Alliance, Aeras, PATH Malaria Vaccine Initiative (MVI) and the Drugs for Neglected Diseases Initiative (DNDi) – are united in mandating of all their partners including industry that any therapeutics produced as a result of their collaborations must be made accessible and affordable to those who need them. That is, for the first time in decades, these PDPs are making serious attempts to shift proprietary practices in drug and vaccine development to protect low rather than high prices, and to tether pharmaceutical investment strategies to the social and medical needs of the global poor. By doing so, health and healthcare inequities are highlighted, but so too is the travesty of 'the unglamorous misery of impoverished people dying from curable disease', to borrow a poignant phrase from Peter Redfield in his book *Doctors Without Borders* (2013, 107).[1]

Spearheading a divergent model of therapeutic production thus means revisioning markets, patents and consumers. It also means expanding the logic of responsibility and community–government relations typical of mainstream commercial pharmaceutical production. Because the goal of PDPs is not only to develop new drugs and vaccines but also to get these to the people who need them, they see their operations encompassing more than laboratories and production facilities to include the governments, scientists and select communities of countries their technologies are designed to benefit. This, in turn, means that PDPs are not just engines of the technical fix. The broader collaborative institutional relations within which new tuberculosis and malaria therapeutics occur blur the boundaries between technical and nontechnical interventions because PDP approaches encompass, among other things, community outreach, infrastructural development, job training, scientific network enhancements and regulatory agency strengthening, thereby expanding considerably the social economies of biomedical intervention.

This does not mean, however, that PDPs necessarily transcend inequitable social and political relations that have long characterised scientific exchanges between Europe or the USA and lower income countries. Yet, even here, there are hopeful signs that the geopolitics of exchange will be shifting in the future towards greater equity in how and what kinds of scientific knowledge production and technology development happen in these partnerships. In the rest of this chapter, based on interviews, international conference proceedings, pharmaceutical facility tours and a clinical trial site visit, I elaborate on the agglomerative effects of malaria and tuberculosis vaccine and drug production, arguing that these techno-logies' traces are multiple, highly variable, yet productive not just in potentially diminishing long-standing burdens of disease, but in galvanising broader social, economic and geopolitical benefits in targeted communities.

The economic and biomedical milieux of malaria and tuberculosis

Tuberculosis and malaria remain two of the most significant causes of global morbidity and mortality in lower income countries. Tuberculosis kills close to one and a half million people a year, newly infects nine million, and costs the global economy an estimated US$380 million a year in lost wages, treatment and hospit-alisation (WHO, 2012a; TBVI, 2013). Malaria in turn caused an estimated 584,000 deaths with 198 million cases in 2013 (WHO, 2014). Both of these diseases disproportionately affect poor people in low-income countries, which means that pharmaceutical companies have not pursued vaccines or drug treat-ments for them because these would not be lucrative enough to warrant the millions of dollars it would take to develop them. Commercial pharmaceutical production today is highly geared towards markets: what gets developed typically is what will earn robust returns on investment, not what will help the most people. This bottom line does not preclude the development of life-saving vaccines and drugs when this matches up with a sufficient, and sufficiently financed, consumer base: the hypertension, diabetes and cancer drugs developed in recent years are powerful testament to that. It is thus not inaccurate to state, as one large pharma-ceutical company does on its website, that they 'are dedicated to improving the quality of human life by enabling people to do more, feel better, live longer' (gsk. com). The question is: What constituencies are they aiming to make feel better and live longer? The London and New York Stock Exchange share prices listed on the same web page for their investors and 'updated every 15 and 20 minutes, respectively' are a clue to answering that question (ibid.). Publicly traded pharma-ceutical companies – which encompasses all of the major ones – are beholden first and foremost to their shareholders and thus to a return on dollars invested. Consumers in higher income countries who have sufficient insurance or income to pay what the market can bear for drugs are the ones the pharmaceutical industry is making feel better and live longer, not the poor in low-income countries (Kesselheim, 2011; GAO, 2006; Dumit, 2012).

Notwithstanding this reality, new treatments are needed for tuberculosis and malaria for multiple reasons. BCG, the current tuberculosis vaccine, came into use in the 1920s and is still the most widely used vaccine in the world, yet this is despite its highly variable efficacy. Although the vaccine confers some degree of protection against pulmonary tuberculosis (TB of the lungs) in infants, it confers no protection against other forms of tuberculosis, and no protection for pulmonary TB in later childhood. How much protection the BCG vaccine confers varies widely, and seemingly geographically, with rates ranging from zero to around 80 per cent and which variability is still inadequately understood. Adults and adolescents are not protected at all (Dye, 2013). Although the BCG is still in wide use, then, it is widely acknowledged that a much better vaccine is needed for the prevention of infection or prevention of disease. Vaccines also need to be found for those tens of thousands co-infected with HIV, since BCG cannot be used for those with HIV or AIDS, or with compromised immune systems (Global Vaccines Forum, 2013).

The primary tuberculosis drugs in use today were developed 40 years ago. Nevertheless, the issue is not effectiveness but the long duration of treatment, and increasing drug resistance. For drug susceptible tuberculosis (DS TB) – tuberculosis that is treatable by these primary or 'first-line' drugs – the average length of treatment is six to nine months using four different drugs (Barry, 2011). Adherence can be arduous and all drugs are not always consistently stocked. For these reasons and others, resistance is occurring to two primary drugs – isoniazid and rifampin – producing what is called multi-drug resistant tuberculosis (MDR TB). MDR TB in turn can be transmitted directly to others, contributing to what many researchers fear is an explosion of cases. While still technically treatable, it takes up to 24 months with multiple 'second-line' drugs, including one drug that typically has to be injected daily for six months. These second-line drugs have severe side-effects, including hearing and renal impairment, making them very challenging to adhere to. They are also exorbitantly expensive, from US$5000 to US$53,300 for full treatment (Marks *et al.*, 2014; Motsoaledi, 2014), making tenuous at best an adequate and consistent supply in the context of underfunded national health budgets (Leinhardt, 2012; Barry, 2011). TB Alliance is thus attempting to research and develop better drugs that will shorten considerably the treatment time for all tuberculosis patients. As their website states, a two- to four-month drug regimen is in development, but their vision is a seven- to ten-day regimen for both DS and MDR TB patients (tballiance.org/about/mission). With enough new drugs that work differently on the tuberculosis bacterium, TB Alliance and their partners in fact hope to dissolve the distinction between drug-sensitive and drug-resistant tuberculosis.

The need for new malaria treatment stems primarily from the fact that parasite resistance has occurred for each subsequent malaria treatment introduced – quinine, chloroquine and its derivatives, artemisinin and its synthetic derivatives, mefloquine, amodiaquine and others. Virtually every malaria drug available today has some resistance to it in an endemic region of the world. Because of this, emphasis is now on combination regimens consisting typically of two drugs, an approach that can hopefully curtail the rate at which resistance develops, and can thus sustain decreases in malaria transmission over a longer period of time. Malaria, more than tuberculosis, also presents significant social and ecological challenges in containment. Mosquito vectors spreading malaria in endemic areas have highly differentiated habits in terms of flight patterns, reproduction and feeding. They multiply easily and spread quickly, making it difficult to sustain mosquito reductions. Yet reduction of mosquito populations and the malaria parasites they harbour is an important partner to drug treatment in order to stop persistent parasite reinfection. Most containment campaigns are thus multi-pronged, including facets of mosquito reduction (i.e. spraying), protection from mosquitoes (i.e. treated bednets) and drug treatment for those infected (Webb, 2009; Packard, 2007; Carter, 2012).

A malaria vaccine has never been developed, in part because of the scientific complexity involved in doing so. As Ashley Birkett, Director of PATH MVI, told me, viruses may have a dozen genes, whereas parasites have over 5000. Determining which of the 5000 genes to hone in on – that is, which of the parasite's mechanisms of reproduction or infection a vaccine could most effectively target – presents a huge logistical, financial and temporal challenge (personal communication, 2010). Until the Gates Foundation and USAID made serious funding commitments to such an endeavour, research towards a malaria vaccine simply did not get very far.

PDPs and the social economies of drug production

PDPs are part of a larger category called Public Private Partnerships for Global Health (PPPs), a rubric which as the name suggests encompasses collaborations of private entities and non-profit or nongovernmental agencies working together usually to mitigate infectious diseases of the Global South. Under Gro Harlem Brundtland, the Director General of the WHO from 1998 to 2003, PPPs and their subunits, PDPs, came into favour in part because the WHO's diminished budget necessitated creative arrangements for addressing health problems, and PPPs 'could bring together dissimilar partners and stakeholders . . . to find the most effective combination of agents to address a particular health problem' (Cueto, 2013, 39). Which agents constituted these combinations was not haphazard. The Bill and Melinda Gates Foundation by the early 2000s was pouring funding into vaccine and drug development for low-income regions, launching and continuing to sustain PDPs like the TB Alliance, MVI and Aeras. Private industry is another component considered essential given the financial and infrastructural resources pharmaceutical companies have to offer, and given that many companies have compounds in their pipelines, acquired often through mergers, that are potentially effective against tuberculosis or malaria.

The rise of PDPs also coincides with a moment when much of the pharmaceutical industry is renegotiating business models in a post-blockbuster era when profits from the sale of new drugs alone is declining. Many companies are also avidly pursuing goodwill endeavours in efforts to combat increasingly negative publicity from recent drug safety concerns, exposure of unethical clinical trials practices, and the global spotlight in 1999 on pharmaceutical companies' attempts to keep affordable generic antiretroviral drugs from South Africans living with AIDS. Not all commercial pharmaceutical companies are joining PDPs, and in fact in recent years three major pharmaceutical companies – Pfizer, AstraZeneca, and Novartis – have withdrawn from their infectious disease research and development efforts (Daniels, 2014; Frick, 2015). However, they still constitute an essential part of PDPs. Although I focus only on tuberculosis and malaria PDPs in this chapter, PDPs currently exist for most of the infectious diseases persisting in low-income countries, including tuberculosis, malaria, Chagas disease, filarial diseases, leishmaniasis and human African tripanosomiasis.

TB Alliance, Aeras, MVI and DNDi function differently in important specifics, but all four PDPs are unquestionably about finding biotechnical solutions to what all see as the travesty of continued suffering from preventable infectious diseases. DNDi, for example, arose as an offshoot of Médecins Sans Frontières (Doctors Without Borders), at a moment in the AIDS epidemic when 'the moral economy of access' (Redfield, 2013, 201) became an overwhelming motif in medical humanitarian practice: too many people were dying of AIDS in poor areas when others geopolitically more fortunate stayed alive with newly available antiretrovirals. The same fundamental humanitarian assumption that all individuals no matter where they live should have access to therapies they need drives TB Alliance, Aeras, MVI and DNDi. Yet addressing such a moral economy of access has to be innovative because, by default, these PDPs largely decouple therapeutic research and production from profit incentives and shareholder demand, meaning that they are forging new territory as they proceed. This is why they work collaboratively with philanthropists like the Gates Foundation and the Wellcome Trust, academics and select pharmaceutical companies, but also with governments and global health organisations such as the WHO. Despite similar mandates, how PDPs forge new territories of pharmaceutical production and what precise scientific, political and material relations they cultivate and with whom diverge in sometimes significant ways.

MVI, TB Alliance and Aeras have more similar approaches than DNDi in how they go about developing and disseminating new technologies. All three of them are Gates Foundation-funded enterprises based in the USA and staffed primarily by American scientists. For all three of these agencies, early-stage research – that is, research to discover new molecular compounds with promising capabilities in targeting disease, and early human trials of these promising compounds and vaccine candidates – is part of what they do, and it tends to occur in the USA, the UK or Europe. In the context of global health interventions it is not typical to talk about capacity building in countries of the Global North, but it is important to note that this does happen, and in important ways. GlaxoSmithKline, for example, has built a separate, state-of-the-art facility outside of Madrid dedicated to diseases of the developing world (DDW), where scientists research treatments for tuberculosis, malaria and kinetoplastids (protozoa causing diseases such as African sleeping sickness, Chagas' disease and leishmaniasis). TB Alliance has funded a number of researchers full time to work with GSK scientists at the DDW campus finding new compounds which show promise against the tuberculosis bacterium. GSK also founded the non-profit Open Foundation, embedded within the DDW facility and working to facilitate collaboration among scientists across disciplines and institutions, as well as outside of proprietary constraints (Barros-Aguirre,

2014). MVI, for their part, are able to carry out early-stage safety and efficacy tests of their malaria vaccines in Maryland where PATH is based. In controlled environments with effective drugs on hand, volunteers can be challenged with malaria parasites and then given the vaccine to monitor responses; scientists at MVI, in turn, deepen their understandings of the malaria parasite and its functioning in the human body (Birkett, 2010).

All three organisations are also heavily involved in later stage clinical trials however, and it is in this area that social economies of innovation are perhaps at their most visible. It has been so long since any tuberculosis or malaria vaccine or tuberculosis drug has been tested that no sites were available when these PDPs were ready to begin testing the efficacy of their new therapeutics. Clinical trial sites require the juxtaposition of high rates of disease – in this case tuberculosis or malaria – with well-equipped clinical facilities, laboratories, researchers and lab statisticians. And though both tuberculosis and malaria take huge global tolls of death and disease annually, only a few sites have sufficiently high concentrations of either disease to conduct large Phase II and Phase III clinical trials. One of those sites for tuberculosis is located in the town of Worcester, outside of Cape Town, South Africa. As Peg Willingham, former director of External Affairs of Aeras, first told me in 2010, Aeras was invested in more than one sense in developing the site in Worcester through partnering with the South African Tuberculosis Vaccine Initiative (SATVI), at the University of Cape Town. They did not simply channel financial resources into developing bare basics at the site; in fact they first made preliminary forays in the form of a town hall meeting in the area to test the level of political will behind getting a tuberculosis vaccine. As Lewellys Barker, Senior Medical Advisory for Aeras, noted, that needs to happen with every community they work in if trials are going to be successful in recruiting and retaining participants, and if participants are going to be convinced that their country and community will be beneficiaries of any successful product tested (personal communication, 2010).

With the thumbs-up on political will came the second step, which was finding the actual rate of tuberculosis in Worcester, so that any subsequent clinical trial would have a baseline against which to compare any drug or vaccine's efficacy. In the case of tuberculosis exact rates are not typically known, since many never come in for testing because diagnostic tests take a long time and thus lose potentially positive cases to follow up, and because the so-called 'gold standard' test, mycobacterium culture, is not reliable in determining tuberculosis in children (Mulenga *et al.*, 2011). To address this gap in knowledge, two preliminary trials determining rates of tuberculosis were run between 2001 and 2006. The first enrolled around 6000 infants, while the second enrolled 6000 adolescents, following them over the course of two years to not only test levels of tuberculosis, but also immune responses in those developing TB versus those who did not (Hanekom, 2011). The rate of tuberculosis proved more than adequate in these constituencies and this, then, gave the green light to turn Worcester into a clinical trial site.

Site development consisted subsequently of building clinic and laboratory infrastructure, and training various staff for clinical trial support. As explained by

Marijke Geldenhuys, former professional development and quality control manager for SATVI, training needed to start from the ground up given that most of the staff at Worcester came from the community and did not have research backgrounds. For Geldenhuys, the more everyone knew about tuberculosis and about clinical trials, the better everyone could do their particular jobs and understand how these fitted within the broader picture of clinical trial process and function. So, with the initial support of Aeras, Geldenhuys developed an approach towards training that brought everyone regardless of background to the same approximate knowledge level. Whether individuals were drivers, cleaners or investigators, starting in 2003 they went through the same basic course on tuberculosis, HIV and malaria (the main diseases in South Africa), the history of clinical research, where Good Clinical Practice[2] came from, and how everyone fitted together in the broader clinical trial enterprise. Given that some staff such as recruiters would have to explain concepts such as randomised trials or incidence rates of tuberculosis, other modules such as biostatistics and epidemiology were added as well (personal communication, 2011). This model of across-the-board staff training was then used by Aeras in developing other sites in countries like Kenya, answering concerns of standardisation but also acknowledging that theirs was a successful and – according to Geldenhuys – relatively unique model of clinical trial site development (ibid.).

TB Alliance also have extensive community engagement programmes in the areas in which they work, developing TB educational outreach to high-burden regions while gaining feedback on the design of clinical trials and community preferences in modes of treatment. The bottom line is the desire to improve clinical trial recruitment and retention, but as their website proclaims, 'without informed and engaged communities, clinical research is not possible' (www.tballiance.org/access/engaging-communities.php). TB Alliance thus establishes community advisory boards (like Aeras) to act as liaisons between community members and researchers, and sponsors regionally specific workshops, training on TB drug research, education and awareness campaigns, and broad-scale surveys determining 'what countries want' in terms of kinds and forms of drug regimens, National Tuberculosis Programme capabilities and physicians' attitudes towards acceptance of new regimens (2009). Most noteworthy of TB Alliance's recent trials includes a Phase III trial called REMox, testing whether moxifloxacin, an established antibacterial whose efficacy in tuberculosis has never been formally tested, could shorten treatment from six to four months when substituted for one of the main first-line drugs used currently in standard treatment of drug-susceptible tuberculosis (i.e. isoniazid or rifampicin). The trial failed in that moxifloxacin did not show the ability to shorten treatment by two months. Yet as TB Alliance points out, the trial succeeded in establishing robust trial sites across nine countries that meet Good Clinical Practices standards. It also netted a biobank of blood specimens providing material for furthering current understanding of which factors are predictive of the outcomes of clinical trials (tballiance.org).

PATH MVI's efforts in developing malaria vaccine candidates have similarly involved multiple facets of capacity building in high-burden countries. It assesses country-level objectives in what a new malaria vaccine should look like, such as what kind of delivery system (inhalant versus injection) is preferred; it determines manufacturing capabilities, and ensures that quality control mechanisms are in place; it works on cost-effectiveness analyses for country-level decision-makers; and also works with Ministries of Health in high-burden countries, ensuring that they have the data needed on vaccine candidates to make decisions on country-wide uptake, including the ability to integrate a new malaria vaccine into already existing childhood vaccine programmes (Botting, 2010). PATH MVI also partnered with GSK in 2001 to further develop GSK's malaria vaccine candidate, RTS,S. In 2009 this vaccine went into Phase III trials across 11 sites in seven high-burden countries in sub-Saharan Africa, enrolling 15,460 infants. Before this could happen, GSK and MVI needed to conduct laboratory, clinical and staff development similar to Aeras' and TB Alliance's efforts in order to create sites that could meet Good Clinical Practice standards (MVI, n.d.).

DNDi's structure and mission is slightly different. They are not funded by the Gates Foundation and have consciously avoided receiving money from major philanthropic foundations where funding typically comes with directives, and in the case of the Gates Foundation, significant representation in committees and decision-making processes.[3] DNDi was founded by Médecins Sans Frontières, the UNICEF-UNDP-World Bank-WHO Special Programme for Research and Training in Tropical Diseases (TDR), and five publicly funded research organisa-tions: the Malaysian Ministry of Health, the Kenya Medical Research Institute, the Indian Council of Medical Research, the Oswaldo Cruz Foundation in Brazil and the Institute Pasteur in France. They receive most of their funding from governments, MSF and industry (Pécoul *et al.*, 2008). As an organisation they do not conduct their own research, but instead 'capitalize on existing fragmented R&D capacity' enhanced by additional expertise where needed (ibid., 82). In the case of malaria, then, DNDi looked to create two new artesunate-containing fixed-dose combinations from already existing malaria drugs. Artesunate is one of many quasi-synthetic analogues of artemisinin, a Chinese herb long known for its ability to cure malaria. The WHO had recently recommended the abandonment of the widely used malaria drug chloroquine in favour of artemisinin-based combin-ation therapies (ACT) given the worsening patterns of drug resistance to the former (ibid.). The hope was that combining artemisinin or its derivatives with one other drug could slow down the development of resistance and provide longer term effectiveness against the malaria parasite. DNDi thus turned to astesunate and amodiaquine (ASAQ) to make one combination for regions in Africa and Asia; and artesunate and mefloquine (ASMQ) for a second combination aimed at Latin America and Southeast Asia (Wells *et al.*, 2013).

With its partner the TDR, DNDi worked primarily within the Global South from the beginning, a strategy marking a second significant difference with the other PDPs highlighted here. DNDi creates spaces for collaboration less in early-stage research than in technology transfer and pharmaceutical infrastructure and expertise enhancement in the geographic regions designated for their new drug combinations. As Jean-René Kiechel, DNDi's Senior Pharmaceutical Adviser and Product Manager, put it, 'you need to know the world of the disease in which you want to intervene', so you partner with scientists experienced in disease and development in their own countries who know what it takes to 'transform ideas into product' (personal communication, 2013). For ASAQ, DNDi collaborated with Universiti Sains Malaysia, Oxford University, Mahidol University in Thailand and the Centre National de Recherche et de Formation sur le Paludisme in Burkina Faso (Pécoul *et al.*, 2008). Since 2004 they have also partnered with Sanofi, a major French pharmaceutical company, to carry out pre-clinical and clinical studies using available data on the drug combination. In what DNDi argues is unprecedented, Sanofi and DNDi agreed that ASAQ would be produced as a 'non-exclusive, not-patented, not-for-profit public good' (ibid., 2). As such, third parties could submit simplified applications to manufacture generic versions of the drug. By 2007, ASAQ was registered in 17 African countries (ibid.).

For ASMQ, DNDi again worked with several research institutes as well as the WHO, and this time partnered with Farmanguinhos/Fiocruz, a Brazilian government-owned pharmaceutical company. Although these drugs separately already had proven records of safety and efficacy, new trials of the combination pill needed to be conducted, including among pregnant women and children; and new formulations and quality control methods had to be developed (Wells *et al.*, 2013). The Brazilian regulatory agency approved the ASMQ FDC for use in 2008. In order to make the new combination pill readily available to Asian populations with malaria, however, a technology transfer agreement – the first South–South agreement – was made between Farmanguinhos and the Indian generic pharmaceutical company Cipla. By March 2012, the Malaysian regulatory agency had approved ASMQ fixed-dose combination for use among those with uncomplicated forms of malaria; and by September 2012 the WHO had prequalified Cipla's ASMQ combination, making it a source for agencies to bulk buy at low cost for resource-limited settings (ibid.).

Although working with locally based pharmaceutical companies is important to DNDi, as are South–South technology transfers, Kiechel was frank about the challenges in doing so. In the case of ASMQ, they lost a year and a half because Farmanguinhos had a hard time consistently obtaining high-quality active pharmaceutical ingredients (APIs) – the main component of drugs – for the combination pill. Cipla was experienced in knowing how to find and sustain the best product, but their Brazilian counterpart was not. Farmanguinhos thought they had found a supplier at one point, but the company stopped supplying the active ingredient and Farmanguinhos had to start the search all over again. In the meantime, production of the product was held up. As Kiechel also noted, being a smaller enterprise competing with major pharmaceutical companies for contracts with API suppliers was difficult in general because API-producing companies did not treat DNDi as a partner 'worthy of being groomed'. They were only interested in a few hundred kilograms of active ingredient, not in the much weightier amounts required by large pharmaceutical companies (personal communication, 2013).

Beyond binaries

Many scholars have made the argument already that drug regimens and vaccines are not simply technical interventions. Instead, they have 'social lives' (Whyte *et al.*, 2002) that always 'go beyond the body, affecting and potentially reshaping interpersonal, family, and community domains' (Petryna and Kleinman, 2006, 8). PDPs like TB Alliance, MVI, DNDi and Aeras recognise that the technologies already available for tuberculosis and malaria have particular and often negative impacts on the social, emotional and economic lives of those with or at risk of these two diseases and their families. First-line drugs for tuberculosis are tedious, inconvenient and not always consistently available over the six to nine months they have to be taken. Second-line drugs for MDR-TB are highly toxic, putting individuals at risk of permanent hearing loss, isolating them from family members and diminishing household income over the long course of treatment. Variable and often low levels of protection with the BCG vaccine mean that families in high-burden areas live with the knowledge that tuberculosis is a constant possibility for themselves and their children. Without any malaria vaccine and with most endemic regions displaying drug resistance, families in malaria-plagued regions live with the constant presence of the disease, aware that they or their children can come down with debilitating cases and that their children especially are at risk of dying as a result of infection.

As suggested earlier, the critiques of the current trend towards technical interventions targeting specific diseases point to the disproportionate attention technological fixes receive in global health policy and funding organisations. One result of such trends, these critics argue, is that broader social and economic interventions that might mitigate patterns of infectious disease transmission such as better housing, nutrition, employment and sanitation, are neglected. In other words, those conditions of poverty that place individuals or populations at higher risk of disease remain in place even after drugs or vaccines become available, diminishing the effects that these technologies are likely to have (Biehl and Petryna, 2013; Farmer, 2004; Adams, 2013). Yet too often these arguments overlook the fact that particular drugs and vaccines already exist for specific diseases like tuberculosis and malaria, and that these can have multiple and deleterious social, physical, financial and psychological impacts on families. What TB Alliance, MVI, DNDi and Aeras propose to do first and foremost is to turn these impacts around by improving upon available technologies.

Yet the broader impacts of their approaches to technology development should not be ignored. Arduous recruitment practices and community engagement programmes, for example, help form reciprocal channels of knowledge exchange, with community members learning more about the technicalities of tuberculosis, and researchers and health personnel learning more about community perceptions of, and interventions into, tuberculosis and malaria as well as attitudes towards healthcare and clinical trials. They also provide opportunities for skilled and semi-skilled employment for those in and around the increasing number of clinical trial sites. Although the ultimate goal remains one of recruiting participants into trials, the broader reach of this process becomes, as Kelly and Beisel state in the case of malaria eradication projects (2011 73), 'a better way to connect landscapes of innovation with landscapes of well-being'. Ensuring high-quality supply and manufacturing channels also means enhancing pharmaceutical sectors in high-burden countries and the consequent 'downstream' enhancements in employment, education, expertise and infrastructure. Meaningful technology transfer agreements similarly entail strengthening biotechnology and academic research sectors; increasing opportunities for scientists, biostatisticians, lab technicians, nurses, physicians, and lay health workers within their own countries and communities; and assisting pharmaceutical regulatory channels to become more efficient and/or harmonise into robust regional agencies.

DNDi, Aeras, TB Alliance and MVI in other words take seriously the myriad roles drug and vaccine regimens will assume and the relations they will mobilise at every level of society in the countries where they will be adopted. They are well aware that simply producing a drug or vaccine is useless; it would amount to pouring time, expertise and capital into molecular compounds and vaccines with little meaning or utility. Doing the extensive work upstream and downstream to get new drugs or vaccines into relevant bodies is what makes them life-saving technologies, and it is achieving this that galvanises a broad set of logistical, regulatory and financial factors. As stated by William Wells (2012), Director of Market Access for TB Alliance,

> Once you get a product through Phase III trials and it gets regulatory approval, what happens next? How does everything line up so that it gets to people? Financing, global and country decisions as to what they want [in a product], what information do they want, what is the regulatory strategy, or pharmacovigilance? What is the rollout strategy after regulatory approval?

Working in the geographic regions they do, and driven by their mission of disease mitigation, PDPs employ practices and procedures that go beyond strict definitions of 'product development' to encompass social and economic facets, including regional perspectives regarding drugs and vaccines, consumer preferences on delivery methods (e.g. pills versus capsules), physicians' knowledge levels and national supply networks.

To be clear, my argument is a relatively constrained one in contesting the accuracy as well as the remit of so-called 'technical' interventions and its cousin, vertical interventions. The latter is criticised for focusing on a single disease – which most PDPs do – rather than broader 'horizontal' facets such as employment, education or nutrition levels that together create patterns of vulnerability to a range of diseases (Biehl, 2011). As practised by the PDPs highlighted in this chapter, developing new drugs and vaccines and getting them to high-burden populations across the globe are neither strictly technical endeavours nor are they devoid of horizontal facets. Recognising the variability of practices, techniques and approaches to developing new drugs and vaccines for infectious diseases means moving away from the construction of either/or dichotomies of global health interventions and replacing these with more productive questions about what, exactly, happens or does not happen in the process of therapeutic development and rollout. Are local and national healthcare systems strengthened or overloaded in the incorporation of new vaccines or drug regimens? Are regulatory agencies made more efficient, and in ways that will aid approval of drugs, diagnostics and vaccines beneficial to local populations? Does strengthening local pharmaceutical manufacturing and supply networks mean better availability of other needed drugs in the future? What are the micro-politics of community participation and the macro-politics of scientific knowledge exchange in producing new therapeutics? In other words, what are the precise and sometimes extensive social economies of biomedical interventions and are they primarily beneficial? And can they in turn open up channels to further needed interventions?

Answering these and similar questions leads to more productive discussions on the variability, complexity and impact of particular interventions, rather than on their categorisation. This in turn generates questions about the received understandings, assumptions or approaches shaping the contours of health interventions and illuminating the means towards improvements where necessary. Answering these questions, for example, highlight caveats to the work of TB Alliance, Aeras, MVI and DNDi in benefiting communities, scientists and public health infrastructures. One is that though regulatory and public health systems as a whole may be strengthened by PDP efforts, clinical trial sites invariably become points of exceptional clinical care in larger settings of deprivation and scarce healthcare resources and access. These sites may produce technologies beneficial to high-burden countries as a whole, and they train staff in areas of expertise needed in many geographic settings. Yet they cannot replicate nationwide the quality of clinical facilities and staffing found on site. This, then, creates patterns and politics of healthcare access that take on particularly poignant tensions in regions of widespread resource scarcity.

Two other caveats have to do in different ways with the temporal structure of pharmaceutical development. The first is that clinical trials are on timelines: they may last for two years or so, but then they are over and so are paid staff positions. Several more trials are being or will be conducted at the Worcester site, for example, but trials will not necessarily be staged uninterrupted. However, and in the meantime, it is expensive to continue paying staff in between trials and funds are typically inadequate in tuberculosis or malaria research to cover times of hiatus (Checkley and McShane, 2011; Tameris, 2013). The individuals working at the Worcester trial site are not immune to these concerns, even though the training they receive at SATVI brings with it somewhat greater potential than staff at some trial sites for finding employment off site. Training, however, is never the only consideration in searching for and acquiring new jobs. And the qualifications which staff members receive with their training are likely to mean that alternative jobs will be well outside of Worcester given the paucity of other clinics and laboratories.

Second, the kind of pharmaceutical production which MVI, Aeras, TB Alliance and DNDi undertake is also promissory: that is, it portends a brighter future for millions once better technologies are developed and broadly disseminated. This promise is speculative however, in that the rewards for all but DNDi's malaria drug combinations remain in the distant future, yet MVI, Aeras and TB Alliance are capitalising on individuals' bodies in the here and now in their clinical trials. And the promise is high risk given how many therapies fail even in late-stage clinical trials. This is not meant as criticism of TB Alliance, Aeras or MVI but rather suggests the overwhelming difficulty of developing new vaccines and drugs with limited resources and for diseases that have been ignored for so long that scientific understandings of them remain inadequate. For example, too little is known of what immune responses the tuberculosis bacterium and malaria parasite stimulate in the body, and which reactions signal efficacy of new drug compounds or vaccines. In the case of tuberculosis, animal models are also not particularly predictive. What this means in the latter case is that later stage clinical trials can fail at higher than average rates because even strenuous animal modelling does not always predict what will happen in humans. And in the former case, it means that trials need to be longer for both diseases because participants have to be followed for typically two years to see if they come down with the disease, rather than researchers being able to determine efficacy through what are called 'biomarkers'; that is, things like antibodies whose presence in the blood can indicate much sooner the success or failure of a new drug or vaccine.

The final caveat I will highlight here is that in different ways all four PDPs too closely mirror unequal geopolitical relations of scientific exchange and knowledge production long-standing between the Global North and Global South. The impetus to develop new biotechnologies aimed at tuberculosis and malaria came primarily not from high-burden countries but from research centres in the USA and the UK, the WHO, and from Bill and Melinda Gates. Money for all four PDPs comes from the Gates Foundation, USAID, MSF, the pharmaceutical industry and various European governments. The advisory boards, committees and many of the scientists are also from the USA, Europe and the UK.

For MVI, TB Alliance and Aeras, scientists and staff in high-burden countries do not enter the picture typically until promising compounds and vaccines are ready for testing in later stage clinical trials, but even here these scientists are often following directives coming from the USA or the UK rather than participating more fully in designing clinical trial protocols. In addition, though outreach to communities and the formation of Community Advisory Boards aids in communicating across lines of clinical trial sponsors, investigators and participants, there is nevertheless room for improvement there as well. At a Community Engagement workshop at the 2013 International Conference on Lung Health in Paris, for example, a senior researcher for SATVI pointed out that sometimes sponsors (not necessarily Aeras) gave clinical trial protocols – the formal blueprint for trial design and conduct – to SATVI with only a few weeks to finalise them, making meaningful feedback from community members or even SATVI scientists next to impossible. At the same workshop, TB researchers also expressed frustration that community members and the Community Advisory Boards that represented them were not being adequately drawn into the actual design of clinical trials, but rather were asked to communicate concerns after the trials were implemented (Hamilton, 2013). As Johanna Crane argues in her book *Scrambling for Africa*, scientific exchanges of any kind with low-resource countries encompass not only present inequalities, but also those of a colonial past.

> In other words, in a postcolonial context, the power dynamics and hierarchies of 'normal science' take on additional meaning and complexity, since they are inevitably infused with the politics of national autonomy, 'Western' political and economic hegemony, and (often) race.
>
> (Crane, 2013, 112)

Yet these inequalities, among scientists as well as among community members, have galvanised productive conversations at international conferences and funding agencies. Notably, the European and Developing Countries Clinical Trials Partnership (EDCTP) is working to expand opportunities for African scientists by strengthening capacity for more African-led clinical trial design and research. Charles Mgone, Executive Director of EDCTP, outlined several areas where he is working to move EDCTP towards expanding African-initiated research and getting more equal African involvement in projects. In the area of clinical trials, Mgone is advocating for the inclusion of local partners in discussions of clinical trial design while looking to implement broader training to make clinical trial staff in participating African countries employable in multiple kinds of clinical trials and scientific projects. Within and across African countries, Mgone is also supporting better networking among scientists at clinical trial sites. Rather than each trial site communicating with the European or American sponsor, as is the current norm, Mgone is moving towards communication networks among the participating trial site scientists. EDCTP also gives out networking grants to allow scientists to share data they are gathering, discuss problems or concerns, and exchange students or site monitors across countries and trial sites. And for the many scientists returning from abroad after earning their Ph.D., EDCTP offers grants for creating their own projects and research teams rather than working on northern-led projects (personal communication, 2012). African members are now full partners in EDCTP, meaning they will also have a greater voice in determining funding decisions, with implications that more trials with African sponsors and principle investigators will be supported.

Conclusion

It remains unclear whether PDPs in the long run will achieve their goals of mitigating malaria and tuberculosis – for the latter, the 'zero deaths by 2015' that TB activists insisted upon during the 2012 International Lung Health Conference in Malaysia has obviously not been realised. Nevertheless, DNDi, Aeras, MVI and TB Alliance among other PDPs are tethering public health needs of the global poor to therapeutic research and development, a movement that is part of the latest political impetus to address high burdens of infectious diseases in low-income countries. Much of this recent impetus has focused on new vaccines and drug therapies, what more than one medical historian has pointed out is the latest in a series of attempts across many decades to diminish the scourge of infectious disease through science and technology (Packard, 2007; Webb, 2009; McMillen, 2015). Yet while technical approaches to mitigating disease burdens deserve scrutiny like all other approaches, the point of this chapter has been to move the scrutiny away from categorical distinctions and the delimited set of questions which such pigeonholing generates. Getting beyond a dichotomous categorisation means that whether an intervention focuses on so-called technological fixes such as new vaccines and drug regimens – as do the PDPs highlighted here – or on so-called socio-economic interventions such as nutritional programmes or small business loans, the point is twofold: first, to recognise that many if not most interventions contain elements of both the technical and the social; and second, to examine each for the opportunities they open up, the agglomerative benefits they accrue, and the ways in which they do or do not improve the lives of the populations they target.

DNDi has already succeeded in getting new fixed-dose combination drugs on the market at affordable prices to thousands in regions where malaria continues to thrive. MVI, TB Alliance and Aeras have yet to succeed in getting new vaccines or drug therapies produced, though they continue in their efforts to do so. All four organisations, however, have helped forge social economies of therapeutic innovation that move well beyond the 'technical' to touch upon the lives of clinical trial participants, the staff and communities where these are located; national healthcare systems; regional pharmaceutical sectors; regulatory agencies and beyond. They go towards what Anne-Emanuelle Birn (2005) argues is the need to adopt multiple approaches simultaneously in order for any approach to work. Having new drugs alone does not sufficiently improve individuals' lives when their living conditions remain destitute and their prospects for acquiring sufficient food, adequate housing, employment or potable water is in doubt. Conversely, having enough food and water and holding down a job remain precarious when an individual is suffering from tuberculosis and has no or insufficient access to appropriate drug therapies.

PDPs do not address explicitly the multiple unmet needs that chronic deprivation has produced in the populations they target. They are not meant as a singular answer to enduring poverty and the health problems that invariably come with it, and they have areas where they need improvement within the goals they have set for themselves. Nevertheless, creating better healthcare in the many clinical trial sites they maintain – however inadequate and enclaved – provides thousands of individuals with well-equipped clinics and consistent drug supplies where otherwise there would be none. Their staff training – though not labelled 'employment enhancement programmes' – provides individuals with education, experience and skills that do in fact enhance their income-generating opportunities. Local scientists are getting more opportunities to run studies, and to acquire further training in areas of health and disease relevant to themselves and their home countries. The remit of these PDPs is, in other words, an encompassing one. Should they succeed in also getting effective and affordable new pharmaceuticals to populations in high-burden areas, they will have relieved the suffering of millions already afflicted with incapacitating disease, and saved millions of others from infection down the road.

Notes

1 Redfield was describing the everyday experiences of MSF doctors in the field, but as part of a larger discussion of MSF's controversial decision to turn towards drug access issues, a decision that resulted in DNDi, or the Drugs for Neglected Diseases initiative.
2 This, as well as Good Laboratory Practice (GLP) and Good Manufacturing Practice (GMP), is a standard requirement for regulatory approval by the FDA or its European counterpart, the European Medicines Agency (EMA).
3 An example of this is when Bill and Melinda Gates announced their push to eradicate malaria rather than to diminish it, MVI had to scrap those vaccine candidates already in the research and development pipeline that were geared towards preventing clinical disease rather than intervening in transmission (Birkett, 2010).

References

Adams, Vincanne. 2013. Evidence-based global public health: subjects, profits, erasures. In Joao Biehl and Adriana Petryna, eds, *When People Come First: Critical Studies in Global Health*, Princeton, NJ: Princeton University Press, pp. 54–90.

Adams, Vincanne. 2010. Against global health? Arbitrating science, non-science, and nonsense through health.l In J. Metzel and A. Kirkland, eds, *Against Health: How Health Became the New Morality*, New York: New York University Press, pp. 40–58.

Barros-Aguirre, David. 2014. Head of Drug Discovery, Tuberculosis DPU, GlaxoSmithKline DDW. Personal communication, 17 June.

Barry, Clifton. 2011. Lessons from seven decades of antituberculosis drug discovery. *Current Topics in Medicinal Chemistry* 11: 1216–1225.

Biehl, Joao. 2007. Pharmaceuticalization: AIDS treatment and global health politics. *Anthropological Quarterly* 80(4): 1083–1126.

Biehl, Joao. 2011. When people come first: beyond technical and theoretical quick-fixes in global health. In R. Peet, P. Robbins and M. Watts, eds, *Global Political Ecology*, New York: Routledge, pp. 100–130.

Biehl, Joao and Adriana Petryna. 2013. Critical global health. In Joao Biehl and Adriana Petryna, eds, *When People Come First: Critical Studies in Global Health*, Princeton, NJ: Princeton University Press, pp. 1–22.

Birkett, Ashley. 2010. Director, PATH Malaria Vaccine Initiative. Personal communication, 13 December.

Birn, Anne-Emanuelle. 2005. Gates' grandest challenge: transcending technology as public health ideology. *The Lancet* 366(9484): 514–519.

Botting, Carla. 2010. Director, Product Development and Access, PATH MVI. Personal communication, 3 December.

Buse, K. and A. Harmer. 2007. Seven habits of highly effective global public–private health partnerships: practice and potential. *Social Science and Medicine* 64(2): 259–271.

Buse, K. and G. Walt. 2000. Global public–private partnerships: part I, a new development in health? *Bulletin of the World Health Organization* 78.

Carter, Eric. 2012. *Enemy in the Blood: Malaria, Environment, and Development in Argentina*, Alabama, OH: University of Alabama Press.

Checkley, Anna and Helen McShane. 2011. Tuberculosis vaccines: progress and challenges. *Trends in Pharmacological Sciences* 32(10): 601–606.

Crane, Johanna Tayloe. 2013. *Scrambling for Africa: AIDS, Expertise, and the Rise of American Global Health Science*, New York: Cornell University Press.

Cueto, Marcos. 2013. A return to the magic bullet? Malaria and global health in the twenty-first century. In J. Biehl and A. Petryna, eds, *When People Come First: Critical Studies in Global Health*, Princeton, NJ: Princeton University Press, pp. 30–53.

Daniels, Colleen, TAG. 2014. Overcoming the challenges in TB R&D. Presentation at the 45th International Lung Health Conference, Barcelona, Spain, 31 October.

Dumit, Joe. 2012. *Drugs for Life: How Pharmaceutical Companies Define Our Health*, Durham, NC: Duke University Press.

Dye, Christopher. 2013. Vaccination and the prospects for elimination. Presentation at the Global TB Vaccines Conference, Cape Town, South Africa, 25 March.

Farmer, Paul. 2004. *Pathologies of Power: Health, Human Rights, and the New War on the Poor*, Berkeley: University of California Press.

Frick, Mike, TAG. 2015. 2014 Report on tuberculosis research funding trends, 2005–2013, 2nd Edition, Treatment Action Group.

Geldenhuys, Marijke. 2011. Professional Development and Quality Control Manager, SATVI. Personal communication, 6 April.

Global TB Vaccines Forum. 2013. Cape Town, South Africa, 25–28 March.

GAO (Government Accounting Office). 2006. New drug development: science, business, regulatory, and intellectual property issues cited as hampering drug development efforts. GAO-07-49. www.gao.gov.

Hamilton, Carol. 2013. Engaging communities in research design. Workshop on Community Engagement, 44th International Lung Health Conference, Paris, France, 31 October.

Hanekom, Willem, Former Co-Director, SATVI. 2011. Personal communication, 7 February. Kelly, Ann H. and Uli Beisel. 2011. Neglected malarias: the frontlines and back alleys of global health. *Biosocieties* 6(1): 71–87.

Kesselheim, Arron. 2011. An empirical review of major legislation affecting drug development: past experiences, effects, and unintended consequences. *Milbank Quarterly* 89(3): 450–502.

Kiechel, J-R. 2013. Senior Pharmaceutical Advisor and Product Manager, DNDi Malaria. Personal communication, 29 May.

Latour, Bruno. 2005. *Reassembling the Social: An Introduction to Actor-Network-Theory*, Oxford: Oxford University Press.

Leinhardt, Christian. 2012. Research activities of the Stop TB Partnership: need for new tools. Presentation at the *42nd International Lung Health Conference*, Lille, France, 28 October.

McMillen, Christian. 2015. *Discovering Tuberculosis: A Global History 1900 to the Present*, New Haven, CT: Yale University Press.

Marks, S., J. Flood, B. Seaworth, Y. Hirsch-Moverman, L. Armstrong, S. Mase, K. Salcedo, P. Oh, E. Graviss, P. Colson, L. Armitige, M. Revuelta, K. Sheeran, and the TB Epidemiologic Studies Consortium. 2014. Treatment practices, outcomes, and costs of multidrug-resistant tuberculosis, United States, 2005–2007. *Emerging Infectious Diseases* 20(5).

Mgone, Charles. 2012. EDCTP Executive Director. Personal communication, 19 July.

Motsoaledi, Aaron, Minister of Health, South Africa. 2014. The importance of the Global Plan to stop TB in the post-2015 strategy. Presentation at the 46th International Lung Health Conference, Barcelona, Spain, 28 October.

Mulenga, H., S Moyo, L. Workman, T. Hawkridge, S. Verver, M. Tameris, H. Geldenhuys, W. Hanekom, H. Mahomed, G. Hussey and M. Hatherill. 2011. Phenotypic variability in childhood TB: implications for diagnostic endpoints in tuberculosis vaccine trials. *Vaccine* 29(26): 4316–4321.

MVI. n.d. RTS,S Fact Sheet. Available at www.malariavaccine.org.

Packard, Randall. 2007. *The Making of a Tropical Disease: A Short History of Malaria*, MD: Johns Hopkins Biographies of Disease.

Pécoul, B., Sevcsik, A-M., Amuasi, J., Diap, G. and Kiechel, J-R. 2008. The story of ASAQ: the first antimalarial product development partnership success. *Health Partnership Review*. Global Forum for Health Research: 77–83.

Petryna, Adriana and Arthur Kleinman. 2006. The pharmaceutical nexus. In A. Petryna, A. Lakoff and A. Kleinman, eds, *Global Pharmaceuticals: Ethics, Markets, Practices*, Durham, NC: Duke University Press, pp. 1–32.

Redfield, Peter. 2013. *Life in Crisis: The Ethical Journey of Doctors Without Borders*, Berkeley: University of California Press.

Rose, Nikolas. 2012. Democracy in the contemporary life sciences. *Biosocieties* 7(4): 459–472.

Tameris, Michele. 2011. Principle Investigator, SATVI. Personal communication, 24 March.

Tameris, Michele. 2013. Principle Investigator, SATVI. Presentation for the Community Engagement Workshop at the 44th International Lung Health Conference, Paris, France, 31 October.

TB Alliance. 2009. What countries want: the value proposition of existing and new first-line regimens for drug-susceptible tuberculosis.

TB Alliance. 2013. TB Alliance licenses late-stage TB program to CISR-OSDD. News release, 20 March.

TBVI (Tuberculosis Vaccine Initiative). 2013. TB vaccine business case: lifesaving TB vaccines feasible, 11 June. Available at www.tbvi.eu/news (last accessed 25 June 2013).

Webb, James. 2009. *Humanity's Burden: A Global History of Malaria*, Studies in Environment and History Series, Cambridge: Cambridge University Press.

Wells, Susan, Graciela Diap and Jean-René Kiechel. 2013. The story of artesunate-mefloquine (ASMQ), innovative partners in drug development: case study. *Malaria Journal* 12(68): 1–10.

Wells, William. 2012. Director of Market Access, TB Alliance. Personal communication, 25 April.

WHO. 2012a. Tuberculosis fact sheet. Available at www.who.int.

WHO. 2012b. World Malaria Report 2012. Fact sheet. Available at www.who.int.en/malaria/publications.

Whyte, Susan Reynolds, S. Van der Geest and A. Hardon. 2002. *The Social Lives of Medicines*, Cambridge: Cambridge University Press.

Willingham, Peg. 2010. Director of External Affairs, Aeras. Personal communication, 16 June.

6 Living well with parasitic worms

A more-than-human geography of global health

Jamie Lorimer

Worms

This is a chapter about worms. More specifically it is about a group of helminths – parasitic worms that inhabit the intestines of all vertebrate animals. Our ancestors evolved with helminths and the majority of people in the world are still infected by them. A heavy burden of worms is understood to harm physical and intellectual development and productivity. The global control of parasitic worms is a long-standing and ongoing public health priority. Deworming programmes have significantly diminished human helminth infections around the world, but they remain prevalent in parts of the Global South, especially in impoverished rural areas in Africa. Efforts to 'deworm the world' have recently been stepped up at the World Health Organisation as part of a global effort to tackle 'neglected tropical diseases' (Hotez, 2013).

However, there is a small but growing movement of scientists and urban citizens in North America and Western Europe who argue that a wormless world may also be pathological. Their thinking is informed by the 'hygiene' or 'old friends' hypotheses, which link the recent rises in non-communicative and autoimmune diseases to the absence of components of the human microbiome. Here, 'missing microbes' (Blaser, 2014) are believed to underpin contemporary 'epidemics of absence' (Velasquez-Manoff, 2012). Studies in animals suggest that helminths can 'modulate autoimmune and allergic inflammatory responses and improve metabolic dysfunction' (Wammes *et al.*, 2014, 1). Clinical trials are underway to test the efficacy of reintroducing worms to tackle various conditions – including allergies, inflammatory bowel diseases (IBDs), multiple sclerosis, rheumatoid arthritis and autism (Wammes *et al.*, 2014).

In parallel to these trials, citizens are devising and experimenting with 'helminth therapies' (Khan and Fallon, 2013). Here, worms have been reinvented as 'gut buddies'[1] and human 'symbionts' (Parker, 2014). They have been returned or introduced as a valuable commodity in a quasi-legal 'hookworm underground' (Velasquez-Manoff, 2012), while regulatory agencies, such as the US Food and Drug Administration, scramble to address a risk of resurgence (Young, 2014). Advocates present this reworming as a form of 'biome reconstitution' (Parker and

Ollerton, 2013): the controlled reintroduction of microbial lifeforms to recalibrate bodily processes. It can be situated within a wider interest in forms of 'biotherapy' (Grassberger *et al.*, 2013), which include practices of bacteriotherapy like fecal transplants (De Vrieze, 2013).

This chapter attends to this seeming paradox – of concurrent programmes to de- and reworm the world – to ask questions of the dominant discourses and spatial imaginaries of global health. After briefly outlining helminth parasitology and providing some more details on programmes to 'deworm' and 'reworm' variegated worlds, the chapter identifies three broad contributions to developing a geographical approach to global health. It first positions this story within a growing body of literature in anthropology and animal studies that explores health and disease as 'more-than-human' (Whatmore, 2006) or 'multispecies' phenomena. This literature traces the entangled relations between people and myriad other lifeforms to flag the manifold agencies and political ecologies that shape human health.

Second, the chapter examines the implications of this ontology of entanglement for understanding the biopolitics of global health. Here, worms become a source of concern in situations of pathological abundance *and* as a result of their absence. Tactics for dealing with situations of abundance are fairly well analysed in the literatures on the history and social studies of medicine. These have explored the 'antibiotic' practices of hygiene, public health and disease eradication, and their social and ecological consequences (Anderson, 2006; Latour, 1988; Stepan, 2013). Attending to absences allows us to tell a slightly different story, in which concerns for the salutary significance of 'life in us' leads to a challenge to modern cartographies of health premised on the hygienic purification of the human body. Drawing upon recent work on the 'microbiopolitics' of living well with microbial life (Paxson, 2008), this chapter examines reworming as a 'probiotic' mode of biopolitics. This involves the selective introduction of 'keystone species' to calibrate dysfunctional bodily systems. Here, the human body is conceived ecologically as a super-organism. This analysis draws on recent work on immunity – in both the natural sciences and biophilosophy – to better specify the practices and relations of de- and reworming.

This analysis informs a third and final contribution. The story of worms provides a unique lens to explore the entangled and unequal spatial relationships between diseases of poverty and affluence in ways that trouble prevalent geographical imaginations of global health. The story of worms does not conform to familiar linear accounts (and associated maps) of international development as an index of absent infection. Instead, this chapter offers a topological reading of the spatial biopolitics of health (after Hinchliffe *et al.*, 2012) that conceives hookworm disease and epidemics of absence as emergent from the intensities of interspecies relations. This approach identifies thresholds and tipping points in disease emergence, linking the incidence of variegated worm-related diseases to both the long histories of colonialism and the pursuit of 'lively capital' (Rajan, 2012) in contemporary biomedicine and hygiene practices.

Helminth parasitology

Parasitologists have recorded over 300 species of helminth that parasitise humans. Many of these are rare or accidental, but about 90 species are commonly found in human bodies (Cox, 2010). Few helminths are host-specific. Instead, many of our parasites are zoonotic – transmissible from vertebrate animals to humans and vice versa. Polyparasitism is also common. Humans evolved and still largely live in a 'wormy world' (Stoll, 1999). As a species we are 'riddled with life' (Zuk, 2007), entangled in a range of multispecies gift economies.

Helminths have three main life cycle stages: eggs, larvae and adults. Adult worms infect definitive hosts (those in which sexual development occurs) whereas larval stages may be free-living or parasitise invertebrate vectors and intermediate hosts. Unlike other forms of life in us (e.g. viruses, bacteria, protozoa and fungi), helminths do not proliferate within host bodies. After infection they grow, moult, mature and then produce offspring, which are voided from the host to infect new hosts or reinfect the original host. The four main modes of transmission by which the larvae infect animals (including humans) are faecal-oral, transdermal, vector-borne and predator-prey.[2] This brief outline gives some sense of the diverse, intimate and visceral ways in which helminths entangle us with other lifeforms and ecologies.

In this chapter I focus primarily on one parasitic worm: the human hookworm. There are two species of hookworm that colonise humans. *Necator Americanus* is generally known as the 'New World' hookworm and predominates in the Americas, sub-Saharan Africa and Southeast Asia. *Ancylostoma duodenale* – the 'Old World' hookworm – predominates in the Middle East, North Africa, India and (formerly) in Southern Europe. Paleoparasitologists believe that humans began to host hookworm about 12,000 years ago during the process of domesticating dogs (Palmer, 2009). The human hookworm is now primarily found in us and is one of the world's most common parasitic helminths (Schneider *et al.*, 2011). *Necator Americanus* (Figure 6.1) is the hookworm species subject to both de- and reworming.

The life cycle and parasitology of the hookworm is shown in Figure 6.2. Humans first acquire hookworm when the infective larval stages living in the soil penetrate the skin – generally between the toes of a bare foot. After entering the host, the larvae migrate through the blood vessels to the right side of the heart and then to the lung. They break out of lung capillaries and ascend the throat when they are coughed and swallowed. From here they enter the gastrointestinal tract where they develop to the adult stage. They take up residence and feed on blood from the walls of the intestine. Approximately five to eight weeks pass from the time that they first infect humans until they reach sexual maturity and mate. Hookworms live in the human intestine for an average of three to ten years with a maximum lifespan of 18 years. Each female produces thousands of eggs daily, which exit the body in faeces. When deposited in soil with adequate warmth, shade and moisture, the eggs hatch within hours and give rise to new larvae. And so the cycle continues (taken largely from Brooker *et al.*, 2004).

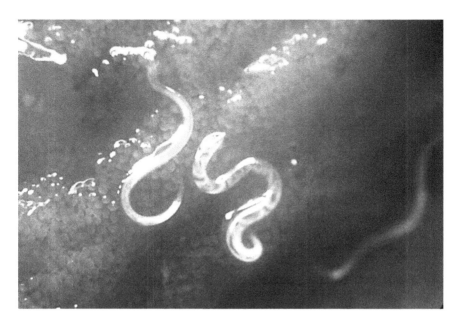

Figure 6.1 The human hookworm (*Necator Americanus*).

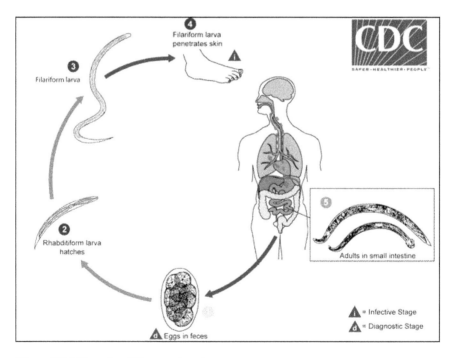

Figure 6.2 Life cycle of *Necator Americanus.*
Source: Centres for Disease Control and Prevention (http://phil.cdc.gov/).

By virtue of their need to reproduce outside of their host, hookworm popula-tions tend to develop slowly in vertebrate bodies. After an initial, generally unsuc-cessful effort to shift the worms, the body learns to tolerate a bearable wormload, with the result that most infections are modest and asymptomatic. Hookworm produce an entirely different 'immune response profile' to microbial (i.e. bacterial) pathogens (Allen and Maizels, 2011). As a result of a long history of human co-evolution, 'helminths have evolved to dampen, rather than disable, the immune system of their hosts' (ibid., 384). Recent work in immunology identifies a 'helminth-induced immune regulatory environment' (Helmby, 2009) or 'network' (Wammes *et al.*, 2014) through which worms enter into a 'continuing dialogue' (Allen and Maizels, 2014, 385) with the human immune system to enable permanent residence. People do not generally develop immunity to helminths (in the sense of securing a human self against a foreign invader). Instead human bodies learn to be affected by worms, calibrating immune systems through an ongoing molecular exchange. Helminths can also manipulate the microbial popu-lation (of their host) for their own ends (ibid.).

Mortality as a direct result of 'hookworm disease' (Necatoriasis) – which scientists differentiate from 'hookworm infection' (Schneider *et al.*, 2011) – is rare. But populations of hookworm can accumulate among populations with poor nutrition, high levels of exposure and/or a particular genetic disposition. Necatoriasis can lead to protein deficiency and anaemia as well as affecting cognitive function and development, especially among children (Brooker *et al.*, 2004). Co-infection is common. Hotez (2013) describes hookworm as part of the 'unholy trinity' of soil transmitted helminths, comprising hookworm, roundworm and whipworm. Together these are responsible for the most prevalent 'neglected tropical disease' of helminthiasis. The immunosuppression associated with helminths can also exacerbate malaria and TB infections (Brooker *et al.*, 2004).

Deworming the world

Human hookworm and other helminths were the target of some of the first major international public health campaigns. 'Eradicating' hookworm in the south of the USA was the founding concern of the Rockefeller Foundation's Sanitary Commission. This grew into the Rockefeller International Health Division (IHD), which ran an international deworming programme in the early twentieth century. After the Second World War the IHD morphed into what is now the World Health Organisation (Farley, 2003). The international deworming activities of the IHD are well recorded by historians of medicine (e.g. Anderson, 2006; Palmer, 2009; Trujillo-Pagan, 2013).

Their accounts tend to position hookworm control within broader colonial and capitalist geographies whose principal aim was to secure the productivity of the labour force in the fast expanding US economies of tropical agriculture and resource extraction. During the latter half of the nineteenth century hookworm was known (among colonial elites) as the 'germ of laziness' due to its effects upon labour productivity (Ettling, 2013). Deworming efforts were largely targeted at plantations, railways and mining enterprises. *Unhooking the hookworm*, to use the title of an IHD public information film,[3] involved practices of what Warwick Anderson terms 'excremental colonialism' (Anderson, 1995): a somewhat obsessive and highly moralised focus on hygiene and sanitation among foreign doctors and administrators targeted at the management of human waste to prevent cycles of reinfection. Such interventions were coupled with the distribution of vermicides to kill off resident worm populations.

However critical, such accounts tend to rely on the archival records of those involved with deworming. We learn less about the lived experience and cosmologies of those who are made the subject of such hygiene practices. There is a limited literature in African medical anthropology that examines local perceptions of worms (Geissler, 1998a, 1998b; Parker *et al.*, 2008; Moran-Thomas, 2013) often conducted in association with deworming campaigns and driven by a desire to explain local resistance. For example, in a two-paper account entitled 'Worms are our life', Wenzel Geissler (1998a, 1998b) examines perceptions of worms and their role in the body in a Luo village in Western Kenya. He explores how adults and children navigate between a 'traditional' and a 'biomedical' understanding. The former 'acknowledged worms as positive agents of both digestion and illness and aimed at maintaining a balanced relationship with them. The latter saw worms as dangerous intruders into bodily order and demanded their expulsion' (1998a, 63). Both models were used side by side according to individual preference or specific context.

Hookworm was successfully controlled in the US, Europe and Australia in the twentieth century, though it has not been eradicated in the absolute sense implied by this term (Stepan, 2011). There have recently been significant decreases in Asia and Latin America due to control and sanitation programmes (Pullan and Brooker, 2012). Today, about 700 million people are infected with human hookworm, primarily in disadvantaged rural communities in tropical and subtropical regions. There are 200 million infected people in sub-Saharan Africa and 200 million in China (see Figure 6.3). It has been estimated that hookworm causes a global 'disease burden' of 1.5 to 22.1 million disability-adjusted life years (Hotez *et al.* 2010).

Interest and investment in controlling hookworm and other helminth infections declined towards the end of the twentieth century when compared with international health investments in treating malaria, HIV and TB. However, in the past ten years, hookworm disease has regained some prominence as a result of its classification as one of a number of 'Neglected Tropical Diseases'. The Global Network for Neglected Tropical Diseases was launched in 2006 at the Clinton Global Initiative. This is an advocacy network run from the Sabin Vaccine Institute. 'Neglected Tropical Diseases' has become an extremely successful fundraising brand, raising more than US$1 billion dollars since its creation (Nordrum, 2015). Significant funding has been channelled to hookworm control, including a new initiative to 'deworm the world'[4] through the school-based delivery of vermicides, often donated by manufacturers. This scheme has been promoted as a 'best buy for development' (J-PAL Bulletin, 2012), though there is

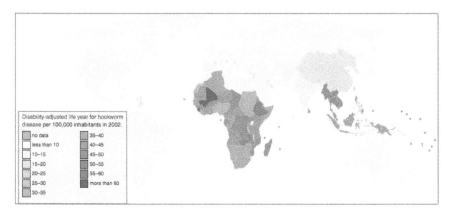

Figure 6.3 Hookworm disease world map, showing DALY from WHO (2002) data.
Source: Lokal_Profil; licensed under CC BY-SA 2.5 via Wikimedia Commons.

some debate about the efficacy of such programmes (Hawkes, 2013), which was not established in a recent Cochrane review (Taylor-Robinson *et al.*, 2012).

The potential of drug-based deworming is limited when infectious larvae remain in the soil enabling immediate reinfection. There is some evidence of growing resistance to the available drugs and research, and development for replacements is limited (Hotez *et al.*, 2008), such that the principal sources of new drugs are the more lucrative markets in agriculture and the pet industry (ibid.). The Sabin Vaccine Institute is seeking to develop a hookworm vaccine (Hotez *et al.* 2013) and received more than US$50 million from the Gates Foundation for this enterprise between 2000 and 2014 (Sabin, 2015). Antigens have been identified and clinical trials are underway. The Brazilian government has offered to manufacture any proven vaccine. This remains some way off and the hookworm does not look like being eradicated anytime soon.

Reworming the world

The desirability of hookworm eradication has begun to be questioned by a growing body of scientific theory, evidence and vernacular practice. This is concerned with the health consequences of the absence of hookworm and other parts of the human microbiome. Epidemiologists have noted for some time an association between declines in infection and the increase in susceptibility to certain autoimmune and allergic diseases. In a much cited paper, Bach (2002) notes that the increase in past decades in the developed world of allergic diseases (e.g. asthma, rhinitis and atopic dermatitis) and autoimmune diseases (e.g. multiple sclerosis, type 1 diabetes and Crohn's disease) is 'concomitant with' a decrease in the incidence of many infectious diseases (Bach, 2002, 911). Epidemiological research on helminths has identified that 'allergic diseases are rare in areas with high helminth parasite exposure and common where helminth exposure is lacking or significantly reduced, such as urban areas of developing countries and industrialized nations' (Feary *et al.*, 2011, Flohr *et al.*, 2009, abstract). The spatial patterns of allergic and autoimmune disease and absent infection correlate with multiple individual, social, economic and environmental factors, and would seem to defy singular causal explanation.

In 1989 David Strachan offered a 'hygiene hypothesis' to account for these broad trends. This has been refined in recent years into the 'old friends' or 'biodiversity' hypotheses (Rook, 2009, 2012; Hanski *et al.*, 2012,). These suggest that changes in the composition of the human microbiome and encounters with the microbial ecologies with which people evolved unsettle basic bodily systems that enable processes like metabolism and immunity. The causes of such changes are manifold but attention has come to focus on a set of reproductive, demographic and ecological shifts often celebrated as fundamental to being hygienic, developed and modern. These are summarised in Table 6.1.

The 'old friends hypothesis' has informed a wide range of epidemiological and laboratory research using existing human populations or animal models to try to track or simulate the incidence and effects of human microbiotic changes on allergic and autommune disease (Blaser, 2014). This research has involved attending as much to the absence of specific organisms and internal ecologies as to the presence of particular pathogens. Absences and ecologies are often harder to detect and measure within the prevalent knowledge practices and assemblages for medical science. One way of researching absence is to return the organism of interest. A number of clinical trials are underway to first test the safety of reintroducing hookworm and other helminths and then to explore their effects upon allergies and inflammatory conditions. These have shown that it is safe to host worms, but have otherwise produced mixed and unclear results (Wammes *et al.*, 2014). Further research and trials are underway. One company (Coronado Biosciences) has patented the production process for producing the ova of the pig whipworm that is commonly used in clinical trials.

Table 6.1 Hygiene practices understood to affect 'human ecology'

Change	Consequence
Clean water	Reduced faecal transmission
Increase in caesarean sections	Reduced vaginal transmission
Increased use of pre-term antibiotics	Reduced vaginal transmission
Reduced breastfeeding	Reduced cutaneous transmission and a changed immunological environment
Smaller family size	Reduced early life transmission
Widespread antibiotic use	Selection for a changing composition
Increased bathing, showering and use of antibacterial soaps	Selection for a changing composition
Increased use of mercury-amalgam dental fillings	Selection for a changing composition

Source: Adapted from Blaser and Falkow (2009, 889).

In parallel with these scientific developments, and in part in frustration at their slow progress, a variety of patients, citizen scientists and health providers have been experimenting with forms of 'biotherapy' (Grassberger *et al.*, 2013). This involves the selective reintroduction of parasites (now recast as 'human symbionts') alongside shifts in lifestyle practices. Hookworms are among these organisms and are used by patients suffering from a range of allergies and inflammatory disorders to try to replicate the 'helminth-induced immune regulatory environment' described above. Interest in hookworm therapy seems to have mushroomed in the past decade (Velasquez-Manoff, 2012) and helminths are now being reintroduced through a variety of economic arrangements.

One of the early advocates was Jasper Lawrence, a British entrepreneur. As a result of a positive experience of participating in an early clinical trial in the early 2000s, Jasper took himself off to rural Cameroon to walk in some latrines in the hope of picking up hookworm to cure his hay fever. He got the wrong worm, but after a further trip to Guatemala he established his own worm colony (Velasquez-Manoff, 2012). He started up a company called *Autoimmune Therapies* breeding, selling and infecting his worms into visiting paying customers. As it is currently illegal to bring hookworm into the USA outside of a human body or to distribute them in a country, Jasper based himself initially in Mexico. It is perfectly legal to cross the border to Tijuana to get infected. At the time of writing there were four commercial providers of hookworm, all of whom now operate through the Internet and will post larvae to anywhere outside of the USA. Several also sell human whipworm.

Another organisation called *Biome Restoration* borrows heavily from the thinking of William Parker, who coined the concept from which the organisation takes its name (Parker and Ollerton, 2013). Their director, Don Donahue (a North American radiologist by training), systematically reviewed the parasitology literature to identify the ideal human 'symbiont'. He settled on Hymenolepis diminuta cysticercoids (which they abbreviate to HDC) – the larval stage of a rat tapeworm. HDC was once common in the food supply, does not take up residence in the human body (necessitating a bi-weekly top-up) and has a low risk of returning into the food system. It is easily farmed and shipped from the organisation's laboratory in the north of England. Biome Restoration's website presents HDC as a probiotic food supplement and suggests that it should be taken as part of every healthy diet, not as a specific therapy.[5] Their strapline is 'exercise your immunity'. Their thinking echoes other commentators who suggest that the 'introduction of parasites as a preventive measure in early life would (seem to) be the most effective way to control inflammatory diseases' (Wammes *et al.*, 2014, 8).

There is limited social science research on this movement. The work that exists (e.g. Strosberg, 2014), and my own preliminary interviews and social media analysis, suggests that users are generally well-educated citizens, suffering from a range of allergies and autoimmune conditions, engaged with mainstream medicine but despairing at the inefficacy and unpleasantness of the treatment options currently available. Velasquez-Manoff (2012) writes of an online 'hookworm underground' of support groups, advocates and enthusiasts sharing knowledge, technologies and organisms. The most visible members of this network on social media are concentrated in North America, Western Europe and Australia. Empowered by online resources and their own experiments, some users have learned to raise their own hookworms. They use worms originally purchased from Lawrence or other commercial providers, or those sourced from participation in clinical trials. They harvest new stock from their faeces in various domestic laboratories and keep others supplied to negate the need to purchase replacements. There is a communitarian ethos to this online world, whose patrons largely remain anonymous for fear of future liability.

Global health in a wormy world

A somewhat paradoxical situation is therefore at large, in which two different groups of scientists, healthcare practitioners and citizens are seeking to simultaneously deworm and reworm their worlds. These groups are largely discrete, though there is some cross-over in the form of scientists examining (or conducting field experiments on) the health effects of eliminating worms (Wammes *et al.*, 2014). In the following analysis I would like to draw out three points of interest from this story for understanding the geographies of global health.

Health as a more-than-human achievement

The first point relates to the agencies of worms within this story and the need to develop a 'more-than-human' (Whatmore, 2006) account of disease, illness and health. By this I mean an account which recognises that being and staying 'human' is a multispecies achievement premised upon and threatened by a host of nonhuman organisms. This helps us theorise the variegated ways in which worms (and other parasites and components of the human microbiome and 'virome') can affect human illness (the lived experience of disease). The risky agencies of 'germs', viruses and their animal vectors are well known and are the subject of extensive work in medical anthropology and geography (see Nading (2013) for a review). This literature explores illness as emergent from entangled multispecies relations configured within particular and uneven geographies and political ecologies (about which I will say more below). Overabundant worms matter here as potential pathogens.

There is an undoubted charisma to human helminths and their visceral, intimate ecologies. In her 'salvage ethnography' of Guinea worm eradication, Moran-Thomas describes the worm as a 'grotesquely photogenic nemesis' (2013, 219) that provides a powerful symbol of poverty and decay and an objectifiable target for global health interventions (see commentary in Biehl and Petryna, 2013). But what makes this worm story most interesting from a more-than-human perspective on health is the importance it affords nonhuman absence (as well as presence). *If* (and it is still a big if) the rise in allergy and autoimmune disease associated with modern, urban living has a nonhuman, ecological signature, then this demands a radical rethink of the prevalent role afforded microbes in our understandings of health. Here, geographies of absence can be as pathogenic as those of presence.

A concern with microbiotic absence can be linked to the recent wider interest in the composition and dynamics of the human microbiome in the life and social sciences (Turnbaugh *et al.*, 2007). Developments in genetic sequencing (metagenomics) have made possible the identification of intimate microbial forms and functions invisible to traditional methods of microbial culture. In short, we are learning that a lot of 'us' is not actually 'us' – in any simple sense of being human – and that the human may best be conceived as a 'super-organism', whose microbiome is part inherited, part gleaned from local environmental and social relationships. It is argued that the composition and shifting dynamics of this life *in us* can have important consequences for human and environmental health. Some commentators have suggested that the findings of this research are driving a revolution in contemporary biology, supplementing the 'modern synthesis' with its focus on discrete genetic individuals and intergenerational heredity and evolution, with a consideration of the microbial composition of lifeforms and their symbiotic and epigenetic relationships with each other and the wider environment (Gilbert *et al.*, 2012; Guthman and Mansfield, 2013). As Haraway (2008, 12) remarks, 'we have never been human': we co-evolved with our parasites, symbionts and gut buddies. We are entangled with them, and novel forms of entanglement and disentanglement risk the human super-organism unravelling.

This understanding has allowed scientists to propose a case that worms (and other parasites) make us different, generating a range of health geographies mapped by diverse variables. For example, immunologists argue that differential histories of human co-evolution with helminths create 'genetic loci' that account for the reduced incidence of immunopathological diseases in helminth-endemic locations and an increased likelihood of developing these diseases in Western countries and urban areas in the developing world (Allen and Maizels, 2011). Our gut buddies have left an inheritable trace. Psychiatrists and others have hypothesised that the presence and absence of worms has an affective signature. For example, recent work has linked the absence of helminths to the incidence of depression, anxiety, autism and other cognitive disorders (Rook, 2009; Siniscalco and Antonucci, 2013). There is an established literature in evolutionary psychology that claims a link between high levels of 'parasite-stress' in a country and a greater incidence of homicide, child mistreatment and 'autocractic' social behaviours (Thornhill *et al.*, 2009; Eppig *et al.*, 2010; Thornhill and Fincher, 2011). In these diverse and sometimes incommensurable accounts, it is argued that worms can keep us sane, as well as make us inhuman.

Perhaps the only thing that is clear from this research is that there is a 'double-edged sword' to helminthic infections (Helmby, 2009, 121): problems can arise with and without them. Hoshi and Medzhitov (2012) note that one of the most pressing issues in current work on the microbiome is to begin to specify the intimate geographies of how, where and when an organism becomes a symbiont or a pathobiont: 'a microorganism that can be part of the normal microbiota in healthy hosts but that can cause disease when some aspect of host-microbial homeostasis is disrupted' (Hoshi and Medzhitov, 2012, 654). Hookworm has the potential to be both.

Microbiopolitics

Thinking health through an entangled, more-than-human ontology of necessary presence could have profound implications for understanding the 'microbiopolitics' of global health. It raises pressing questions for the recently reinvigorated enthusiasms for global disease eradication (Stepan, 2013). I borrow the term microbiopolitics from Heather Paxson (2008) for whom (developing Foucault and Latour) it describes: 'the creation of categories of microscopic biological agents; the anthropocentric evaluation of such agents; and the elaboration of appropriate human behaviors vis-a-vis microorganisms engaged in infection, inoculation, and digestion' (Paxson, 2008, 17). In the grand narrative of the moderns, made famous in Latour's account of pasteurisation (Latour, 1988), microbiopolitics involves science coupled to medicine, engineering and governance. It enables the domestication of nature, the elimination of risks and the securitisation of the human through a range of antibiotic practices.

Critics of these programmes document the violence, partialities and inefficacies of these initiatives, but recent thinking on 'epidemics of absence' further troubles a modern linear narrative and its imagined geographies of development. Rethinking the fundamental modern processes listed in Table 6.1 as pathological brings into question many of the central tenets of the model of 'excremental colonialism' and moral hygiene at the heart of public health discourse. As Paxson (2008) notes with her work on raw-milk cheese, the recognition of the salutary potentials of the microbiome moderates prevalent modern anxieties about our corporeal vulnerability to nonhuman life and offers different, 'post-Pasteurian' concept of hygiene.

The story of reworming illustrates some such post-Pasteurian modes of microbiopolitics, which we might understand as 'probiotic'. The term 'probiotic' is largely associated with contested claims in the food industry where it tends to refer to discrete microbes or bacterial mixes commodified for bodily restoration through repeat dosage. Reworming is 'post-Pasteurian' in more transformative and ecological ways than these interventions. Specific species of worm are (re) introduced in known quantities to (re)calibrate bodily systems (Parker *et al.*, 2012) through a process targeted towards restoring desired systemic properties. Worms become 'gut buddies' because they have powerful ecological leverage, enabling them to deliver immunity or metabolism, for example.

In framing such probiotic interventions, advocates draw upon ecological theory and make comparisons with interventions in the macrobiome. For example, worms are presented as 'keystone species'. This term describes species with disproportionate agency capable of transforming their constituent ecologies. An obvious analogy is with the recent reintroduction of wolves to rewild the ecologies of North American National Parks. Here, wolves are valued for their ability to address 'trophic cascades' – dramatic shifts in the abundance of species down the food chain as a result of their absence. The presence of wolves and the 'ecologies of fear' (Ripple and Beschta, 2004) they engender have caused landscape scale shifts in grazing dynamics and vegetation composition. We are encouraged to imagine worms exerting similar systemic traction.

For some advocates, reworming involves the restoration of our wild immunity through a return to a dirtier, messier past. This represents a somewhat anti-Pasteurian sensibility and requires a rather gung-ho embrace of the premodern microbiome and a 'paleo' lifestyle. Witness, for example, the writings of Jeff Leach, an anthropologist who runs the 'Human Food Project'. Leach recently went native, giving himself a transplant of the faeces of a Hadza hunter-gatherer within whom he was living in Tanzania (Eakin, 2014). For others, like William Parker, we need to rework our science and technology, domesticating our parasites or synthesising their secretions to selectively and strategically intervene in complex systems. 'Resilience', 'functionality' and 'adaptability' are the buzzwords in a discourse somewhat akin to that of ecological modernisation in the macrobiome.

Even in their extreme, neo-primitivist incarnations, a probiotic approach reworks (rather than abandons) the antibiotic logics associated with the antimicrobial practices of public health and hygiene – exemplified in this story by the search for a 'magic bullet' hookworm vaccine. The modern target of securing the human and the hygienic population is not giving way to a deep ecological, anti-humanist release of the vital potentials of life. With good reason, the biopolitics of human–helminthic relations remains fixed on securing certain human life in individual and aggregate forms often at the expense of certain nonhuman/animal commensals, but the story of worms suggests that new practices are emerging.

We can understand these developments in the context of wider enthusiasms for probiotic approaches to health – including forms of bacteriotherapy (like faecal transplants) and general enthusiasms for dirt (Pollan, 2013) – and can situate this probiotic approach with a rapidly expanding literature in the social and natural sciences that has developed metaphors of (auto)immunity to critically examine contemporary forms of politics (Esposito, 2011; Napier, 2012). The practice of reworming clearly departs from the binary model of immunity premised on the separation of self–other that has been much criticised – both by scientists (Anderson and Mackay, 2014) and by social scientists concerned with its traffic into broader social discourse (Cohen, 2009). To use Scott Gilbert's (Gilbert *et al.*, 2012) terms, reworming shifts the dominant metaphor of human–nonhuman relations from 'war', through 'tolerance', to 'active recruitment'. The subject of this recruitment is not an intentional human mind, but a super-organism emergent from a collaboration amidst its microbial denizens in an entanglement that flags the salubrious properties of infection, symbiosis and multispecies community.

Topologies of health

An immunological analysis of diseases related to hookworm presence and absence also draws attention to the spatial dimensions of global health and the practices of disease control and eradication. On the one hand, the North–South and Urban–Rural gradients in hookworm abundance map familiar regional cartographies of global health (see Figure 6.3). Here, hookworm presence and absence can be mapped as an index of international development: a mosaic of nations in strategically shaded blocks of colour. While such maps are interesting and politically important, they fail to convey the spatial connections and intensities that would appear to configure the diseases of hookworm presence and absence.

In recent work on biosecurity and immunity, Steve Hinchliffe and his colleagues develop a topological geography of 'folded life' (Hinchliffe *et al.*, 2012, Hinchliffe and Ward, 2014) that is helpful for mapping the human–nonhuman entanglements illustrated in the practices of de- and reworming. This is a geography of relations, connections and intensities that attends to porous bodies, leaky boundaries and the promiscuous natures of multispecies' molecular and viral exchanges. This topological model offers a geography that complicates linear narratives of development, hygiene and becoming modern that lie at the heart of global health (Hinchliffe, 2015).

Thinking the geographies of hookworm topologically helps us attend to the entangled spatial and political ecologies of its parasitology. Hookworm is spread by humans: the African slave trade introduced hookworm into North America (Coelho and McGuire, 2006), while the export of indentured labour from India during the nineteenth century spread hookworm around the British empire (Palmer, 2009). Palmer suggests that hookworm flourished in the topologies of colonial capitalism, whose political ecologies pushed hookworm infections past a tipping point. He argues that 'simmering among rural peoples around the world, [hookworm] boiled over not so much in "the tropics" as in the liminal zones of nineteenth-century world capitalist expansion – in temperate Europe as well as in the colonial and national tropics' (2009, 678). He notes that:

> Hookworm disease was a sickness of ecological, economic, and cultural displacement and recombination; its virulent appearance along these teeming trenchworks of modernity went hand in hand with the increasing density and speed of the globe's road, rail, and ocean connections. A close relative of nineteenth-century capital, the hookworm parasite thrived in heated frontier regions where vulnerable bodies were amassed for hard labor, and it became potent through accumulation.
>
> (Palmer, 2009, 679)

The 'trenchworks of modernity' were the tropical mines, tunnels, railroad beds and plantation soils of nineteenth-century colonial capitalism. These were worked by high densities of exploited and undernourished labour, which created the ideal conditions for hookworm disease.

This analysis of a hookworm disease crossing a threshold or tipping point is similar to Hinchliffe and colleagues' (2012) diagnosis of the pathological nature of the contemporary intensive global food system, whose intensive relations of mobile, concentrated and immune-compromised animal bodies generate the conditions for viral evolution and epidemic emergence. Understood this way, hookworm is not a disease of underdevelopment, but a consequence of the intensity of exploitative socio–ecological relations. High wormloads were not (and will not be) addressed without investments to research the intensities that tip hookworm infection into hookworm disease. Sanitation, nutrition and wider healthcare, coupled with rural to urban migration, are ultimately what drive hookworm control.

The seeming spatial paradox is that historic (and generally commendable) efforts to address unsanitary ecologies have propelled microbial ecologies past a different tipping point. Here, the absence of parasite ecologies and their associated intensities of 'immunological exercise' have driven a further refolding of the human microbiome and its interspecies relations. This is a topology marked by absence; a disequilibrium created by the successful eradication of forms of difference now understood to be integral to the stability and functioning of human identity. In the analysis of biophilosophers like Esposito, the absence of relations is symptomatic of 'autoimmunity' and suggests a system with a pathological unease with difference – in this case the nonhuman difference that keeps us human.

Subsequent efforts to engineer intensities and difference back into interspecies relations are taking contrasting political ecological forms. For example, worms have become a frontier for 'lively capital' (Rajan, 2012) in Jasper Lawrence's entrepreneurial bioprospecting return to the source, or in Coronado Biosciences' privatised whipworm ova TSO™. The promise of commodifiable immunity is at the heart of current excitement about the sequencing of the hookworm genome and the 'veritable pharmacopoeia' (Tang *et al.*, 2014, 268) of synthetic (and thus patentable) anti-inflammatory molecule secretions it might deliver. In contrast, the hookworm underground seeks to circulate 'hookworm without borders' through a communitarian biosociality of exchange. Here, knowledge, support and materials are delivered at cost or through the work of volunteer enthusiasts and advocates.

In place of an antibiotic model of health, Hinchliffe and Ward suggest that genuine biosecurity, or what they call 'the making of safe life', 'is constituted through an ability to work with rather than against a complex microbial environment' (2014, 136). They propose 'living with' as an approach to 'immunology management' akin to the probiotic approaches outlined above. Here,

> [L]iving with . . . becomes a matter of working alongside others, and with those people who appreciate the complexities of health and illness, the dimensions of pathological life, and, in doing so shifts the debate from securing territories (be they national states, corporate or animal bodies) and towards more nuanced immunological registers (and thus geographies).
>
> (Hinchliffe and Ward, 2014, 138)

For hookworm, a geography of inside–outside/self–other might be replaced with a topology of absence–presence; of conjoined alterity and interspecies entanglements requiring conversation, moderation (perhaps even agonism) with the life in us for the maintenance of human health.

Conclusions

In this chapter I have offered a geography of worms, examining the contemporary paradox of concurrent programmes to deworm and reworm the world. This analysis identifies the need to understand the geographies of global health as multispecies achievements, where both the presence and the absence of nonhuman organisms and relations can be pathogenic. Attending to geographies of microbial presence and absence helps identify the significance of microbiopolitics – the governance of circulating populations of microbes and people to secure desired systemic functions. Hookworm illustrates anti- and probiotic tendencies in modern forms of microbiopolitics, which confound prevalent linear models of hygiene and development. Thinking hookworm disease and epidemics of absence topologically flags the political ecologies responsible for driving disease intensification and autoimmunity.

The geographies and microbiopolitics for living well with worms are not well understood – timings, composition, dosage and symbiotic/parasitic co-infections all make a difference to immune response. These are currently the subject of a range of laboratory research projects, clinical trials and citizen science experiments. What is clear however is that they pose far-reaching questions for the modernist dreams of some dimensions of global health, not least ongoing efforts to 'deworm the world' through the development of a hookworm vaccine. While this is sincerely promoted as an 'antipoverty' vaccine (Hotez, 2013), in the words of one commentator, it could 'lead to the emergence of inflammatory and metabolic conditions in countries that are not prepared for these new epidemics' (Wammes *et al.*, 2014, 1), permanently immunising populations against the salutary potentials of helminthic gut buddies.

Notes

1 This is the title of a blog recounting personal experiences of using helminths to treat IBD. See http://gut-buddies.com/wordpress/. See also http://coloncomrades.wordpress.com/.
2 Much of this overview is taken from the Australian Society of Parasitology's website at http://parasite.org.au/para-site/contents/helminth-intoduction.html,
3 See www.youtube.com/watch?v=aqBoT_DyOsI.
4 See http://evidenceaction.org/deworming/. Cherie Blair is one of the supporters of this initiative and was persuaded to dress up as a hookworm at the 2008 Davos Summit and accost the global elite to draw attention to deworming (Hawkes, 2013).
5 See https://www.biomerestoration.com/.

References

Allen, J.E. and R.M. Maizels (2011). Diversity and dialogue in immunity to helminths. *Nature Reviews Immunology* 11(6): 375–388.

Anderson, W. (1995). Excremental colonialism: public health and the poetics of pollution. *Critical Inquiry* 21(3): 640–669.

Anderson, W. (2006). *Colonial Pathologies: American Tropical Medicine, Race, and Hygiene in the Philippines*, Durham, NC: Duke University Press.

Anderson, W. and I.R. Mackay (2014). *Intolerant Bodies: A Short History of Autoimmunity*, Baltimore, MD: Johns Hopkins University Press.

Bach, J-F. (2002). The effect of infections on susceptibility to autoimmune and allergic diseases. *New England Journal of Medicine* 347(12): 911–920.

Biehl, J. and A. Petryna (2013). *When People Come First: Critical Studies in Global Health*, Princeton, NJ: Princeton University Press.

Blaser, M. (2014). *Missing Microbes: How Killing Bacteria Creates Modern Plagues*, London: Oneworld Publications.

Blaser, M.J. and S. Falkow (2009). What are the consequences of the disappearing human microbiota? *Nature Reviews Microbiology* 7(12): 887–894.

Brooker, S., J. Bethony and P.J. Hotez (2004). Human hookworm infection in the 21st century. *Advances in Parasitology* 58: 197–288.

Bulletin., J-P.P. (2012). *Deworming: A Best Buy for Development*, Cambridge, MA: Abdul Latif Jameel Poverty Action Lab.

Coelho, P.R.P. and R.A. McGuire (2006). Racial differences in disease susceptibilities: intestinal worm infections in the early twentieth-century American South. *Social History of Medicine* 19(3): 461–482.

Cohen, E. (2009). *A Body Worth Defending: Immunity, Biopolitics, and the Apotheosis of the Modern Body*, Durham, NC: Duke University Press.

Cox, F.E.G. (2010). *History of Human Parasitology*, New York: John Wiley & Sons.

De Vrieze, J. (2013). The promise of poop. *Science* 341(6149): 954–957.

Eakin, E. (2014). The excrement experiment. *New Yorker*, December.

Engel, S. and A. Susilo (2014). Shaming and sanitation in Indonesia: a return to colonial public health practices? *Development and Change* 45(1): 157–178.

Eppig, C., C.L. Fincher and R. Thornhill (2010). Parasite prevalence and the worldwide distribution of cognitive ability. *Proceedings of the Royal Society B: Biological Sciences* 277(1701): 3801–3808.

Esposito, R. (2011). *Immunitas: The Protection and Negation of Life*, Oxford: Polity Press.

Ettling, J. (2013). *The Germ of Laziness: Rockefeller Philanthropy and Public Health in the New South*, Cambridge, MA: Harvard University Press.

Farley, J. (2003). *To Cast Out Disease: A History of the International Health Division of Rockefeller Foundation (1913-1951)*, New York: Oxford University Press.

Feary, J., J. Britton and J. Leonardi-Bee (2011). Atopy and current intestinal parasite infection: a systematic review and meta-analysis. *Allergy* 66(4): 569–578.

Flohr, C., R.J. Quinnell and J. Britton (2009). Do helminth parasites protect against atopy and allergic disease? *Clinical & Experimental Allergy* 39(1): 20–32.

Geissler, P.W. (1998a). 'Worms are our life', part I: Understandings of worms and the body among the Luo of western Kenya. *Anthropology & Medicine* 5(1): 63–79.

Geissler, P.W. (1998b). 'Worms are our life', part II: Luo children's thoughts about worms and illness. *Anthropology & Medicine* 5(2): 133–144.

Gilbert, S.F., J. Sapp and A.I. Tauber (2012). A symbiotic view of life: we have never been individuals. *Quarterly Review of Biology* 87(4): 325–341.

Grassberger, M., R.A. Sherman, O.S. Gileva, C.M.H. Kim and K.Y. Mumcuoglu (2013). *Biotherapy – History, Principles and Practice: A Practical Guide to the Diagnosis and Treatment of Disease using Living Organisms*, New York: Springer.

Guthman, J. and B. Mansfield (2013). The implications of environmental epigenetics: a new direction for geographic inquiry on health, space, and nature–society relations. *Progress in Human Geography* 37(4): 486–504.

Hanski, I., L. von Hertzen, N. Fyhrquist, K. Koskinen, K. Torppa, T. Laatikainen, P. Karisola, P. Auvinen, L. Paulin, M.J. Makela, E. Vartiainen, T.U. Kosunen, H. Alenius and T. Haahtela (2012). Environmental biodiversity, human microbiota, and allergy are interrelated. *Proceedings of the National Academy of Sciences* 109: 8334–8339.

Haraway, D.J. (2008). *When Species Meet.* Minnesota, MN: University of Minnesota Press.

Hawkes, N. (2013). Deworming debunked. *British Medical Journal* 346: 8558.

Helmby, H. (2009). Helminths and our immune system: friend or foe? *Parasitology International* 58(2): 121–127.

Hinchliffe, S. (2015). More than one world, more than one health: re-configuring inter-species health. *Social Science & Medicine* 129: 28–35.

Hinchliffe, S. and K.J. Ward (2014). Geographies of folded life: how immunity reframes biosecurity. *Geoforum* 53: 136–144.

Hinchliffe, S., J. Allen, S. Lavau, N. Bingham and S. Carter (2012). Biosecurity and the topologies of infected life: from borderlines to borderlands. *Transactions of the Institute of British Geographers* 38(4): 531–543.

Hoshi, N. and R. Medzhitov (2012). Germs gone wild. *National Medicine* 18(5): 654–656.

Hotez, P.J. (2013). *Forgotten People, Forgotten Diseases: The Neglected Tropical Diseases and Their Impact on Global Health and Development,* New York: ASM Press.

Hotez, P.J., A. Fenwick, L. Savioli and D.H. Molyneux (2009). Rescuing the bottom billion through control of neglected tropical diseases. *The Lancet* 373(9674): 1570–1575.

Hotez, P.J., J.M. Bethony, D.J. Diemert, M. Pearson and A. Loukas (2010). Developing vaccines to combat hookworm infection and intestinal schistosomiasis. *Nature Reviews Microbiology* 8(11): 814–826.

Hotez, P.J., P.J. Brindley, J.M. Bethony, C.H. King, E.J. Pearce and J. Jacobson (2008). Helminth infections: the great neglected tropical diseases. *Journal of Clinical Investigation* 118(4): 1311–1321.

Hotez, P.J., D. Diemert, K.M. Bacon, C. Beaumier, J.M. Bethony, M.E. Bottazzi, S. Brooker, A.R. Couto, M. da Silva Freire, A. Homma, B.Y. Lee, A. Loukas, M. Loblack, C.M. Morel, R.C. Oliveira and P.K. Russell (2013). The human hookworm vaccine. *Vaccine* 31: B227–B232.

Khan, A.R. and P.G. Fallon (2013). Helminth therapies: translating the unknown unknowns to known knowns. *International Journal for Parasitology* 43(3–4): 293–299.

Latour, B. (1988). *The Pasteurization of France.* Cambridge, MA: Harvard University Press.

Moran-Thomas, A. (2013). A salvage ethnography of the guinea worm: witchcraft, oracles and magic in a disease eradication program. *When People Come First: Critical Studies in Global Health*: 207–240.

Nading, A.M. (2013). "Humans, animals, and health: from ecology to entanglement. *Environment and Society: Advances in Research* 4(1): 60–78.

Napier, A.D. (2012). NONSELF HELP: how immunology might reframe the Enlightenment. *Cultural Anthropology* 27(1): 122–137.

Nordrum, A. (2015) How three scientists 'marketed' neglected tropical diseases and raised more than $1 billion. *International Business Times,* 14 May. Available at www.ibtimes.com.

Palmer, S. (2009). Migrant clinics and hookworm science: peripheral origins of international health, 1840–1920. *Bulletin of the History of Medicine* 83(4): 676–709.

Parker, M., T. Allen and J. Hastings (2008). Resisting control of neglected tropical diseases: dilemmas in the mass treatment of schistosomiasis and soil-transmitted helminths in north-west Uganda. *Journal of Biosocial Science* 40(2): 161–181.

Parker, W. (2014). The 'hygiene hypothesis' for allergic disease is a misnomer. *British Medical Journal* 349: 5267.

Parker, W. and J. Ollerton (2013). Evolutionary biology and anthropology suggest biome reconstitution as a necessary approach toward dealing with immune disorders. *Evolution, Medicine, and Public Health* 2013(1): 89–103.

Parker, W., S.E. Perkins, M. Harker and M.P. Muehlenbein (2012). A prescription for clinical immunology: the pills are available and ready for testing. A review. *Current Medical Research and Opinion* 28(7): 1193–1202.

Paxson, H. (2008). Post-pasteurian cultures: the microbiopolitics of raw-milk cheese in the United States. *Cultural Anthropology* 23(1): 15–47.

Pollan, M. (2013). Some of my best friends are germs. *New York Times*, 15 May. Available at http://www.nytimes.com/2013/05/19/magazine/say-hello-to-the-100-trillion-bacteria-that-make-up-your-microbiome.html (accessed 21 September 2016).

Pullan, R.L. and S.J. Brooker (2012). The global limits and population at risk of soil-transmitted helminth infections in 2010. *Parasites and Vectors* 5(1): 81–95.

Rajan, K.S. (2012). *Lively Capital: Biotechnologies, Ethics, and Governance in Global Markets*, Durham, NC: Duke University Press.

Ripple, W.J. and R.L. Beschta (2004). Wolves and the ecology of fear: can predation risk structure ecosystems? *BioScience* 54(8): 755–766.

Rook, G.A.W. (2009). Review series on helminths, immune modulation and the hygiene hypothesis: the broader implications of the hygiene hypothesis. *Immunology* 126(1): 3–11.

Rook, G.A.W. (2012). Hygiene hypothesis and autoimmune diseases. *Clinical Reviews in Allergy and Immunology* 42(1): 5–15.

Sabin (2015). Human hookworm vaccine: history. Available at www.sabin.org.

Schneider, B., A.R. Jariwala, M.V. Periago, M.F. Gazzinelli, S.N. Bose, P.J. Hotez, D.J. Diemert and J.M. Bethony (2011). A history of hookworm vaccine development. *Human Vaccines* 7(11): 1234–1244.

Siniscalco, D. and N. Antonucci (2013). Possible use of Trichuris suis ova in autism spectrum disorders therapy. *Medical Hypotheses* 81(1): 1–4.

Stepan, N.L. (2013). *Eradication: Ridding the World of Diseases Forever?* London: Reaktion Books.

Stoll, N.R. (1999). This wormy world. *The Journal of Parasitology* 85(3): 392–396.

Strachan, D.P. (1989). Hay fever, hygiene, and household size. *British Medical Journal* 299(6710): 1259–1260.

Strosberg, S.A. (2014). *The Human Hookworm Assemblage: Contingency and the Practice of Helminthic Therapy*. M.Sc. thesis, Department of Geography, University of Kentucky.

Tang, Y.T., X. Gao, B.A. Rosa, S. Abubucker, K. Hallsworth-Pepin, J. Martin, R. Tyagi, E. Heizer, X. Zhang, V. Bhonagiri-Palsikar, P. Minx, W.C. Warren, Q. Wang, B. Zhan, P.J. Hotez, P.W. Sternberg, A. Dougall, S.T. Gaze, J. Mulvenna, J. Sotillo, S. Ranganathan, E.M. Rabelo, R.K. Wilson, P.L. Felgner, J. Bethony, J.M. Hawdon, R.B. Gasser, A. Loukas and M. Mitreva (2014). Genome of the human hookworm Necator americanus. *Nature Genetics* 46(3): 261–269.

Taylor-Robinson, D., N. Maayan, K. Soares-Weiser, S. Donegan and P. Garner (2012). Deworming drugs for soil-transmitted intestinal worms in children: effects on nutritional indicators, haemoglobin and school performance. *Cochrane Database of Systematic Reviews* 11.

Thornhill, R. and C.L. Fincher (2011). Parasite stress promotes homicide and child maltreatment. *Philosophical Transactions of the Royal Society B: Biological Sciences* 366 (1583): 3466–3477.

Thornhill, R., C.L. Fincher and D. Aran (2009). Parasites, democratization, and the liberalization of values across contemporary countries. *Biological Reviews* 84(1): 113–131.

Trujillo-Pagan, N.E. (2013). Worms as a hook for colonising Puerto Rico. *Social History of Medicine* 26(4): 611–632.

Turnbaugh, P.J., R.E. Ley, M. Hamady, C.M. Fraser-Liggett, R. Knight and J.I. Gordon (2007). The Human Microbiome Project. *Nature* 449(7164): 804–810.

Velasquez-Manoff, M. (2012). *An Epidemic of Absence: A New Way of Understanding Allergies and Autoimmune Diseases*, New York: Scribner.

Wammes, L.J., H. Mpairwe, A.M. Elliott and M. Yazdanbakhsh (2014). Helminth therapy or elimination: epidemiological, immunological, and clinical considerations. *The Lancet Infectious Diseases* 14(11): 1150–1162.

Whatmore, S. (2006). Materialist returns: practising cultural geography in and for a more-than-human world. *Cultural Geographies* 13(4): 600–609.

Young, K.A. (2014). Of poops and parasites: unethical FDA overregulation. *Food and Drug Law Journal* 69(4): 555–574, ii.

Zuk, M. (2007). *Riddled with Life: Friendly Worms, Ladybug Sex, and the Parasites that Make Us who We are*, New York: Harcourt.

7 Resistant bodies, malaria and the question of immunity

Uli Beisel

Introduction

The eradication of malaria is a long-standing quest in global public health. Over the past decade, rising malaria case numbers, the inclusion of malaria in the Millennium Development Goals, and an interest in the disease by key philanthropic actors in global health have not only increased funding for malaria control and research but also reinvigorated the disease eradication agenda. In 2008, world leaders endorsed an ambitious *Global Malaria Action Plan*, involving a US$3 billion commitment to reduce the number of malaria deaths to near zero. The new drive towards the eradication of malaria began in 2007, when the Bill and Melinda Gates Foundation (BMGF), which quickly rose to paramount importance in global health following its establishment in 1999, announced their focus on malaria eradication. After the failure and abandonment of the first eradication campaign in 1969, the WHO advocated malaria management and control over the intervening decades. The move of BMGF led to a return to eradication in international policies, resulting in a substantial realignment of funding and disease control policies (Kelly and Beisel, 2011).

But soon after the announcement, the revived eradication campaign was met with more sobering evidence that, by all accounts, should have tempered the overwhelming optimism that characterises a policy of malaria eradication. The news came in late 2008 from Pailin, a town in Western Cambodia close to the border with Thailand. Long-held fears were confirmed in a letter published by the *New England Journal of Medicine* reporting evidence for artemisinin-tolerant parasites in this area (Noedl *et al.*, 2008). Although artemisinin is still effective against malaria in the region, in many places it is at a much slower pace. This slower pace can already decide over life or death in a seriously ill patient; more time for the parasites to live and multiply within the bloodstream can be deadly for a weak body. Moreover, if artemisinin loses its effectiveness, the success of malaria treatment is endangered worldwide. Artemisinin tolerance has now spread across the Mekong Subregion (WHO, 2014). This development is all the more threatening, since it happened before: in the 1960s, parasites became resistant to chloroquine. Since its discovery in the late 1930s, chloroquine was popular as the first-line malaria treatment all over the world. It was not only highly effective but also a cheap treatment with only minor side-effects. However, after the development of resistance, chloroquine had to be phased out in malarious countries. It was replaced by artemisinin-combined therapy, the treatment currently threatened by emerging resistance.

Resistance pushes us to ask if humans are really as much in control as policy narratives might suggest, or instead might nature rather be 'inhumane' (Clark, 2011)? Emerging resistance and its spread shows that life is not easily separable in human and other-than-human processes; in the development of malaria *Plasmodium* parasites sneak into our body, penetrate our red blood cells and make us ill. Blood-seeking *Anopheles* mosquitoes are the vehicle that parasites not only use to travel from human to human, but in whose mid guts they also fulfil one part of their reproductive cycle, while the other half of multiplying happens in the human blood. Resistant parasites redefine what malaria treatment means and they force humans to rethink control measures. Human and nonhuman organisms, social and biological processes are inescapably intertwined in the emergence of malaria. The human/nonhuman distinction is done actively through certain practices and gets blurred through other practices and experiences – be that human or other-than-human practices.

A recent turn towards multispecies understandings in human–animal relations has emphasised entanglements rather than modernistic binary divisions (Haraway, 2008; Whatmore, 2002; for mosquito-related research see Nading, 2014; Kelly and Lezaun, 2014; Beisel, 2010). However, although many scholars seek to understand aggression and violence between humans and nonhumans (The Animal Studies Group, 2006; Ginn *et al.*, 2014), the turn to multispecies entanglements nevertheless has a romantic thrust, aimed at understanding and bringing to the fore our more-than-human vitality that gets lost in antagonistic environmental politics and mastery of nature tropes. This chapter asks if multispecies understandings might also help us to open up new ways of advancing less innocent, survival-focused thinking. After all, malaria and its control is a game of intervention and response, following the motto of 'who can bite back faster?' (Beisel, 2010). For in the end, survival is never innocent but always violent, as it carries power and requires sacrifice. Emily Yates-Doerr and Annemarie Mol make this point nicely recounting a scene at a Spanish butchery, where Emily was buying meat while carrying her baby:

> While the butcher praised the flavours of milk-fed lambs, the mother held on tightly to her charge. For all of a sudden she sensed the similarity between one kind of flesh (lamb turned into meat) and the other (boy that definitely should not be eaten). The similarity was striking, the difference shaky. . . . How, then, to differentiate between boy and lamb? Does the first have an interior, a soul, and the second not? Or might this difference be rather more practical. One belongs to a species – a kind, a group, a clan – that has organized itself so as to cultivate and kill the other. The other is just a lamb. Its mother carries no money and no butcher's knife. Its father has long since been slaughtered. Its body is not particularly strong

but strikingly tasty. As the human boy must be fed with yet more milk, the human mother needs to eat, and therefore it is the lamb's fate to be eaten.

(Yates-Doerr and Mol, 2012, p. 60)

In this chapter I focus on the question of species survival and what taking the different agencies of humans, mosquitoes and parasites may seriously entail. In the malarial game of infection, survival and death, 'resistance' plays a vital role for all involved. It is not only parasites that become resistant: recent scientific efforts to decrease human infection and increase survival chances have focused on the development of a malaria vaccine. Here, the desired effect of immunity is to shut the parasites out, to keep them from multiplying in our body and so prevent disease – immunity means that our bodies learn to *resist* the parasites. While parasite resistance and human immunity are biologically similar processes of adaptation to a threat for species survival, we employ two different terms: while humans develop 'immunity' to parasites, parasites develop 'resistance' to drugs attempting to kill them. The dominant notion of resistance suggests that one actant actively and violently resists another, while immunity suggest a legitimate process of closing oneself off from violence.

I discuss the development of a malaria vaccine, the rise of malaria drug-tolerant parasites, as well as vernacular logics of negotiating partial immunities in order to investigate the survival strategies and practices of humans and parasites alike.[1] I read these practices of humans and parasites through the concept of 'immunity', and so aim to reintroduce a form of symmetry in the analysis I propose, enabling us to see both practices as a struggle for survival. I suggest that thinking resistance through immunity allows us to slow down and suspend the normative judgement the notion of 'resistance' presumes. Indeed, reading what is usually understood as resistance as immunity might open up new ways of thinking about human–mosquito-parasite entanglements, the prospects of eradication and the biopolitical registers at play in malaria prevention and treatment in global health today. I argue that interrogating malaria policies and ecological disease dynamics through the notion of immunity draws attention to the 'folded geographies' (Hinchliffe and Ward, 2014) of the three species that constitute malaria – to the complex topologies at play in the entanglements of humans, mosquitoes and parasites.

It is these complex and sometimes contradictory multiple immunities of malaria that I attend to in the following sections. In the next section I introduce how the concept of immunity has shifted in immunology from understandings of cells at war to complex and non-linear relations between different types of organisms. I then move on to discussing visions of vaccination, mutating and moving parasites, as well as how humans acquire partial immunity to malaria. In short, this chapter is an attempt to rethink malaria and its control in a way that explicitly aims to – in the words of Donna Haraway (2010) – 'stay with the trouble' of the politics of opening and closing our bodies to micro-organisms rather than to simply negate or indeed try to eradicate the other.

Bioecologies, resistance and immunity

The complex interplay between malaria eradication on the one hand and the development of mosquito and parasite tolerance on the other is often framed in terms of war. In this war, mosquitoes and parasites are humans' adversaries; developing tolerance to drugs or insecticides is conceived of as a cunning move, which puts 'them' a few steps ahead. But in the name of health and progress humans must press on, be even faster and develop new means to beat 'them'. Military metaphors in malaria control have a long history, dating back to the first malaria eradication phase in the 1950/1960s and before. They were initially used predominantly in entomology, namely in attempts to eliminate the malaria vector, and were intended to serve the purpose of attracting and sustaining funding for the campaign (Brown, 1997, pp. 135–136; Beisel and Boëte, 2013). In the recently renewed eradication 'fight against malaria' such military metaphors are present again in attempts to 'shrink the malaria map' (Feachem *et al.*, 2010), 'invest in the future, defeat malaria' (World Malaria Day theme, 2015) or to 'count malaria out' (World Malaria Day theme, 2009, 2010; see http://www.worldmalariaday.org).

In her study on immunity in American culture, Emily Martin shows that war metaphors also pertain to another domain; they are used in popular culture to characterise the immune system, comparing our bodies to a 'nation state at war' (Martin, 1994). She argues that not only does this language 'domesticate violence', but it also perpetuates a model of biology that is marked by an ideal of internal purity (ibid., p. 417). A similar case can be made for malaria, where war metaphors underplay the significance of the coevolution of humans, mosquitoes and parasites. This renders malaria control as a temporally and spatially delineated fight, rather than drawing attention to constant calibrations of microenvironments in control practices (Kelly and Beisel, 2011).

Immunology, on the other hand, has moved on from war metaphors towards emphasising the flexibility and complexity of immune reactions. As Martin shows, such new understandings of 'flexible bodies' resemble late capitalist language, but Martin cautions against a developing new social Darwinism. Similarly, however, in a more hopeful mode, for Haraway, contemporary immunology bids farewell to binary battlefields, when it draws the body as a network and so, Haraway suggests, literally opens the body up (Haraway, 1991). And indeed, contemporary scientific understandings of the immune system are based on complexity, specificity and non-linearity. Hinchliffe and Ward, for instance, discussing farm agriculture, emphasise that the same bacteria which cause disease can also engender health (Hinchliffe and Ward, 2014). Equally, the distinction between self and non-self is shifting, even dissolving in some cases, as Napier puts it:

> [W]e now know that defending the body against a viral 'attack' is nothing like defending it from invading organisms. Viruses need cells to achieve vitality, and cannot attack without the life that autogenous, 'self-made' cells (ones made by our own bodies) bring to each and every viral encounter.
>
> (Napier, 2012, p. 125)

Indeed, as Donna Haraway also argues, our bodies lack clear distinctions between Self and Other, they are to an overwhelming majority other, sustained by millions of bacteria (see e.g. Hararway, 2008), rendering us into a 'strategic assemblage called self' (Haraway, 1990, p. 212). Immunity then is a practice of complex bodily multispecies coordination that takes work to be sustained. Moreover, this is one that may well break down once in a while during the course of our lives, leading in extreme cases to the immune system turning against our own bodies (Anderson and Mackay, 2015). Much remains unknown about the causes of autoimmunity: despite decades of intensive scientific research no clear causes have been established with 'precision or authority' (ibid., p. 144). As Jacques Derrida has pointed out, autoimmunity seems to pertain to its own logic, it is characterised by contradiction and 'undecidability' (Derrida, 1996, quoted in Anderson and Mackay, 2015, p.145).

Other philosophers have pondered on the relation between (auto)immunity and community. Peter Sloterdijk (2004) observes that immunisation as a cultural practice has expanded in contemporary societies through the pressures of globalisation. However, he states that immunisation comes with new insecurities, and thus may turn into societal forms of autoimmunity. Building on this insight, Mutsaers argues that mainstream biosecurity interventions to control Swine and Avian Flu threats have resulted in what Sloterdijk calls 'exaggerated immunisation' responses, where nature is caste as bioterrorist: 'the practice of pre-emptive immunisation as applied to infectious diseases thus appears to convey a militaristic approach' (Mutsaers, 2015, p. 127). Roberto Esposito also reflects on the relation between immunisation and society. Immunity, in his reading, is to be thought with the notion of community, or com-munus (Esposito, 2011). The Latin *munus* comes from *onus* (obligation) and *officium* (office), and *donum* (the gift). To Esposito, immunity is a gift that combines the former two, making it into a much more intense form of the gift: it is 'the gift that one gives, not the gift that one receives', 'the gratitude that demands new donations' (Esposito, quoted in Campbell, s.a., p. 7). As Campbell explains, for Esposito community and immunity are complexly interlinked: 'immunity presupposes community, but also negates it, so that rather than centred on simple reciprocity, community doubles upon itself, protecting itself from a presupposed excess of communal gift-giving' (ibid., p. 8). In other words, someone who is *immunitas* enjoys the privilege of being freed from communal responsibilities and is therefore singled out from the community: 'the condition of immunity signifies both "not to be and not to have in common" ' (ibid.). However, if a society protects itself too much through *immunitas,* the link to community, *communitas*, becomes too weak. This to Esposito signifies 'the constitutively exposed character of living' (Esposito, quoted in in Campbell and Esposito, 2006, p. 51). *Immunitas* and *communitas* thus are opposites, but need to be in balance; 'immunitas in high doses entails the sacrifice of the living' (ibid.). While community and immunity are opposites they are thus also inextricably linked – community and *immunitas* are made possible through (opposition to) each other; immunity encompasses difference and belonging at the same time.

In contrast to this understanding, much conventional and applied work on immunity and biosecurity often presumes distinct boundaries between self and other, risk and benefit, or good and bad circulations (see also Mutsaers, 2015). However, as I discussed above, these boundaries do not hold true with regard to how immunity is established and nourished. Approaches to immunity as complex and, in part, unpredictable then caution against binary war and eradication approaches in multispecies communities. If we attempt to eradicate too many viruses, bacteria and parasites from our multispecies community, we may – following Esposito — also loosen the link to the communities that sustain us. Furthermore, it is important to keep in mind that resistance is not a phenomenon developing independently from human action. As Hannah Landecker reminds us, antimicrobial resistance is not the result of natural bioterrorists, but of the medical-industrial complex: 'Through the industrial-scale growth of microorganisms to harvest their metabolic products' humans have fostered bacteria evolution. Resistance may thus be understood as 'the physical registration of human history in bacterial life' (Landecker, 2015, p. 1). As we will see in the following sections, the development of malaria drug resistance also emerges from the actions and entangled practices of humans, parasites and mosquitoes.

Following these current understandings of immunity and resistance, then, it is not that easy to separate our enemies and allies in the war for health. However, attempts at disease eradication and binary war rhetoric prevail for a good reason, as malaria continues to make millions of people sick on this planet every year; it also kills a good share, and tragically the majority of deaths are children under 5 years of age (WHO, 2014). Nevertheless, I would like to suggest that it is worth pausing, stepping back from this war rhetoric and to think through the socio-ecological entanglements underlying human attempts to 'win the war'. In the spirit of Isabelle Stengers (2010) and Nick Bingham (2008), I will use the following pages to 'slow down', and begin to rethink how we may understand the techno-scientific politics of malaria differently.

In order to do this, I will discuss the development of biological tolerance and resistance of parasites. I suggest that – for mosquitoes, parasites and humans alike – these represent attempts to create a form of 'immunity'. I use this term not necessarily in order to establish some simplistic form of symmetry between the actions of mosquitoes, parasites and humans (although I do think a certain amount of humbleness from the side of humans is helpful), but first and foremost in order to take the complex entanglements of local biologies and global ecologies of malaria seriously. As Latour has pointed out, the notion of symmetry in actor-network theory was intended to do this kind of work (but has often been misunderstood):

> ANT is not, I repeat is not, the establishment of some absurd 'symmetry between humans and nonhumans'. To be symmetric, for us, simply means *not* to impose a priori some spurious *asymmetry* among human intentional action and a material world of causal relations.
>
> (Latour, 2005, p. 76)

Thus, I use immunity as an analytical lens which starts from the premise that we are – for better and for worse – profoundly entangled in our worldings. This is a conceptual move that Donna Haraway would call the non-innocent politics of companion species (Haraway, 2003, 2008). In what follows I attempt to carve out the complex movements between symbiosis and parasitism, or between mutuality and suffering in human and parasite malaria practices and politics.

The multiple immunities of malaria

Visions of vaccination

Speaking of malaria and immunity, the most obvious question raised is about vaccines against malaria. The first remark here needs to be that up until today, no vaccine against any parasitic disease exists, largely owing to the high biological complexity of parasites (in comparison to bacterial or viral organisms). Research on a vaccine against malaria started as early as the beginning of the twentieth century (Desowitz, 1991), but despite many scientific efforts no vaccine has yet proven to be both effective and non-toxic for humans. Over recent years, however, new scientific prospects have arisen from the possibility of mapping the genomes of humans and parasites, or as Ntoumi *et al.* call it, the possibility of 'mining the human and parasite genome:

> The sequencing of the human genome provides a new opportunity to determine the genetic traits that confer resistance to infection or disease. The identification of these traits can reveal immune responses, or host–parasite interactions, which may be useful for designing vaccines or new drugs. . . . The malaria parasites are well known for their ability to undergo antigenic variation, and in parallel to cause a diverse array of disease syndromes, including the severe syndromes that commonly cause death. Genome-based technologies are being harnessed to relate gene and protein expression levels, or genetic variation, to the parasite forms that are targets of protective immunity.
>
> (Ntoumi *et al.*, 2007, p. 270)

Indeed, advances in scientific knowledge such as these have led to about 30 potential malaria vaccine candidates that are currently under development. One of these vaccines, called RTS,S/ASO2A, is the first malaria vaccine candidate to have concluded stage III of clinical trials and is currently under consideration for licensure. The vaccine was initially developed in GlaxoSmithKline's laboratories in Belgium; systematic development goes back to the year 1984, and the active compounds that would be known as RTS,S were first combined in 1987 (GSK MVI, 2010). The vaccine went through initial test phases in Belgium and at the Walter Reed Army Institute in the USA in the 1990s (ibid.), as well as a first proof-of-concept study test in The Gambia and later Mozambique, where it was tested on 2022 children aged 1 to 4 years in a double-blind, randomised, controlled trial (Alonso *et al.*, 2004; Aponte *et al.*, 2009). Vaccine development and trials started to accelerate substantively from 2001, when the public–private partnership PATH Malaria Vaccine Initiative (MVI) started to finance and coordinate the development and trials. Funded by the Gates Foundation, MVI's general aim is 'to accelerate the development of promising malaria vaccines and ensure their availability and accessibility in the developing world' (MVI Factsheet, 2008). MVI alone has invested approximately US$220 million in RTS,S/ASO2A. GSK invested US$300 million up until the end of 2012 and estimated that another US$100 to 200 million in development costs will be necessary (MVI interview). There were also other, smaller investments in RTS,S/ASO2A, for instance, through the Walter Reed Army Institute. In general, the investment costs in RTS,S/ASO2A exceed US$500 million, which correlates with the estimated general costs of vaccine development (ibid.).

In addition, although GSK has invested a great deal in RTS,S/ASO2A, it was indeed mainly the foundation of MVI that enabled the clinical trials phase II and III in seven African countries conducted between 2007 and 2014. The malaria vaccine trials were among the first large-scale vaccine trials conducted on the African continent in history. In order to adhere to international standards of trial regulation, a capacity-building component has been important to the international consortium conducting the trials: funding from the Gates Foundation enabled the establishment of a Malaria Clinical Trial Alliance (MCTA), which is run under the umbrella of the INDEPTH Network, a Ghana-based organisation. MCTA and MVI conduct 'Good Clinical Practice' training for health workers involved in all stages of the trials – from doctors, nurses, fieldworkers, malaria microscopists to trial management staff. These trainings of, for instance, malaria microscopists were highly valued by participants and offered local laboratory workers a rare opportunity to participate in international training and networking (Interviews at malaria vaccine trial sites in Ghana, 2008). Trial locations have also benefited from new infrastructure, such as better equipment for laboratories. Such capacity building is an advantage for the participating hospitals, and has contributed to the building of biomedical capacity in the trial sites of the seven participating countries (Interviews at malaria vaccine trial sites in Ghana, 2008). However, such investments in selected hospitals are tied closely to research-trial institutions, which re-enforces unequal geographies of healthcare infrastructure and provision in developing countries, and creates what has been called 'archipelagos of science' on the African continent (Rottenburg, 2009; Geissler, 2013).

In 2014 the RTS,S/ASO2A malaria vaccine candidate completed phase III of clinical trials, and it has become clear that RTS,S/ASO2A will not have the protective effect that many were hoping for. The aim of the vaccine was never that the vaccine will provide full protection from malaria, but that it will offer a partial immunity of around 60 per cent, meaning the immunity levels of naïve individuals will be pushed up to the level of having successfully lived through a malaria infection. Sixty per cent is considered significant in public health logic, as it would avert six out of ten malaria infections (Interview, Vaccine Scientist, 2012). Considering that the large majority of malaria deaths occur in immunologically naïve children under 5, it is assumed that this would have a significant impact on malaria mortality. However, the latest clinical trial results indicate that while for children in the age group 5 to 17 months the protection was 45.1 per cent over 14 months (RTS,S Clinical Trials Partnership, 2011), protection for 6- to 12-week-old babies was disappointing with 31.3 per cent (RTS,S Clinical Trials Partnership, 2012). In 2014 the RTS,S Clinical Trials Partnership reported that the vaccine efficacy against clinical malaria in infants was 27 per cent, 'with no significant protection against severe malaria, malaria hospitalization, or all-cause hospitalization' (RTS,S Clinical Trials Partnership, 2014). Furthermore, initial protection rates decline quickly, making a four-dose vaccination regime necessary (RTS,S Clinical Partnership, 2015).

In 2012 an editorial in the *New England Journal of Medicine* suggested that the vaccine's efficacy results were 'disappointing', and it remains doubtful whether the vaccine will be licensed at the end of the trial (e.g. Daily, 2012). Other commentators were more optimistic and expect a positive licensing decision by the World Health Organisation. The decision was expected in 2015, but the World Health Organisation's 'Strategic Advisory Group of Experts on immunization (SAGE)' has recently pushed back the decision and called for implementation studies. This was the committee's reasoning:

> [O]ne primary outstanding question with regard to RTS,S/AS01 use in 5–17 month old children is the extent to which the protection demonstrated in the Phase 3 trial can be replicated in the context of the routine health system because of the challenge of implementing a four-dose schedule that requires new immunization contacts.
>
> (WHO/SAGE, 2015)

WHO rightly worries that a four-part routine immunisation is neither practical nor affordable in many contexts in sub-Saharan Africa.

However, regardless of this important political and economic question, one may ask: Why has the development of a malaria vaccine been so challenging? This is a question that the editorial in the *New England Journal of Medicine* answers as follows:

> [V]accine developers are faced with an organism that resides in the peripheral-blood compartment and that boldly circulates alongside immune cells and proteins to facilitate further transmission. *The success of this pathogen is related to prolonged coevolution with humans, allowing the development of cunning biologic strategies to resist immune-system clearance.*
>
> (Daily, 2012, p. 1, emphasis added)

In other words, whether we humans like it or not, plasmodium parasites are not only 'cunning', they also have a long and successful history of cohabiting with humans, which makes it rather tricky to 'defeat' them. Indeed, as historians of medicine suggest:

> [I]t is reasonable to suppose that it is older than we, that our primate ancestors were recognisably malarious before they were recognisably human, that the parasite, which causes the fever and the mosquito, which transfers it from one person to another have accompanied us throughout the Darwinian descent.
>
> (Harrison, 1978, p. 1)

Additionally, as studies in mice models have shown, a partially effective vaccine may at best 'buy us time', as it would considerably increase evolutionary pressure in Plasmodia, which has resulted in the emergence of more virulent parasites in mice models (Mackinnon and Read, 2004). Considering this, the high investment which vaccine development requires, and the fact that visions of vaccines have already failed to deliver their promise for decades, one might wonder if this hope for immunity in human bodies is the best way to limit the deadly circulations among humans, mosquitoes and parasites. Before dwelling on this question in more detail, the next section will discuss how immunity also develops in parasite bodies – as so-called tolerance of or resistance to malaria drugs.

The (dangerous) wanderlust of an Asian plasmodium falciparum parasite

A region in the borderlands between Cambodia and Thailand has been singled out in the international press coverage on malaria. This interest is based on the news that artemisinin-tolerant plasmodium parasites have been developing and spreading in Southeast Asia. In late 2008 a letter in the *New England Journal of Medicine* reported first evidence for artemisinin-resistant malaria; the study team found that of 60 patients treated with artesunate (monotherapy) four patients had recurring parasitemia, and two of those patients could be characterised as having artemisinin-resistant infection (Noedl *et al.*, 2008). Today, it is now present in five countries of the Greater Mekong sub-region: Cambodia, Laos, Myanmar, Thailand and Vietnam. Scientifically, plasmodium parasites are not resistant against artemisinin, but *tolerant*, as resistance would mean 100 per cent efficacy loss. However, artemisinin is still efficacious in the affected regions, but clears parasites from the bloodstream at a much slower pace. In a recent comparative study, the half-lives of parasite clearing times ranged from 1.9 hours in the Democratic Republic of Congo to 7.0 hours at the Thailand–Cambodia border. In other words, artemisinin is still capable of treating malaria, but requires prolonged courses of drug administration (Ashley *et al.*, 2014). Resistance is thus not an absolute but a gradual phenomenon. Nevertheless, WHO and all major malaria initiatives –such as the US President's Malaria Initiative (PMI) and the Bill and Melinda Gates Foundation – have expressed severe concern and identified the need for urgent action. As WHO put it on their webpage:

The spread of artemisinin resistance to other regions, or its independent emergence in other parts of the world, could trigger a major public health emergency. Urgent action is therefore required by endemic countries and development partners to prevent the situation from worsening.

(WHO/SAGE, 2015)

The WHO devised a 'global plan for artemisinin resistance containment' (WHO, 2011), as well as a framework for 'emergency response to artemisinin resistance in the Greater Mekong subregion' (WHO, 2013). Malaria drug resistance is all the more threatening, since it has happened before with chloroquine in the 1960s. And, as the history of resistance against chloroquine teaches us, newly configured parasites slowly but steadily broaden their borders. Figure 7.1 shows the travel itinerary of chloroquine-tolerant parasites 60 years ago.

Resistance was first reported in the late 1950s along both the Panama–Colombia and Thai–Cambodian borders, and radiated slowly and inexorably outward from these two foci, taking ten years to advance across Thailand to Burma, reaching central India by the late 1970s. Resistance more rapidly disseminated throughout the Amazon region, crossing southward across Bolivia in the early 1960s and extending to the Atlantic coast of French Guiana and Surinam by the early 1970s. Chloroquine resistance appeared in East Africa in 1978 and moved westward across the continent in a less well-documented pattern owing to limited surveillance in Central and West Africa (Plowe, 2009, p. S12).

Rather than a third mutation emerging in Africa, it has been demonstrated that the mutations leading to resistance in Asia and Africa are genetically identical (ibid.). Thus, the resistant parasites must have travelled from Asia to Africa. This

Chloroquine resistance

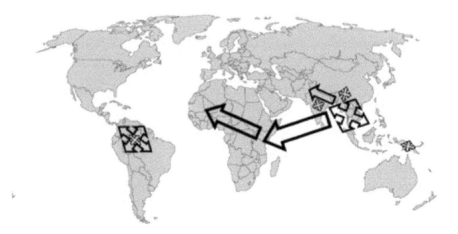

Figure 7.1 Spread of chloroquine resistance
Source: Plowe (2009, p. S12).

is believed to have happened not through mosquitoes that hitched a ride on a plane or a boat, as happened in the 1930s when *Anopheles gambiae* travelled on warships from West Africa to Brazil (Killeen *et al.*, 2002, p. 620), or from Sudan to Egypt (Mitchell, 2002, p. 22). Rather, chloroquine resistance presumably travelled from Asia to East Africa in humans. It is likely that the parasite hitched a ride with Southeast Asian workers, who came to East Africa in the 1970s to build a railway from Beira in Mozambique to Kinshasa in the Democratic Republic of Congo (then Zaire) (Campbell *et al.*, 1979). The workers unknowingly helped transmit resistant parasites to Africa. From East Africa, resistance broadened its borders slowly but significantly, continuing to travel overland, reaching West Africa last. So, while resistance emerges in parasites through a mutation of its genome, it travelled in mosquitoes and humans. Understanding the emergence and patterns of spread of resistance requires us to understand the socio-ecological entanglements of the three species.

For malaria patients, chloroquine resistance meant that first-line malaria treatment worldwide had to be replaced by another antimalarial drug, artemisinin. Since its discovery in the late 1930s, chloroquine was popular as first-line malaria treatment all over the world; it was not only highly effective but also a cheap treatment with minor side-effects. However, following the development of resistance, chloroquine had to be phased out in malarial countries, plummeting malaria control into crisis. Shortly after chloroquine, treatment with sulfadoxine-pyrimethamine, another common antimalarial drug, started to fail as well, and, as the history of malaria has shown us, this trend is also likely to happen with artemisinin-tolerant parasites. Thus scientists argued that early containment of resistance is vital, given the region's history and the parasite's wanderlust:

> Chloroquine and sulfadoxine-pyrimethamine resistance in *P. falciparum* emerged in the late 1950s and 1960s on the Thai–Cambodian border and spread across Asia and then Africa, contributing to millions of deaths from malaria. . . . Measures for containment are now urgently needed to limit the spread of these parasites from western Cambodia and to prevent a major threat to current plans for eliminating malaria.
>
> (Dondorp *et al.*, 2009, pp. 466–467)

Resistant parasites have a survival advantage over non-resistant ones and hence will multiply and spread. Thus a different version of malaria is created – a version of malaria to which there is no known cure so far. A version that is not only created by vicious parasites, but is helped into being by a confluence of complex factors in Pailin and worldwide. The resistance against chloroquine has so far been explained by a failed state intervention, while the emergence of artemisinin resistance tends to be blamed on unruly citizens using artemisinin as monotherapy, or, worse, producing counterfeit malaria drugs that foster resistance (Dondorp *et al.*, 2004). However, this explanation is rather unconvincing since both phenomena appear in many regions of the world, particularly the African continent (Bate *et al.*, 2008). According to James Scott's study (2009), the highlands in Southeast Asia have for centuries been populated by people actively evading state structures in the lowlands. Scott states that '*escape agriculture*: forms of cultivation designed to thwart state-appropriation'" (ibid.) were an integral part of autonomy-seeking practices. Since *Artemisia annua* grows especially well in the highlands we can speculate that it has circulated in the region for centuries, and was part of Scott's 'escapist crops'. Did the introduction of mass-produced artemisinin constitute an ecological tipping point, and lead to the emergence of resistance? No comprehensive study exists so far, but a convincing explanation of the rise of resistance would need to integrate patterns of human, parasite and mosquito behaviour and include sociohistorical, environmental and political processes. Ultimately though, this new version of artemisinin-resistant malaria was created by tiny, mutated protozoan parasites, a eukaryote – just like the symptoms of the disease itself. The parasite genome invents and reinvents malaria. But it is not the parasite alone that creates and defines malaria, it does so in interaction with mosquitoes and humans. Human practices are also crucial to understanding the bioecologies of malaria. So, how might humans negotiate disease and (partial) immunities?

Negotiating partial immunity: living *with* malaria

While plasmodium parasites develop drug tolerance to artemisinin, *Anopheles* mosquitoes also become increasingly tolerant to insecticides, and a malaria vaccine that conveys immunisation is not yet in sight, what do people in Ghana (and other low-income areas with malaria transmission) do to protect themselves from falling ill and to prevent severe disease when infected with malaria? The first thing to say is perhaps that most people in endemic areas routinely live with malaria. Although nicknaming (as some do) the disease as 'the African cold' dangerously underplays the severity of the disease, it does draw attention to the fact that most people in endemic areas suffer from malaria regularly. But let me begin with a short fieldwork encounter from Ghana:

Walking along a busy shopping street in Accra I often bumped into Kwaku – an artist and street vendor, who tried to sell me his artwork. Kwaku and I frequently engaged in friendly small talk, and once this involved malaria. I asked him about his malaria treatment habits, and he told me that he usually buys artesunate when he feels feverish (artesunate is an artemisinin-based monotherapy to treat malaria). He would not go to the hospital, since he says he knows how malaria feels. For him, he says, it is a particular pain in the belly that comes together with fever. Kwaku's guts know how to diagnose malaria. Other people describe different symptoms to me that they specifically associate with malaria. But what everyone seems to agree on is that malaria can be identified easily; you know how it feels in your body after you have had it once. A body that is familiar with malaria does not need clinical or laboratory diagnosis, Kwaku would argue; one knows how to self-diagnose malaria. Thus, Kwaku – like most people who have grown up with malaria – is aware of his own malaria symptoms. To him there is no need to spend precious money (and time) in the hospital for a diagnosis, where – as he complains – the doctor or nurse would often not do a blood test for him and just prescribe malaria medication. And amodiaquine (the nationally recommended first-line drug), no – he does not like it, he says, it makes him too weak. So Kwaku ends up buying artesunate monotherapy in a pharmacy, which – in 2008, when this conversation occurred – was readily available in Accra and he is happy with the effectiveness of the treatment in his body.

Currently this is a good choice for Kwaku's body, but as was discussed in the previous section, this has changed already in Southeast Asia and artemisinin-tolerant parasites may eventually develop or arrive in Ghana. But not only do parasites develop resistance; Kwaku's body also displays a form of resistance. Through regular bodily encounters with the plasmodium parasite it is likely that Kwaku is partially immune to malaria. Being partially immune means that human bodies are less likely to develop severe forms of malaria (for instance, cerebral malaria), and so convey partial protection. Partial immunity develops in places where malaria is endemic. Malaria in Ghana is holoendemic, meaning transmission rates are so high that every person living in a determined area is affected by the disease, albeit with unequally distributed vulnerabilities. Research in Ghana showed that parasites are routinely present in approximately 58 per cent of the population (Owusu-Agyei *et al.*, 2009). The people taking part in this study did not show any symptoms of disease; they were randomly chosen and then tested for parasite prevalence. In other words, in areas with high malaria transmission people cohabit with parasites most of the year without necessarily developing malaria symptoms. This is due to an acquired specific immunity (Marsh, 2002), which humans develop through continued exposure to malaria parasites and lived-through malaria infections. Specific immunity is mainly present in adults living in areas with constant, high malaria transmission. Specific immunity is partial, meaning it does not prevent all malaria infections, but makes malaria episodes less frequent and conveys some protection for people to fall severely ill from the disease. In this regard, naturally acquired specific immunity is quite similar to the immunity the RTS,S/ASO2A vaccine provides (RTS,S Clinical Partnership, 2011, 2012, 2015). This, or so epidemiologists argue, could be a life-saving intervention for children under 5 years old whose immune system is still developing and who have not had the opportunity to develop specific immunity as yet. However, even for these groups infection with parasites does not necessarily lead to disease. As malariologist Kevin Marsh points out, 'even during the period of maximum susceptibility to severe disease, children spend the majority of their time parasitized but healthy' (Marsh, 2002, p. 256).

When I asked one of the principal investigators of the malaria vaccine trials in Ghana, a local medical doctor, why he thinks I as an immunologically naïve person still did not develop malaria after spending over eight months in the country and getting bitten by mosquitoes regularly, he responded with a shoulder shrug and this strikingly simple explanation: 'maybe your liver works well and flushes all parasites out.' And indeed, notwithstanding much research on the topic, the concrete factors that make an individual vulnerable to developing malaria in a body are still unclear and a recurrent topic of scientific studies (Marsh,

2002, 2010). We know that people who have never lived through a malaria infection are more vulnerable, but still, the rate, frequency and severity of disease varies greatly among individuals. We know that the immunity to malaria which a body can develop is only partial, that furthermore this immunity is particular to subspecies of the plasmodium parasite and thereby local. We know that humans lose this partial immunity after not being exposed for some time. Haemoglobin variations (most prominently sickle-cell anaemia) and other genetic polymorphisms have been explained in terms of an adaptation to malaria (mainly based on their biological mechanism, and the correlation of occurrence and malaria prevalence). The development of general anaemia and malaria is also assumed to be entangled, with anaemic people being more vulnerable to developing malaria; in turn malaria contributes to and can cause anaemia. Furthermore, the development of Burkitt's lymphoma is arguably due to an interaction between plasmodium falciparum and the Epstein-Barr virus (Marsh, 2002, pp. 252–267). So disease interactions and adaptations are manifold but what remains unclear is which factors *exactly* make a human body vulnerable to malaria, or offer protection against it.

This uncertainty is also expressed in people's reasonings and disease prevention practices that are based on their bodily and observed experiences with fever, as one of my co-researchers reflected on our interviews in Ghana:

> One man among the opinion leaders present for the workshop said 'everyone is bitten by mosquitoes day in day out but those, who are more likely to get malaria, are those who eat a lot of oily food and stay in the sun for longer hours'. Among the pregnant women, there was a wide range of causes for malaria which included mosquitoes, unkempt environment, staying in the sun for long hours, drinking dirty water (from stagnant source), eating a lot of oily food such as groundnut, eating excess sugar, houseflies and working around fire . . . I think it was quite interesting.
>
> (Martin Agyemang, interview, London, 2008)

Such reasoning could of course be dismissed as ignorance and lacking in formal education, as is regularly done in the biomedical literature and in health education approaches, but this does not do justice to what is going on. An unhealthy diet (eating too much sugar or fatty oils) or a weakened immune system (standing too long in the sun, being close to breeding places) may well be factors contributing to someone's vulnerability to malaria. These are triggers of malaria that people observe in their bodies, their lives, their practices. Malaria gets transmitted by mosquitoes, but is not only caused through the presence of parasites in the blood; people are routinely bitten by mosquitoes and cohabit with parasites without becoming ill (see above, Owusu-Agyei *et al.*, 2009). In high transmission areas, then, malaria regularly lingers in our bodies and whether the body falls ill or not is determined by a complex chain of factors.

How then do people navigate this uncertain terrain? How does one live *with* malaria? Kwaku, whose habits are similar to those of many people I chatted to, prefers to treat himself. He buys artesunate monotherapy in a pharmacy, which was readily available in Accra. While artesunate is popular with Kwaku and others because it treats malaria quickly and has few side-effects, monotherapy is problematic from a global perspective, as it may foster resistance more quickly. After all, artemisinin combination therapies were introduced in the hope of slowing down the development of resistance considerably (WHO, 2003). But despite a widely implemented policy change towards combination therapy (globally as well as in Ghanaian health policy), malaria monotherapy and artesunate continue to be widely available and are popular with patients. Artesunate provides fast relief from malaria's symptoms and so gets people back to work and their lives more quickly.

Another example of such self-diagnosis and treatment is Arthur, an employee at a Malaria Vaccine Trial project in Ghana, who tells me that his favourite anti-malarial is still chloroquine. Arthur is well aware of the treatment failures chloroquine has, but for him personally the drug still works fine, he says. He does not experience many side-effects, it is cheap and removes the parasites quickly from his body. Since the introduction of artemisinin combination therapy in 2005, Ghana has been phasing out chloroquine, but –as I learned from the National Malaria Control Programme and the WHO country adviser – this proved to be a slow process. Ghana still had two years of chloroquine supplies when the Head of the National Malaria Control Programme announced in April 2005 that chloroquine was to be phased out within a year (Health News, 2005). In summer 2008, when I ended my fieldwork in Ghana, it was still purchasable. Arthur observed that it became increasingly hard to get, but was still available.

These are two instances where patient logics clashed with public health concerns. What do the examples teach us? First, they make clear that public and indeed global health logics of resistance prevention cannot be equated with individual drug experiences and treatment choices. People too do not (although some might) make such decisions based on ignorance about malaria and treatment protocols, but as results of their situated everyday and bodily experiences. All this is hardly surprising, but still an important lesson with regard to how the development and spread of drug resistance is thought about in public health. The spread of malaria resistance is mainly explained by 'non-adherence' to treatment protocols; in other words, wrong drug intake. This is – in mainstream conceptions at least – to be answered with health education campaigns, including tools such as behaviour change communication. These are unlikely to succeed, however, if they assume lack in knowledge rather than informed individual decisions as the basis for treatment behaviour.

Second, people of course do much more to prevent against malaria than just take drugs that are recommended by the clinic, government or sold in pharmacies. Herbal medicine, spiritual ceremonies, a variety of protective measures and many more activities represent strategies against fever/malaria. The variety of fever/convulsion diseases overlaps with Western-scientific malaria in complex ways, but are certainly not coextensive.[2] Although herbal medicines or spiritual ceremonies would not treat 'malaria', they may still be aimed at the symptoms that a doctor in the clinic would call malaria, or what the malaria microscopist would visualise as plasmodium parasites. It does not matter much if these diseases could or could not be visualised as malaria under a microscope; it is important to recognise that people through their practices define the disease (Mol, 2002). And it is important to recognise that these practices are knowledgeable, as purposeful tinkering with bodies and their well-being; as Annemarie Mol explains, this tinkering may be seen as what characterises care: 'caring is a question of "doctoring": of tinkering with bodies, technology and knowledge – and with people too' (2008, p. 12).

What is common to all these logics of treatment is that people who regularly live with malaria have developed their own ways to negotiate living well and staying free of malaria parasites, or treating infections quickly and effectively. As I have shown in this section, crucial to this is the negotiation of a life–health balance if you like. In Kwaku's case, self-diagnosis artesunate monotherapy is what works, as it saves him both time in the health centre (and thus he gains time to earn money) and the side-effects of the nationally recommended first-line drug. Arthur too has developed his own treatment practice to relieve his body quickly and effectively from parasite loads. Malaria thus comes into being differently according to what patients feel and self-diagnose, where they go for support and how they (get) treat(ed) themselves. Patients' prevention and treatment practices engage in negotiating and extending their specific and partial immunity. This might be in harmony with national treatment protocols and global measures to prevent drug resistance or clash with them. In any case, the biomedical disease malaria and the development of immunity and resistance emerge in a relational web that is made up of patients, treatment protocols, clinic personnel, drug formulations, local and global mosquito and parasite behaviour (to name just the obvious).

Malaria, global health and immunity/community

What do we gain from juxtaposing these processes of creating and acquiring tolerance to diseases or drugs in humans and parasites? Why bundle them together under the term 'immunity' and so risk (over)simplifying complex bioecological and technoscientific dynamics? I suggest that bringing human attempts to prevent malaria (through vaccination or everyday treatment and prevention practices) in conversation with parasites' ability to evolve tolerance to drugs might provide us with some purchase on the underlying bioecological complexities and the fragility of technoscientific dreams of mastering disease. Writing both human and parasite practices as 'immunity', as the legitimate struggle of earthly organisms for survival, I hope makes evident that similar processes of species flourishing are at stake. They also make clear that parasites are – to stay with the eradicationists' war metaphors – a worthy sparring partner for humans. However, the short narratives about tricky vaccine development, elusive parasites and tinkering patients also make a dimension of Esposito's concept of immunity visible: the paradoxical relationship between community and immunity. Indeed, the entanglement of mosquitoes, humans and parasites that makes up malaria is characterised by a long, intertwined history, turning us into one multispecies community. Still, this is a 'non-excluding relation with the common opposite' – parasites and mosquitoes spell danger for us, they remain other (Esposito, 2011, p. 17). But although humans would very well flourish without parasites and mosquitoes, their 'stubborn' presence makes us not into simple adversaries, but first and foremost into a multispecies knot that has so far proven impossible to untangle effectively and sustainably. Reading resistance through immunity asks how we might conceive of a malaria control policy that does not aim to win a war, but that starts from the (grudging) acknowledgment of our continued shared presence on this earth. Based on this we can then start to think more about what these more subtle reconfigurations of human-parasite-mosquito entanglements might look like, be and do.

Notes

1   It is beyond the scope of this chapter to include a discussion of mosquitoes, mosquito control and their role in the multispecies entanglement that produces malaria. For related analyses on the dis/entanglements of mosquitoes and humans in malaria control see Kelly and Lezaun (2014) and Beisel (2015).
2   The epistemological relation between different malaria treatments is not the subject of this chapter, but, for instance, Stacey Langwick offers a beautiful, symmetrical exploration of encounters between malaria and the Southern Tanzanian fever disease 'degede' (Langwick, 2007).

References

Anderson, W. and Mackay, I.R. 2015. *Intolerant Bodies: A Short History of Autoimmunity*, Baltimore, MD: The Johns Hopkins University Press.
Alonso, P.L., J. Sacarlal. and J.J. Aponte. 2004. Efficacy of the RTS,S/AS02A vaccine against plasmodium falciparum infection and disease in young African children: randomised controlled trial. *The Lancet* 364(9443): 1411–1420.
Aponte, D., A. Schellenberg, A. Egan, A. Breckenridge, I. Carneiro, J. Critchley, I. Danquah, A. Dodoo, R. Kobbe, and B. Lell. 2009. Efficacy and safety of intermittent preventive treatment with Sulfadoxine-pyrimethamine for malaria in African infants: a pooled analysis of six randomised, placebo-controlled trials. *The Lancet* 374 (9700): 1533–1542.
Ashley, E.A. *et al.* 2014. Spread of artemisinin resistance in plasmodium falciparum malaria. *New England Journal of Medicine*, 371(5): 411–423.
Bate, R., P. Coticelli, R. Tren and A. Attaran. 2008. Antimalarial drug quality in the most severely malarious parts of Africa – a six country study. *PLoS ONE* 3(5): e2132.
Beisel, U. 2010. Jumping hurdles with mosquitoes? Collaborative book review: *When Species Meet*, by D.J. Haraway. *Environment and Planning D: Society and Space* 28(1): 46–49.
Beisel, U. 2015. Markets and mutations: mosquito nets and the politics of disentanglement in global health. *Geoforum* 66: 146–155.
Beisel, U. and C. Boëte, 2013. The flying public health tool: genetically modified mosquitoes and malaria control. *Science as Culture* 22(1): 38–60.

Bingham, N. 2008. Slowing things down: lessons from the GM controversy. *Geoforum* 39(1): 111–122.

Brown, P.J. 1997. Culture and the global resurgence of malaria. In Inhorn, M.C. and Brown, P.J. (eds) *The Anthropology of Infectious Disease: International Health Perspectives*, London and New York: Routledge, pp.119–141.

Campbell, C.C., W. Chin, W.E. Collins, S.M. Teutsch and D.M. Moss. 1979. Chloroquine resistance in plasmodium falciparum from East Africa. *The Lancet* 2: 1151–1154.

Campbell, T. and R. Esposito. 2006. Interview with Roberto Esposito. *diacritics* 36(2): 49–56.

Campbell, T. n.d. Bíos, immunity, life: The thought of Roberto Esposito. Available at http://www.biopolitica.org/ingles/docs/Campbell_Introduction_Bios.pdf.

Clark, N., 2011. *Inhuman Nature: Sociable Life on a Dynamic Planet*, London: Sage.

Daily, J.P. 2012. Malaria vaccine trials – beyond efficacy end points. *New England Journal of Medicine* 367(24): 2349–2351.

Derrida, J., 2003. Autoimmunity: real and symbolic suicides: a dialogue with Jacques Derrida. In *Philosophy in a Time of Terror: Dialogues with Jürgen Habermas and Jacques Derrida*, Chicago, IL: University of Chicago Press, pp.85–136.

Desowitz, R.S. 1991. *The Malaria Capers. Tales of Parasites and People*, New York: W.W. Norton.

Dondorp, A.M., P.N. Newton, M. Mayxay, W. Van Damme, F.M. Smithuis, S. Yeung, A. Petit, A.J. Lynam, A. Johnson, T.T. Hien, R. McGready, J.J. Farrar, S. Looareesuwan, N.P. Day, M.D. Green and N.J. White. 2004. Fake antimalarials in Southeast Asia are a major impediment to malaria control: multinational cross-sectional survey on the prevalence of fake antimalarials. *Tropical Medicine and International Health* 9(12): 1241–1246.

Dondorp, A.M., F. Nosten, P. Yi, D. Das, A.P. Phyo, J. Tarning and K.M. Lwin. 2009. Artemisinin resistance in plasmodium falciparum malaria. *New England Journal of Medicine* 361(5): 455.

Esposito, R. 2011. *Terms of the Political: Community, Immunity, Biopolitics*, New York: Fordham University Press.

Feachem, R.G., A.A. Phillips, J. Hwang, C. Cotter, B. Wielgosz, B.M. Greenwood, O. Sabot, M.H. Rodriguez, R.R. Abeyasinghe, T.A. Ghebreyesus and R.W. Snow. 2010. Shrinking the malaria map: progress and prospects. *The Lancet* 376(9752): 1566–1578.

Geissler, P.W. 2013. The Archipelago of public health. Comments on the landscape of medical research in 21st century Africa. In Prince, R.J. and Marsland, R. (eds) *Making and Unmaking Public Health in Africa: Ethnographic and Historical Perspectives*, Michigan, OH: Ohio University Press, pp.231–256.

Ginn, F., U. Beisel and M. Barua. 2014. Living with awkward creatures: vulnerability, togetherness, killing. *Environmental Humanities* 4: 113–123.

GSK MVI (2010) *Fact Sheet: RTS,S Malaria Vaccine Candidate*. Accessible at http://www.worldmalariaday.org/download/partners/Updated_RTSS_FactSheet_21_April_2010.pdf (accessed 12 October 2012).

Haraway, D.J. 1991. The biopolitics of postmodern bodies: constitutions of self in immune system discourse. In Haraway, D.J. *Simians, Cyborgs and Women: The Reinvention of Nature*, New York: Routledge, pp. 203–230.

Haraway, D.J., 2003. *The Companion Species Manifesto: Dogs, People, and Significant Otherness*, Chicago, IL: Prickly Paradigm Press.

Haraway, D.J. 2008. *When Species Meet*. Minneapolis: University of Minnesota Press

Haraway, D. 2010. When species meet: staying with the trouble. *Environment and Planning D: Society and Space* 28(1): 53–55.

Harrison, G. 1978. *Mosquitoes, Malaria and Man: A History of the Hostilities since 1880*, London: John Murray.

Health News. 2005. Chloroquine not first choice drug for malaria, 5 April. Available at www.ghanaweb.com (accessed 2 January 2009).

Hinchliffe, S. and K. Ward. 2014. Geographies of folded life: how immunity reframes biosecurity. *Geoforum* 53: 136–144.

Kelly, A.H. and J. Lezaun. 2014. Urban mosquitoes, situational publics, and the pursuit of interspecies separation in Dar es Salaam. *American Ethnologist* 41(2): 368–383.

Kelly, A.H., and U. Beisel. 2011. Neglected malarias: the frontlines and back alleys of global health. *BioSocieties* 6(1): 71–78.

Killeen, G.F. 2003. Following in Soper's footsteps: northeast Brazil 63 years after eradication of *Anopheles gambiae*. *Lancet Infectious Diseases* 3: 663–666.

Landecker, H. 2015. Antibiotic resistance and the biology of history. *Body and Society*: 1–34. Published online before print, 13 March, doi:10.1177/1357034X14561341.

Langwick, S. 2007. Devils, parasites and fierce needles. Healing and the politics of translation in Southern Tanzania. *Science, Technology and Human Values* 32(1): 88–117.

Latour, B. 2005. *Reassembling the Social: An Introduction to Actor-Network-Theory*. Oxford: Oxford University Press.

Mackinnon M.J. and A.F. Read. 2004. Immunity promotes virulence evolution in a malaria model. *PLoS Biology* 2(9): e230.

Marsh, K. 2002. Immunology of malaria. In Warrell, D.A. and Gilles, H.M. (eds) *Essential Malariology*, London: Arnold, pp. 252–267.

Martin, E. 1994. *Flexible Bodies: Tracking Immunity in American Culture From the Days of Polio to the Age of AIDS*, Boston, MA: Beacon Press.

Mitchell, T. 2002. Can the mosquito speak? In Mitchell, T. *Rule of Experts: Egypt, Technopolitics, Modernity*, Berkeley: University of California Press, pp.19–53.

Mol, A. 2002. *the Body Multiple: Ontology in Medical Practice*, Durham, NC: Duke University Press.

Mol, A. 2008. *The Logic of Care: Health and the Problem of Patient Choice*, London: Routledge.

Mutsaers, I. 2015. One-health approach as counter-measure against 'autoimmune' responses in biosecurity. *Social Science & Medicine* 129: 123e130.

MVI. 2008. *Fact Sheet: RTS,S/AS Malaria Vaccine Candidate*. Available at www.malariavaccine.org/files/12052008__RTSSfactsheet.pdf (accessed 30 November 2008).

Nading, A. 2014. *Mosquito Trails: Ecology, Health and the Politics of Entanglement*, Oakland: University of California Press.

Napier, D. 2012. Nonself help: how immunology might reframe the Enlightenment. *Cultural Anthropology* 27(1): 122–137.

Noedl, H., Y. Se, K. Schaecher, B.L. Smith, D. Socheat and M.M. Fukuda for the Artemisinin Resistance in Cambodia 1 (ARC1) Study Consortium. 2008. Letter to the Editor: Evidence of artemisinin-resistant malaria in Western Cambodia. *New England Journal of Medicine* 359(24): 2619–2620.

Ntoumi, F., D.P. Kwiatkowski and M. Diakité. 2007. New interventions for malaria: mining the human and parasite genomes. *American Journal for Tropical Medicine and Hygiene* 77(Suppl. 6): 270–275.

Owusu-Agyei, S., K.P. Asante, M. Adjuik, G. Adjei, E. Awini, M. Adams, S. Newton, D. Dosoo, D. Dery, A. Agyeman-Budu, J. Gyapong, B. Greenwood and D. Chandramohan. 2009. Epidemiology of malaria in the forest-savanna transitional zone of Ghana. *Malaria Journal* 8(220): 1–10.

Plowe, C.V. 2009. The evolution of drug-resistant malaria. *Transactions of the Royal Society of Tropical Medicine and Hygiene* 103S: S11–S14.

Rottenburg, R. 2009. Social and public experiments and new figurations of science and politics in postcolonial Africa. *Postcolonial Studies* 12(4): 423–440.

RTS,S Clinical Trials Partnership. 2011. First Results of Phase 3 Trial of RTS, S/AS01 Malaria Vaccine in African Children. *New England Journal of Medicine* 365(20): 1863.

RTS,S Clinical Trials Partnership. 2012. A Phase 3 trial of RTS,S/AS01 malaria vaccine in African infants. *New England Journal of Medicine* 367(24): 2284–2295.

RTS,S Clinical Trials Partnership. 2015. Efficacy and safety of RTS,S/AS01 malaria vaccine with or without a booster dose in infants and children in Africa: final results of a Phase 3, individually randomised, controlled trial. *The Lancet* 386(9988): 31–45.

Scott, J. 2009. *The Art of Not Being Governed: An Anarchist History of Upland Southeast Asia*, New Haven, CT: Yale University Press.

Sloterdijk, P. 2004. *Sphären III. Plurale Sphärologie. Schäume*, Frankfurt am Main: Suhrkamp Verlag.

Stengers, I. 2010. *Cosmopolitics I*, Minneapolis: University of Minnesota Press.

The Animal Studies Group. 2006. *Killing Animals*, Illinois: University of Illinois.

Whatmore, S. 2002. *Hybrid Geographies: Natures, Cultures, Spaces*, London: Routledge.

World Health Organisation. 2003. Access to antimalarial medicines: improving the affordability and financing of artemisinin-based combination therapies, WHO/CDS/MAL/2003.1095, Geneva: World Health Organisation.

World Health Organisation. 2011. *Global plan for Artemisinin Resistance Containment (GPARC)*, Geneva: World Health Organisation. Available at http://www.who.int/malaria/publications/atoz/9789241500838/en/.

World Health Organisation. 2014. *Status Report on Artemisinin Resistance*, January 2014, Geneva: World Health Organisation. Available at http://www.who.int/malaria/publications/atoz/status_rep_artemisinin_resistance_jan2014.pdf?ua=1.

World Health Organisation. 2015. *Containment of Artemisinin Resistance*. Available at http://www.who.int/malaria/areas/drug_resistance/containment/en.

World Health Organisation/SAGE. 2015. *Summary of the October 2015 Meeting of the Strategic Advisory Group of Experts on Immunization (SAGE)*, Geneva: World Health Organisation. Available at http://www.who.int/immunization/sage/meetings/2015/october/sage_report_oct_2015.pdf?ua=1.

Yates-Doerr, E. and A. Mol. 2012. Cuts of meat: disentangling Western natures–culture. *Cambridge Anthropology* 30(2): 48–64.

8   A genealogy of evidence at the WHO

Nele Jensen

Introduction

'The movement towards basing health policy development and advice on rigorous scientific evidence has begun.' This was the proclamation by the World Health Organization's (WHO) then Director-General Gro Harlem Brundtland in 2003. Indeed, with the WHO as an early and influential proponent, 'evidence-based policy' (EBP) has become something of a shibboleth, separating the good from the bad in global health decision-making and indispensable to improving health in what are still commonly referred to as 'developing' countries. Despite an abiding opacity as to what 'evidence' or EBP actually are, demand for both has grown in tandem with pressure to justify and monitor the success of international or internationally funded health programmes with the help of statistical, epidemiological and economic methods, or even their a priori configuration as randomised controlled trial (RCT) models of research interventions (Adams, 2013; Storeng and Béhague, 2014).

Critical global health studies often analyse these pushes for global health evidence as examples of a globalisation of western rationalities and practices. Ethnographic accounts have contrasted the universalising tendencies with the situated effects of globalised evidence-based biomedical research (Petryna, 2009; Geissler and Molyneux, 2011; Brives, 2013), and its ensuing 'evidence' once it is circulated as standardised knowledge across geographical and epistemic boundaries in the form of guidelines or drugs (Timmermans and Berg, 1997; Lakoff, 2005). Others have criticised evidence-based approaches in global health more broadly as the scientised or pseudo-scientific (audit) tools of ever-expanding technocratic forms of governance (Adams, 2013; Storeng and Béhague, 2014). Easily associable with the sprawl of neoliberalism, these emerging configurations are argued to systematically devalue and disqualify those healthcare practices that elude description through discrete measurable indicators.

Still, despite the existence of such varied critiques, little attention has been paid to the specific empirically grounded processes of how and why these demands for global health 'evidence' have emerged and proliferated. The research that forms the basis of this chapter started off as an attempt to address this important gap. Based on an analysis of WHO documents and the wider policy literature, my original aim was to trace the history of EBP at the WHO. As an intergovernmental organisation seeking a coordinating and norm-setting role in international health, the WHO appeared to have been an early advocate of evidence-based public health in the late 1990s. Using the WHO as a case study thus promised to offer some broader insights into the circumstances of the emergence of EBP for global health.

However, two sets of questions arose fairly quickly that have given me quite a headache. First: What does it actually mean to write a history of EBP at the WHO? Should this be a history of a term or a concept? Of a particular epistemology, method or technology? Of the WHO as an institution? Or even a history of 'fields' such as Public Health or Epidemiology or Global Health? Second, but relatedly: Where might one even start? Which documents should be explored, which ones included and which ones left out? In other words, I have been grappling with questions familiar to historians of who sets the boundaries or makes the cut, how, and what are the consequences.

To tackle these questions and reflect further on the issues they raise, this chapter tells two stories of the emergence of evidence-based policy at the WHO; or perhaps two different versions of the same story. My starting point is a particular document, the WHO *Report on Health Systems Performance Assessment* (henceforth the *Report*) introduced by the Brundtland epigraph at the beginning of this chapter. The *Report* presents EBP as the 'natural' result of efforts to make healthcare more scientific. In the first section of this chapter, I briefly follow this history and depict some of its key components. In the subsequent part I aim to re-trace it by paying particular attention to what has been included and excluded from the *Report*'s historical account, and what might be added to it. This results in a different story that challenges the narrative of a deterministic emergence of EBP at the WHO, by situating it as a very specific practice articulated through complex entanglements of particular people, ideas, contexts and technologies – including documents and the (hi-)stories they tell. It also emphasises the performative character of the ways in which knowledge is produced and ordered. In the final part, the chapter will discuss how making visible some of what might be called *evidentiary practices* and the material-discursive spaces in which they are embedded may help to open up new ways of challenging how these spaces are constructed and maintained.

Following narratives of scientific progress

Gro Harlem Brundtland's proclamation of the dawn of a new evidence-based policy era introduces the 2003 *Report on Health Systems Performance Assessment*, edited by Christopher Murray and David Evans and prepared largely by their team from the WHO's Evidence and Information for Policy (EIP) unit. The *Report* itself – with its 962 pages, 61 chapters, 245 figures, 185 tables, and myriad tools, concepts and frameworks – reads rather like a manifesto for these new realities. The *Report*'s aims are two-fold. First, more narrowly, it intends to review and build on the EIP's attempts to develop the 'science' of measuring the performance of health systems (Murray and Evans, 2003, 4, 16). Key to these efforts had been another document, the *World Health Report 2000* (WHR, 2000), and the Murray and Evans *Report* promises to 'openly report' on associated criticism, and to further improve the 'global evidence base on what works and what does not for health systems' (ibid., 16, xxvii).

Second, both *WHR 2000* and the *Report* itself are also held up as catalysts of a much wider development: the progress towards basing health policy on scientific evidence as opposed to ignorance, ideology and opinion (ibid., 4). The *Report* recounts that it was Brundtland who introduced EBP at the WHO upon becoming Director-General in 1998. But it also suggests that the concept of evidence for policy simply represents the logical extension of evidence-based medicine (EBM) to the policy arena and that 'it is *natural* that the focus on evidence has spread from the world of clinical decision-making to public health decision-making' (ibid., 715, emphasis added).

If we were to follow the *Report*'s narrative we could begin in 1991, when the term 'evidence-based medicine' was coined by clinical epidemiologist Gordon Guyatt from Canada's McMaster University (Guyatt, 1991). The following year, Guyatt and his colleagues from the newly established EBM Working Group published an article in the *Journal of the American Medical Association*, arguing that expert judgement and mechanistic reasoning, the traditional pillars of clinical decision-making, were too often biased – and should therefore be largely replaced by objective, transparent and generalisable evidence preferably derived from RCTs (EBM Working Group, 1992). By the end of the 1990s, EBM appeared to dominate much of US/European clinical medicine, a success story that its proponents have attributed to both EBM's common sense (EBM Working Group, 1992) and its epistemologically sound (Howick, 2011) objective to make clinical medicine more scientific. This narrative of a deterministic progress of medical science appears to be the story that Murray and Evans try to tie in with their notion of EBP. Indeed, by the time Brundtland became the head of the WHO there were increasing calls to apply 'evidence-based' principles to decision-making beyond clinical practice (e.g. Ham *et al.*, 1995; Brownson *et al.*, 2009).

Brundtland was approved as WHO Director-General at the 51st World Health Assembly (WHA) in May 1998. Under her new leadership, the WHO embarked upon a process of wide-ranging reforms (Lee, 2009). One of Brundtland's first actions – seemingly in line with the *Report*'s narrative – was the launch of the Evidence and Information for Policy (EIP) unit, the first WHO unit specifically tasked with providing evidence of the best ways to promote health (EIP, 2000). The EIP unit was headed by Julio Frenk and Chris Murray, and comprised five departments in charge of the production and dissemination of evidence for policy. Responsible for evidence production was the Global Programme on Evidence for Health Policy, led by David Evans, and its sub-team Epidemiology and Burden of Disease, headed by Alan Lopez. In addition, the Economic Advisory Service provided macroeconomic evidence of the benefits of investing in health, under the command of Dean Jamison. As part of its evidence dissemination efforts, the EIP was furthermore responsible for the annual publication of the *World Health*

Reports and the WHO flagship journal *Bulletin of the World Health Organization.* The latter was re-launched under Brundtland with Richard Feachem as new editor-in-chief to explicitly promote the link between research evidence and policy-making (Brundtland, 1999; EIP, 2000).

Through its various teams, the EIP became involved in a range of activities and was highly influential in the WHO's direction under Brundtland. One of its first outputs was the 1999 *World Health Report* (*WHR1999*), which enunciated what it presented as Brundtland's vision for a new WHO that combined the organisation's values with 'evidence' to provide global health leadership in the form of norms and standards to improve the health status of poor populations (WHO, 1999, xvi–xvii). At the heart of this vision, the *WHR1999* propositioned four new concepts: (1) the principle of new universalism, based on the idea that 'if services are to be provided for all then not all services can be provided' (ibid., 33); (2) cost-effectiveness analysis (CEA) as the favoured tool to determine which health services should be provided; (3) disability-adjusted life years (DALYs) as a measure to quantify and compare the 'burden' of different diseases; and (4) the analytical basis for a new health systems framework that defined the universal functions and goals of health systems (later published in Murray and Frenk, 2000). A year later, these four components provided the matrix for the EIP's most significant publication, the *WHR2000.* But they also enunciated the notion of EBP promoted by the EIP and WHO under Brundtland more broadly: the burdens of diseases and cost-effectiveness were promoted as key evidence, while the new universalism and health systems framework provided their justification and framing.

This brief tracing of Murray and Evans' account offers a fairly straightforward – if perhaps a little prosaic – history of EBP at the WHO, a (hi)story of scientific progress born from the visions of a few enlightened reformers. In the following I will present an alternative story that aims to describe the emergence of EBP as a much more distributed process. On the one hand, this story will highlight that most of the individuals recruited by Brundtland in 1998 for the EIP unit were medical doctors, epidemiologists and economists associated with a few key institutions, notably Harvard and the World Bank, and that the notion of evidence for global health that they promoted was framed in a very specific and narrow way, linked to key concepts, techniques and tools that they had developed almost ten years earlier. On the other hand, my story also aims to argue that the (in some ways ephemeral, as will be shown later) success of their notion of evidence for policy is less to do with its embodiment of neutral science than with its co-evolution with a particular material-discursive space linked to the emergence of a 'global' health itself.

The beginning of a different story: from counting deaths to calculating health

In 1984, a recent Harvard graduate knocked on the door of WHO epidemiologist Alan Lopez's door and said: 'My name is Chris Murray, and everything you've written about mortality in Africa is wrong' (quoted in Smith, 2013, 74). Murray and Lopez agreed that the WHO's standard way to measure the health of the world's populations was both inconsistent and inadequate – and envisioned an independent team that could objectively provide better data. This encounter in Geneva could thus mark the beginning of a quite different story from the one traced above. Still, this is not meant to be just another hero story (cf. Smith, 2015). While Murray and Lopez arguably play important roles in the history of EBP at the WHO, one needs to place their encounter in the context of an even earlier set of events.

The desire to assess and compare the health of populations over time and across countries has been central to the WHO's mission from its inception. When the WHO constitution was approved in 1946, it included provisions requiring member states to regularly report on 'the progress achieved in improving the health of its people' and to provide respective epidemiological and statistical reports (WHO, 1946, Articles 61 and 64). Plans for the WHO Director-General to publish an annual summary of reports from member states were initially abandoned, but they gave the impetus for the eventual publication of eight *World Health Situation* assessments between 1959 and 1993. While the WHO constitution promoted a definition of health not only as the absence of disease but as a 'state of complete physical, mental, and social wellbeing' (WHO, 1946), these *Situation Reports* largely based their estimations of population health on mortality and morbidity statistics. In early reports these statistics were featured in a 'general survey' section that summarised the world's health status with regard to particular (and predominantly notifiable communicable) 'diseases of major concern', such as malaria and tuberculosis (WHO, 1963, 8–29). There were also attempts to produce rankings of causes of mortality and morbidity to identify potential priorities for national health policies, although these were hampered by a lack of data for most countries (e.g. WHO, 1974).

While efforts to standardise, collect and compare international mortality and morbidity statistics burgeoned, North American researchers in particular also became increasingly interested in developing tools to measure health as such. From the 1960s onward, various summary population health measures were proposed that combined mortality with morbidity or disability data (Mathers, 2007) – in other words, single indicators to count up fatal and non-fatal disease impacts. On the one hand, proponents of these measures argued that these were needed to measure newly emerging problems, especially a rise in chronic diseases and disabilities due to demographic changes, and an 'epidemiological transition' from communicable to non-communicable diseases in developing countries (Gold *et al.*, 2002; Mathers, 2007). As these transitions were also mobilised as characteristic of countries' modernisation from developing to developed nations in developmental stage thinking, attempts to capture population health patterns boomed (Omran, 1971; Jamison *et al.*, 1993; Wahlberg and Rose, 2015). On the other hand, being able to quantify health was increasingly deemed crucial to guide the allocation of health resources. This led to the development of 'quality-adjusted life years' (QALYs) in the late 1960s/early 1970s by teams of US/Canadian doctors, economists and epidemiologists. As a composite measure of health, QALYs could be used as denominators in cost-effectiveness analyses (CEA) to calculate the 'value for money' of competing medical services and procedures (Gold *et al.*, 2002).

At the WHO, too, international expert committees on statistics in the 1960s and 1970s urged the improvement of statistical and epidemiological data to both evaluate and guide healthcare interventions, ideally with the help of a single universally applicable population health measure and cost-effectiveness calculations (WHO, 1971; White, 2007). However, the WHO of the 1970s seemed to try to avoid an emphasis on narrow biomedical interventions, economic considerations and quantifiable targets in favour of a broader approach that linked health and development. Following the 1978 United Nations' Alma-Ata Conference, the WHO adopted its *Global Strategy for Health for All by the Year 2000 (HFA2000)*, which promoted universal access to primary healthcare (PHC) and aimed to put health at the centre of international development strategies and a wider struggle for political, social and economic justice (WHO, 1981b). As one consequence, the 'general survey' section of its *Situation Reports* was renamed 'global analysis' and indeed became increasingly global in purview, focusing on 'global trends' in health development and research (WHO, 1980, 207ff.) and much more than before evoking a collective responsibility of wealthier nations and international institutions to improve health in developing countries (WHO, 1980, 50). In addition, *Situation Reports* shifted their focus from mainly reporting on specific diseases and their control through targeted medical interventions to an analysis of wider socio-economic, environmental and health policy issues that impacted upon health (WHO, 1980). The reports continued to summarise the world's health status based on mortality and morbidity statistics, although cautioning that a lack of reliable data especially from developing countries hampered the ability to discern global health trends; but also that these statistics failed to measure health as defined in the WHO constitution (WHO, 1980, 37, 227).

Despite some initial enthusiasm for *HFA2000,* its perceived lack of tangible goals quickly attracted heavy criticism (Cueto, 2004). As an alternative, major US-based organisations like the Rockefeller and Ford Foundations, USAID, the World Bank and later UNICEF championed selective primary healthcare (SPHC), an approach that more narrowly defined health as the absence of disease, and promoted cost-effective biomedical interventions, target populations identified by mortality and morbidity statistics, and the role of experts to design, implement and assess interventions (Rifkin and Walt, 1986; Cueto, 2004; Birn, 2014). Although the WHO held on to *Health for All* as its guiding strategy, it has been suggested that the adoption of a number of global quantifiable indicators – including the health status indicators based on mortality and morbidity data – to measure the strategy's impact in the early 1980s was in direct response to this criticism (WHO, 1981a; Cueto, 2004).

This is the context that forms the backdrop to the meeting of Murray and Lopez in 1984. The two men shared the conviction that there were two problems with how the WHO measured health. On the one hand, the availability and utilisation of mortality data at the WHO was still fragmented. Accurate estimates for the number of global deaths were hampered by a lack of reliable data for many countries, but also by a lack of standardisation caused by 'different methods, different degrees of rigor and databases of different quality' (Lopez quoted in Smith, 2013, 4). Furthermore, most data were still collected and reported by individual WHO programmes on specific diseases, appearing to lead to double-counting of deaths as programmes focused on their own numbers – often for advocacy purposes – at the expense of an objective 'big picture' of the world's population health (ibid., 4). On the other hand, Murray and Lopez agreed that mortality and morbidity statistics alone could not express the importance of health problems. To properly 'map the landscape' (ibid., 74), the importance of diseases had to be assessed based on a summary measure of the combined fatal and non-fatal impact of different diseases upon people's health, including the impact of chronic diseases, injuries and disabilities (ibid.).

From calculating health to setting policy priorities

After their initial meeting, Murray and Lopez kept in touch. Lopez continued working in various roles at the WHO, while Murray completed a doctorate in International Health Economics at Oxford. Here, Murray started employing existing summary population health measures to produce cost-effectiveness analyses for specific public health interventions (Evans and Murray, 1987). But he also published an article that criticised the WHO, World Bank and other agencies for their publication of fragmentary mortality data that did not allow for the appropriate comparative quantitative analyses of health improvements in developing countries (Murray, 1987).

Murray returned to Harvard as a medical student and member of the School of Public Health, and in the late 1980s he and Lopez reunited as external contributors on the World Bank's *Health Sector Priorities Review* (HSPR) project. The HSPR was tasked with assessing the influence of individual diseases on population health in developing countries and with identifying the most suitable interventions to address them. Other team members included Harvard economist Jamison, as well as trained doctor and public health specialist Frenk, on a sabbatical from a stint as Visiting Professor at Harvard, and Feachem, the former dean of the London School of Hygiene and Tropical Medicine (LSHTM); and WHO economist Andrew Creese. Like Murray and Lopez, these men had all been involved in trying to measure health problems and identify the priorities for and cost-effectiveness of health interventions in developing countries for years (see Jamison, 1992).

It was as part of the HSPR project and its priority-setting aim that Murray and Lopez started to use the summary population measure disability-adjusted life years (DALYs). DALYs resembled QALYs in that they represented a standardised single measure combining mortality and morbidity data. However, unlike QALYs, DALYs did not aim to capture the comparative positive impact upon health of a medical intervention but the comparative negative impact of different diseases in relation to a state of ideal health. The design of DALYs was thus not particularly original. Moreover, a precursor of DALYs had been used to assess the national 'burden of disease' by a team of international researchers in Ghana at the beginning of the 1980s (Ghana Health Assessment Project Team, 1981). What was novel, however, was that the HSPR team used DALYs as a standardised 'burden of disease' denominator for cost-effectiveness analyses of both clinical and public health interventions, and to promote this as the 'rational' way of setting healthcare priorities for developing countries explicitly aligned with the premises of selective primary healthcare (Murray, 1990; Jamison *et al.*, 1993). In other words, DALYs were promoted as a universally applicable measure to express the best value for money of health interventions, which in turn should be the norm to guide health policy on both international (donor) and national (developing country governments) level.

In an even more important development, at the beginning of the 1990s key members of the HSPR – including Jamison, Feachem, Frenk, Creese, Lopez and Murray – became involved in the preparation of the 1993 *World Development Report* (*WDR1993*), the first of the World Bank's flagship publications dedicated entirely to health. The *WDR1993* provided an overview of the world's health status and recommended minimum packages of cost-effective public health and clinical interventions for low-income countries and donors to focus on. Its main message and tools drew heavily upon the HSPR's efforts: priority should be given to those health problems causing high disease burdens and for which cost-effective interventions were available (WDR, 1993, 63). But the report also featured DALYs not only as denominators in CEAs, but also as a summary measure to express the 'global burden of disease' (GBD). DALYs thus underwent a further transformation to become a new composite indicator for population health that permitted the comparison of combined fatal and non-fatal health impacts across a number of health-impairing conditions and populations. By quantifying the geographic distribution of disease burdens, DALYs were hailed as a new technology to produce a global map of ill-health. But as such, they also made visible a new 'global' health space and turned it into a target for interventions.

From priority-setting to evidence

Much of the statistical raw data was provided by various WHO programmes, while a Harvard team led by Murray and Lopez produced the actual 'disease burdens' calculations, which also involved selecting diseases, reconciling vast numbers of mortality and morbidity statistics, modelling estimates in the many cases of missing statistics, and coming up with comparable weighting scores for the 'burden' for different health impairments and different age groups. The huge efforts involved eventually turned the undertaking into a stand-alone project, the Global Burden of Disease (GBD) study. In the mid-1990s, the GBD team published what it referred to as the final and detailed results of their study and its complex methods in three separate volumes (Murray and Lopez, 1996a, 1996b,

1998). Furthermore, summaries of these final results were published in *The Lancet*, which hailed it as a catalyst for new ways to set priorities in international health (The Lancet, 1997).

By then, a number of 'national burden of disease' exercises had been produced for several countries – often involving ex-GBD staff, including the first study for Mexico overseen by Frenk (Lozano *et al.*, 1995) – and the World Bank, WHO and other key aid organisations had started to promote GBD and CEA as tools to guide health sector reform in developing countries (e.g. IDRC, 1993). Yet, proponents of priority-setting based on DALY and CEA complained that, particularly on an international level, donors and organisations still failed to 'rationally' target resources at those 'global health problems' causing the largest disease burdens (WHO, 1996, 29–30).

It was on the back of these developments that at the end of 1996 Murray and Lopez published a *Science* article on the 'Lessons from the Global Burden of Disease Study', calling it an independent, objective and evidence-based approach to health policy-making. As their previous publications had only used the term 'evidence' in a fairly unspecific manner to refer to indications or epidemiological observations, the article signalled two important shifts: on the one hand, it promoted the rhetorical transformation of GBD and CEA from priority-setting tools to 'evidence-based' policy approaches, arguably masking even further that these tools corresponded to a specific concern of wanting to compare and rank causes of ill-health in order to allow economic prioritisation. But the article also helped connote the term 'evidence' with a very specific meaning, namely epidemiological and economic measurements.

During this time another major event occurred that was to prove highly significant: Bill Gates had reportedly read the *WHR1993* more than twice, and its alleged ability to identify top health problems and quantify the 'return of health investments' convinced him to give his first large grant to the Children's Vaccine Program in 1998, marking the beginning of both his forceful engagement with 'global health' issues and his championing of evidence-based approaches to address these issues (Specter, 2005; Smith, 2013).

The WHO: change or die

Both the World Bank's increasingly powerful engagement and Gates' ascent as a lavish and highly influential donor (McCoy *et al.*, 2009; Birn, 2014) played important roles in changing the landscape of international health development in the 1990s. In addition to the World Bank, a number of new 'Global Public–Private Partnerships' had emerged, many focused on biomedical interventions against particular diseases and gaining the support of major funders, including Bill Gates. By contrast, the WHO had become increasingly sidelined – partly due to its unpopular commitment to *Health for All* (Lee, 2009) – and the growing imbalance between the WHO's regular budget compared to voluntary contributions escalated concerns about the independence of WHO decision-making and policies (Godlee, 1994; Brown *et al.*, 2006). These developments were interrelated with what was widely presented as a time of deep crisis at the WHO, brought about by a lack of direction both with regard to its internal organisation and to its role in a new 'global' health arena and a world argued to be rapidly transforming through globalisation (Lee, 2009, 83). As a result, external pressure on the WHO to reform grew and the WHO was claimed to face a situation where it had to either 'change or die' (Smith, 1995).

Discussions on WHO reforms took place externally through an influential series of conferences initiated by Harvard and supported by the Rockefeller Foundation (and attended by key ex-GBD study members). Discussions also took place internally, through mechanisms such as the WHO Working Group on the WHO Response to Global Change. These debates seemingly produced a broad consensus that the WHO had to recoup global health leadership by strengthening its 'global' functions and by setting norms and priorities (WHO, 1993; Al-Mazrou, 1997; Jamison *et al.*, 1998). These debates arguably influenced a number of important developments at the WHO, including the publication of the first *World Health Report* in 1995 as a renewed effort to provide annual global health assessments (WHO, 1995), and a new framework for WHO priority-setting that listed disease burden and cost-effectiveness analyses among the analytical tools to determine priority health problems and interventions (WHO, 1997; see also Lee, 2009, 29; Clift, 2013). Furthermore, *Health For All* was re-launched at the 51st WHA in 1998 as an update to the WHO's commitment to universal access to health, but with a new emphasis on strengthening health systems and health services 'based on scientific evidence' (WHA, 1998, 2). The same assembly confirmed Gro Harlem Brundtland as the WHO's new Director-General. A medical doctor with a degree in Public Health from Harvard and Norway's former prime minister, Brundtland's acceptance speech emphasised the need for more evidence for policy in the form of burden of disease and cost-effectiveness analyses (Brundtland, 1998). One month later, Murray and Frenk were recruited to be in charge of the EIP unit.

Assembling the components

As highlighted at the beginning of this chapter, the key document produced by the EIP unit was the *World Health Report (WHR)* 2000, aimed at providing policy-makers with 'evidence' on how health systems worldwide performed, and how this could be improved (WHO, 2000). As a first component, the *WHR2000* presented a ranking of all 191 WHO member states according to the performance of their health systems, determined based on their combined performance against the set of universal goals from Murray and Frenk's health systems framework. As the key goal, health was measured as disability-adjusted life expectancy (DALE), later renamed health-adjusted life expectancy (HALE). Unlike DALYs that calculated the contribution of any specific disease to a population's health, the newly developed HALEs were designed to quantify the overall morbidity and mortality of populations with the goal of allowing comparisons between, and ranking of, countries (WHO, 2000, 28; Gold *et al.*, 2002). Second, the report proposed that governments could improve population health (and thus their performance ranking) by giving priority to the most cost-effective interventions, with effectiveness measured in DALYs (WHO, 2000, 52–53). As has already been pointed out, Murray and his colleagues hailed the *WHR2000* as a vital step towards evidence-based policy at the WHO (Murray and Frenk, 2000; Murray and Evans, 2003, 3–4). Indeed, the report concretised their very particular notion of 'evidence for policy', namely epidemiological disease burden maps and cost-effectiveness analyses based on population health measures developed by Murray and Lopez ten years earlier.

Coming full circle: stabilising assemblages, making evidence

Taking Murray and Evans' (2003) narrative of the emergence of EBM as its starting point, much of this chapter has aimed to offer an alternative to their tele-ological account of a 'natural' progression from EBM to EBP as the next logical step in the linear progress of the application of a scientific method to healthcare. Instead, I have tried to show that their EBP was apprehended by the WHO as a very specific practice, articulated through and dependent on a spatial–temporally situated assemblage of very particular people, expertise, ideas, concepts, circumstances and technologies, some of which I have sought to (re-)trace in this chapter. I now want to briefly return to Murray and Evans' *Report* to argue that this document itself is one of these technologies.

Far from being passive organisational artefacts, documents have been shown to have ordering functions: from providing the narratives in which discoveries are embedded (Bowker and Star, 1999), to catalysing the production of facts (Latour, 1987), and even the enactment of those realities they reflect upon (Riles, 2006). To analyse the Murray and Evans report under these aspects, it is useful to recall that the report situates itself at a particular time point: at once looking back – reviewing and summarising EBP at the WHO, with a particular focus on the example of evidence for health systems performance assessments – but also forward-looking, heralding the emergence of a wider EBP movement.

What was omitted from both Murray and Evans' history and, so far, in my retelling of it, is the persistent, widespread resistance to GBD and CEA analyses which later turned into substantial unease about their promotion as evidence for policy. Already, the *WDR1993* became subject to heavy criticism, with some critics simply denouncing the report as an ideology-driven attempt by the World Bank to transform international health policy (Lee, 2009, 112). Others, however, specifically targeted their wide-ranging and sustained critiques at the CEA and GBD analyses, especially challenging the large extent of estimations, value judgements and normative prescriptions involved in their 'rational and objective' methodologies (for good summaries see Anand and Hanson, 1997; Paalman *et al.*, 1998; Gold *et al.*, 2002). Similar concerns also appear to have fuelled lingering tensions between the WHO and the World Bank during their collaboration for the *WDR1993*. Archival records suggest that, originally, 'burden of illness' estima-tions by Murray and Lopez were only intended as a background paper or small subsection of the *WDR1993* (Jamison, 1992; Subramanian, 1992a). And at least some WHO staff cautioned that the *WDR1993* should reflect the WHO's commitment to *Health for All*, equity and 'people's perception of priority problems' as opposed to the 'World Bank's view on disease-oriented epidemiological intervention' and cost-effectiveness (Subramanian, 1992b).

Despite these concerns, a global burden of disease analysis not only became a cornerstone of the final *WDR1993,* but GBD and CEA analyses were also widely promoted as the basis for policy-making and priority-setting. Still, both the *WDR1993* and GBD study continued to cause tensions between the World Bank and the WHO (The Lancet, 1997; Lee, 2009, 112ff.). As one result, Brundtland's decision to recruit Murray and many of his *WDR1993* co-authors to establish the EIP unit in 1998 was highly contentious (Lee, 2009, 105; Yamey, 2002). And when the EIP unit published the *WHR2000* it became one of the most controversial *World Health Reports* ever. Adding to concerns levelled at burden of disease and CEA analyses, critics took issue with several other methodological and conceptual aspects of the report. Among other things, they questioned how a standardised single composite performance indicator could adequately deal with the complexity and variation within and between health systems and populations, as well as the report's seemingly implicit assumption that health only depended on (the financing of) targeted health care interventions (Almeida *et al.*, 2001; Navarro, 2000). Furthermore, the legitimacy of the *WHR2000*'s findings was doubted-especially when it emerged that much of the evidence had been computed by Murray and his colleagues with little input from concerned member states or the wider WHO community (Musgrove, 2003)-and so too was the report's assertion that it was the product of objective and neutral science. As Walt and Mills noted: 'Most health policy analysts would support the search for better measures to provide evidence to inform health policy, but few would see this search as an exercise that can be stripped of values and ideology' (Walt and Mills, 2001).

Persistent criticism forced Brundtland, Murray and colleagues to issue several public defences of the *WHR2000* (Murray and Frenk, 2001; Murray *et al.* 2001; Brundtland *et al.*, 2003). But it also prompted the WHO Executive Board to officially request Brundtland to subject the report's methodology to consultations with WHO member countries as well as an external review (WHO, 2001). The Murray and Evans *Report*, however, largely ignores many of the above-mentioned contestations, despite its claim to openly report debates and criticism. Instead, it purports to include appraisals of the *WHR2000* in the form of 'Regional Perspectives', 'Expert Consultations' and a 'Report of the Scientific Review Committee Group'. While requested by the WHO Executive Board to address widespread criticism, these reviews are presented in the *Report* as transparent provisions to 'ensure that the methods continued to develop' (Murray and Evans, 2003, 6). In other words, formal requirements are transformed into exemplary good practice. By incorporating controversies and ruptures in this way, the *Report* manages to control the terms of debates and shape them, casting resistance to its methods as 'strategic rather than scientific' (ibid., 7). In turn, concerns about evidence and EBP are transformed into problems solvable by technical solutions:

doubts become statistical uncertainties that can be measured by numerical intervals, which in turn become part of the 'audit trail' to safeguard data transparency and accountability (ibid., 716–720). As a result, the claims made in the Murray and Evans *Report* are only strengthened by appearing to incorporate and address criticism. Furthermore, the narrative of a *natural* emergence of EBP is reinforced, as doubts become challenges that are gradually solvable by technical/scientific progress. However, these strategies make other things invisible: the concepts of evidence and EBP themselves are increasingly turned into matters of fact that are beyond discussion.

But the Murray and Evans *Report* does even more than this. In its attempt to herald a wider evidence movement, the *Report* introduces 'a common language and approach' for EBP in the future (Murray and Evans, 2003, 718), including a new taxonomy of evidence (ibid., 720), and five general principles for evidence production and dissemination: validity; reliability; comparability; consultation; and explicit audit trail (ibid., 15). Notably, with its consolidation of myriad authors, references, numbers and uncertainty intervals, figures, tables, taxonomies, standardised tools, consultations and audit trails, the Murray and Evans *Report* clearly seems to perform its own principles for the production and appraisal of 'evidence'. As a consequence, the *Report* not only transforms into a piece of evidence itself – into evidence of evidence – but it also tries to determine the 'right' way to do EBP in the future. For example, by adding consultations and an audit trail to its five principles for the production of evidence, Murray and Evans produce new classifications of *who* is allowed to have a voice in EBP debates – countries/regions, policy experts, scientists, peer reviewers. But it also ascribes to them new and distinctive levels of authority: summaries of regional country meetings are included in the report as 'Regional Perspectives' and contrasted with 'Expert Consultations' among WHO staff and selected 'major world experts' (ibid., 109); covering around two-thirds of the whole *Report,* the chapter 'Methods and Empiricism' is written by EIP staff and affiliated (mostly ex-*GBD* study) authors; and the *Report* pinnacles in the 'Scientific Peer Review'. The stacking of these new authority categories strikingly resembles EBM's 'evidence hierarchies' which value meta-reviews over empirical evidence over expert opinion over anecdotal evidence (e.g. Oxford Centre for Evidence-based Medicine, 2009). This has two effects: by surviving increasingly 'scientific' scrutiny, the *Report*'s claims – its various concepts, categories, value judgements, quantitative methodologies and evidence – increasingly appear like scientific matters of fact. Second, the *Report* tries to transfix new norms and regulations of how evidence for policy should be produced and appraised.

In summary, the Murray and Evans *Report* closes the black box on EBP's history (and associated controversies) and thus corroborates and further legitimises a narrative of EBP as linear, scientific progress from which EBP emerges as a matter of fact. As a document, the report actively holds together and stabilises the assemblage of different actors, technologies, concepts and trajectories that underlie their particular notion of EBP at the WHO. But by laying out and consolidating the histories, authorities, technologies and procedures that should be involved, it also draws boundaries around what evidence-based policy should be. As such, it tries to enact a future of global health policy that is 'naturally' governed by epidemiological and economic tools as evidence and appraisal based on the new categories of their evidence-based taxonomy.

The end of one story and the beginning of another: de- and reassembling EBP

As it was, the Murray and Evans *Report* became one of the last outputs of the EIP unit. By the time it was published, Jamison, Feachem and Frenk had already left the WHO to take up other positions. Murray and Lopez left following Brundtland's WHO exit in July 2003. In many ways, this marked the end of Murray and colleagues' notion of EBP at the WHO. But while the EBP future as envisioned in the Murray and Evans *Report* may never have materialised at the WHO, it did elsewhere with perhaps even more far-reaching effects.

Shortly after their departure, Murray and Lopez published an article calling for an independent agency to produce population health measures, arguing that as a political organisation the WHO was unable to produce objective evidence (Murray *et al.*, 2004). In 2007, with a US$105 million donation from Bill Gates and help from Frenk, Murray established the Institute for Health Metrics and Evaluation (IHME) in Seattle. Many of Murray's ex-HSPR and ex-EIP colleagues became associated with the IHME, including Brundtland, Lopez, Feachem and Jamison. The IHME strives to provide policy-makers with a comprehensive global health 'roadmap' in the form of evidence of the world's most important health problems and the best strategies to tackle them (IHME, 2015). At the centre of the IHME's work is an ever-expanding portfolio of global burden of disease and cost-effectiveness analyses, the former regularly showcased in *The Lancet* as 'the strongest evidence-based assessment of people's health problems around the world' (Murray *et al.*, 2012; Lancet, 2012). Indeed, the IHME and their evidence are seen to play an increasingly prominent role in guiding global health advocacy, priority-setting and resource allocations (Levine, 2015).

Meanwhile, the WHO continues to publish its own burden of disease analyses and evidence-for-policy networks have continued to expand, although now largely disassociated from each other. While the WHO is formally a collaborating partner of the IHME, a number of public disagreements and struggles over the authority to produce disease burden estimates have soured the relationship (Cohen, 2012). This has been reinforced under the current WHO leadership of Margaret Chan who has emphasised the limitations of global statistic modelling exercises (Chan, 2012). On the other hand, official WHO terminology has undergone a subtle semantic shift from 'evidence-based' to 'evidence-informed' policy, to reflect an appreciation that policy cannot be based on research evidence alone but is contingent upon other factors, including values and context (Oxman *et al.*, 2009). This has been accompanied by an increasing focus on the systematic appraisal of different types of evidence and their better 'translation' into policy. While perhaps laudable at first impression, these developments still raise a number of important questions. For one, it could be argued that the notion of 'evidence-informed' policy has the curious effect of reaffirming and reinstating the objective/ apolitical/epistemologically pure status of the evidence itself: whereas a focus on the translation of knowledge acknowledges that policy is influenced by contexts, judgements and values, the same factors seem to continue to be firmly located outside of and external to the processes of knowledge production themselves. In other words, values and contexts are accepted to affect the *application* of research evidence, but the *evidence itself* remains unaffected or unsituated (cf. Savransky and Rosengarten (2015) and their critique of the externalisation of contingency underlying the distinction between efficacy and effectiveness RCTs). This, on the other hand, poses a number of questions (albeit for another chapter), including where, by whom and how is this unsituated evidence produced, and what does it look like?

Conclusion: making sense of things

This chapter has aimed to present an alternative to the history of EBP at the WHO as presented by Murray and colleagues, by showing that its emergence was neither natural nor inevitable. It also shows that Murray and colleagues did not simply transfer evidence-based medicine principles to the global health policy arena. This is not to say that their version of EBP does not embrace both similar methods and rhetoric to EBM, or its epidemiological and statistical underpinnings. A closer focus on the question of what these methods or rhetoric are may have resulted in different stories, perhaps situating this EBP within wider historical shifts in statistical and epidemiological styles of reasoning (Hacking, 1990; Wahlberg and Rose, 2015) or quantification and audit cultures (Porter, 1995; Power, 1999; Strathern, 2000; Storeng and Béhague, 2014), linked to new global regimes of biopolitical governance.

What my re-narration has argued, however, is that EBP at the WHO also has its very own spatio-temporally situated and contingent history. In this story, EBP is not the impervious outcome of a coherent operative logic, but emerges with a fragile assemblage of a small but powerful group of advocates, ideas, technologies and circumstances. This 'emerging with' seems key: on the one hand, the shape and form which EBP took and takes has been highly contingent upon the material-discursive space from which it has emerged. On the other hand, EBP has helped bring particular realities into being. At its most ambitious, my story has pointed to such a co-emergence of EBP and the field of 'global health' itself. It suggests that the emergence of DALYs and CEA as macro-level health policy-setting tools and their translation into evidence were at once driven by and contributed to the enactment of very particular problematisations and imaginations regarding global health spaces. These include: problematisations around demographic and epidemiological changes that boosted the development of global population health measures (see also Wahlberg and Rose, 2015); visions of a global strategy to improve a world health that underlay debates over primary healthcare and *Health For All*; the alleged need for global health priority-setting in the 1990s that boosted the uptake of DALYs and CEA and their transformation into 'evidence'; but also the uptake of a notion of EBP that seemed able to reinvigorate the WHO's role as a global health norm-setting institution in a 'dramatically changing' world. These examples have in common their problematisation of a 'global health' space that needs to be mapped and governed, and could thus be described as among the conditions of possibility for EBP.

But in turn, EBP also played a role in turning these problematised abstract spaces into real entities. Didier Fassin recently argued that:

> even if we cannot deny that some problems are unprecedented and some solutions are innovative, it could be that global health is less about new problems (or solutions) but about new 'problematizations', . . . that is new ways of describing and interpreting the world – and therefore transforming it.
>
> (Fassin, 2012, 112–113)

Indeed, a number of recent studies have highlighted how global health knowledge and evidence not just mirror global health realities but co-configure them, such as when international health policy that emphasises quantifiable, economically value-able and 'global' health problems effect the privileging of particular health conditions, interventions, people and norms (McCoy *et al.*, 2013; Storeng and Béhague, 2014; Wahlberg and Rose, 2015), while discounting the particularities and realities that don't fit into the 'statistical straightjacket' (Adams, 2013, 86). These studies thus form an important starting point for further analyses into who, where and how determines what is made to matter in an evidence-based global health.

In this chapter, I have also pointed to the Murray and Evans *Report* as a concrete example of the performative character of knowledge practices in global health. Moreover, I have tried to show that in many ways our stories of these developments are also *evidentiary practices* that share with 'evidence-based' approaches the problem of trying to conscientiously collect evidence to represent a particular reality, while also re-enacting or even bringing these realities into being (Strathern, 1991; Law and Urry, 2004). In my case, 're-tracing' Murray and Evans' history of EBP risks unwittingly reproducing their already dominant narrative (Star, 1990), since – despite hinting at ruptures and possible diversions – too little attention could be paid to (more radically) alternative histories and spaces of evidence, including the question of how global or post-global (Adams *et al.*, 2014) health knowledge might be produced differently. For these reasons my account is very much just one possible (hi)story of evidence-based approaches in global health. But, by resisting the closing down of EBP and opening it up instead as an object of investigation, such histories are critical at a time when EBP and its associated new 'global health' spaces are increasingly inaccessible and impossible to criticise by anyone unable or unwilling to engage with particular technologies or types of expertise.

References

Adams, Vincanne. 2013. Evidence-based Global Public Health. In *When People Come First – Critical Studies in Global Health*, edited by João Biehl and Adriana Petryna. Princeton, NJ: Princeton University Press.

Adams, Vincanne, Nancy J. Burke and Ian Whitmarsh. 2014. Slow Research: Thoughts for a Movement in Global Health. *Medical Anthropology* 33 (3): 179–197. doi:10.1080/014 59740.2013.858335.

Al-Mazrou, Yagob. 1997. A Vital Opportunity for Global Health: Supporting the World Health Organization at a Critical Juncture. *The Lancet* 350(9080): 750–751. doi:10.1016/ S0140-6736(05)62559-7.

Almeida, Celia, Paula Braveman, Marthe R. Gold, Celia L Szwarcwald, Jose Mendes Ribeiro, Americo Miglionico and John S Millar. 2001. Methodological Concerns and Recommendations on Policy Consequences of the World Health Report 2000. *The Lancet* 357(9269): 1692–1697. doi:10.1016/S0140-6736(00)04825-X.

Anand, Sudhir and Kara Hanson. 1997. Disability-adjusted Life Years: A Critical Review. *Journal of Health Economics* 16(6): 685–702. doi:10.1016/S0167-6296 (97)00005-2.

Birn, Anne-Emanuelle. 2014. Philanthrocapitalism, Past and Present: The Rockefeller Foundation, the Gates Foundation, and the Setting(s) of the International/global Health Agenda. *Hypothesis* 12(1). doi:10.5779/hypothesis.v12i1.229.

Bowker, Geoffrey C. and Susan Leigh Star. 1999. *Sorting Things Out: Classification and Its Consequences*. Cambridge, MA: MIT Press.

Brives, Charlotte. 2013. Identifying Ontologies in a Clinical Trial. *Social Studies of Science* 43(3): 397–416. doi:10.1177/0306312712472406.

Brown, Theodore M., Marcos Cueto and Elizabeth Fee. 2006. The World Health Organization and the Transition from 'International' to 'Global' Public Health. *American Journal of Public Health* 96(1): 62–72. doi:10.2105/AJPH.2004.050831.

Brownson, Ross C., Jonathan E. Fielding and Christopher M. Maylahn. 2009. Evidence-based Public Health: A Fundamental Concept for Public Health Practice. *Annual Review of Public Health* 30: 175–201. doi:10.1146/annurev.pu.30.031709.100001.

Brundtland, Gro Harlem. 1998. Dr Gro Harlem Brundtland, Director-General Elect: The World Health Organization: Speech to the Fifty-first World Health Assembly, Geneva, 13 May 1998. World Health Organization. Available at http://apps.who.int//iris/ handle/10665/79896.

Brundtland, Gro Harlem. 1999. Making a Difference. *Bulletin of the World Health Organization* 77(1): 1.

Brundtland, Gro Harlem, Julio Frenk and Christopher J.L. Murray. 2003. Who Assessment of Health Systems Performance. *The Lancet* 361(9375): 2155. doi:10.1016/ S0140-6736(03)13702-6.

Chan, Margaret. 2012. From New Estimates to Better Data. *The Lancet* 380(9859): 2054. doi:10.1016/S0140-6736(12)62135-7.

Clift, Charles. 2013. The Role of the World Health Organization in the International System. Chatham House. Available at http://www.chathamhouse.org/publications/ papers/view/189351.

Cohen, Jon. 2012. Health Metrics. A Controversial Close-up of Humanity's Health. *Science* 338(6113): 1414–1416.

Cueto, Marcos. 2004. The ORIGINS of Primary Health Care and SELECTIVE Primary Health Care. *American Journal of Public Health* 94(11): 1864–1874.

EIP. 2000. Evidence and Information for Policy: Empowering People to Make Better Decisions. World Health Organization. Available at http://apps.who.int/iris/handle/10665/66333.

Evans, Timothy G. and Christopher J.L. Murray. 1987. A Critical Re-examination of the Economics of Blindness Prevention under the Onchocerciasis Control Programme. *Social Science & Medicine* 25(3): 241–249.

Evidence-Based Medicine (EBM) Working Group. 1992. Evidence-Based Medicine. A New Approach to Teaching the Practice of Medicine. *JAMA: The Journal of the American Medical Association* 268(17): 2420–2425.

Fassin, Didier. 2012. The Obscure Object of Global Health. In *Medical Anthropology at the Intersections*, edited by Marcia C. Inhorn and Emily A. Wentzell, pp. 95–115. Durham, NC, and London: Duke University Press.

Geissler, P. Wenzel and Catherine Molyneux. 2011. *Evidence, Ethos and Experiment: The Anthropology and History of Medical Research in Africa.* New York: Berghahn Books.

Ghana Health Assessment Project Team. 1981. A Quantitative Method of Assessing the Health Impact of Different Diseases in Less Developed Countries. *International Journal of Epidemiology* 10(1): 73–80.

Godlee, Fiona. 1994. WHO in Crisis. *British Medical Journal* 309(6966): 1424–1428.

Gold, Marthe R., David Gold, Dennis G. Stevenson and Dennis G. Fryback. 2002. HALYS AND QALYS AND DALYS, OH MY: Similarities and Differences in Summary Measures of Population Health. *Annual Review of Public Health* 23 (11): 115–134.

Guyatt, Gordon H. 1991. Evidence-based Medicine. *APC J Club* 114(A-16).

Hacking, Ian. 1990. *The Taming of Chance.* Cambridge, MA: Cambridge University Press.

Ham, Chris, David J. Hunter and Ray Robinson. 1995. Evidence Based Policymaking. *British Medical Journal* 310(6972): 71–72.

Howick, Jeremy H. 2011. *The Philosophy of Evidence-based Medicine.* Chichester: John Wiley & Sons.

IDRC. 1993. Conference Report: Future Partnership for the Acceleration of Health Development. Ottawa: International Development Research Centre. Available at https://idl-bnc.idrc.ca/dspace/bitstream/10625/13563/1/99451.pdf.

IHME. 2015. Director's Statement. Available at http://www.healthdata.org/about/director-statement.

Jamison, D.T. 1992. Preliminary and Unapproved Draft of WDR 1993. March 1992 [Archival Source], WHO Archives. Geneva: World Health Organization.

Jamison, Dean T., Julio Frenk and Felicia Knaul. 1998. International Collective Action in Health: Objectives, Functions, and Rationale. *The Lancet* 351(9101): 514–517.

Jamison, Dean T., Henry W. Mosley, Anthony R. Meashem and and Jose-Luis Bobadilla. 1993. *Disease Control Priorities in Developing Countries.* 12384. Washington, DC: The World Bank. Available at http://documents.worldbank.org/curated/en/1993/10/698818/disease-control-priorities-developing-countries.

Lakoff, Andrew. 2005. *Pharmaceutical Reason: Knowledge and Value in Global Psychiatry.* Cambridge: Cambridge University Press.

Latour, Bruno. 1987. *Science in Action: How to Follow Scientists and Engineers Through Society.* Milton Keynes: Open University Press.

Law, John and John Urry. 2004. Enacting the Social. *Economy and Society* 33(3): 390–410.

Lee, Kelley. 2009. *The World Health Organization (WHO).* Abingdon, Oxon: Routledge.

Levine, Ruth. 2015. Power in Global Health Agenda-setting: The Role of Private Funding; Comment on 'Knowledge, Moral Claims and the Exercise of Power in Global Health.'

International Journal of Health Policy and Management. Available at http://www. ijhpm.com/article_2976_0.html.

Lozano, Rafael., Chris J.L. Murray, Julio Frenk and Jose-Luis Bobadilla. 1995. Burden of Disease Assessment and Health System Reform: Results of a Study in Mexico. *Journal of International Development* 7(3): 555–563.

Mathers, Colin D. 2007. Epidemiology and World Health. In *The Development of Modern Epidemiology*, edited by Walter W. Holland, Jørn Olsen and Charles du V. Florey, pp. 41–62. Oxford: Oxford University Press. Available at http://www. oxfordscholarship.com/view/10.1093/acprof:oso/9780198569541.001.0001/acprof-9780198569541.

McCoy, David, Gayatri Kembhavi, Jinesh Patel and Akish Luintel. 2009. The Bill & Melinda Gates Foundation's Grant-making Programme for Global Health. *The Lancet* 373(9675): 1645–1653.

McCoy, David, Nele Jensen, Katharina Kranzer, Rashida A Ferrand and Eline L Korenromp. 2013. Methodological and Policy Limitations of Quantifying the Saving of Lives: A Case Study of the Global Fund's Approach. *PLoS Medicine* 10(10): e1001522.

Murray, Christopher J.L. 1987. A Critical Review of International Mortality Data. *Social Science & Medicine* 25(7): 773–781.

Murray, Chris J. 1990. Rational Approaches to Priority Setting in International Health. *The Journal of Tropical Medicine and Hygiene* 93(5): 303–311.

Murray, Chris J. and David B. Evans. 2003. Health Systems Performance Assessment. WHO. Available at http://www.who.int/publications/2003/hspa/en/.

Murray, Chris and J. Frenk. 2001. World Health Report 2000: A Step towards Evidence-based Health Policy. *The Lancet* 357(9269): 1698–1700.

Murray, Christopher J.L. and Julio Frenk. 2000. A Framework for Assessing the Performance of Health Systems/C.J.L. Murray and J. Frenk. *Bulletin of the World Health Organization: The International Journal of Public Health* 78(6): 717–731.

Murray, Chris J. and Alan D. Lopez. 1996a. *Global Health Statistics*. Cambridge, MA: Harvard University Press. Available at http://www.hup.harvard.edu/catalog. php?isbn=9780674354494.

Murray, Chris J. and Alan D. Lopez. 1996b. *The Global Burden of Disease: A Comprehensive Assessment of Mortality and Disability from Diseases, Injuries and Risk Factors in 1990 and Projected to 2020*. Cambridge, MA: Harvard University Press. Available at http://www.who.int/healthinfo/global_burden_disease/publications/en/.

Murray, Chris J. and Alan D. Lopez. 1998. *Health Dimensions of Sex and Reproduction*. Cambridge, MA: Harvard University Press. Available at http://www.hup.harvard.edu/ catalog.php?isbn=9780674383357.

Murray, Christopher J.L., Alan D. Lopez and Suwit Wibulpolprasert. 2004. Monitoring Global Health: Time for New Solutions. *BMJ (Clinical Research Edn)* 329(7474): 1096–1100.

Murray, Chris J., Julio Frenk, David Evans, Kei Kawabata, Alan Lopez and Orvill Adams. 2001. Science or Marketing at WHO? A Response to Williams. *Health Economics* 10(4): 277–285.

Murray, Christopher J.L., Majid Ezzati, Abraham D. Flaxman, Stephen Lim, Rafael Lozano, Catherine Michaud and Mohsen Naghavi. 2012. GBD 2010: A Multi-investigator Collaboration for Global Comparative Descriptive Epidemiology. *The Lancet* 380(9859): 2055–2058.

Musgrove, Philip. 2003. Judging Health Systems: Reflections on WHO's Methods. *The Lancet* 361(9371): 1817–1820

Navarro, Vincente. 2000. Assessment of the World Health Report 2000. *The Lancet* 356 (9241): 1598–1601.

Omran, Abdel R. 1971. The Epidemiologic Transition: A Theory of the Epidemiology of Population Change. *The Milbank Memorial Fund Quarterly* 49(4): 509–538.

Oxford Centre for Evidence-based Medicine. 2009. Levels of Evidence. *CEBM*. Available at http://www.cebm.net/oxford-centre-evidence-based-medicine-levels-evidence-march-2009/.

Oxman, Andrew D., John N. Lavis, Simon Lewin and Atle Fretheim. 2009. SUPPORT Tools for Evidence-informed Health Policymaking (STP) 1: What Is Evidence-informed Policymaking? *Health Research Policy and Systems/BioMed Central* 7(Suppl 1): S1.

Paalman, Maria, Henk Bekedam, Laura Hawken and David Nyheim. 1998. A Critical Review of Priority Setting in the Health Sector: The Methodology of the 1993 World Development Report. *Health Policy and Planning* 13(1): 13–31.

Petryna, Adriana. 2009. *When Experiments Travel: Clinical Trials and the Global Search for Human Subjects*. Princeton, NJ: Princeton University Press.

Porter, Theodore M. 1995. *Trust in Numbers: The Pursuit of Objectivity in Science and Public Life*. Princeton, NJ: Princeton University Press.

Power, Michael. 1999. *The Audit Society: Rituals of Verification*. Oxford: Oxford University Press.

Rifkin, Susan B. and Gill Walt. 1986. Why Health Improves: Defining the Issues Concerning 'Comprehensive Primary Health Care' and 'Selective Primary Health Care.' *Social Science & Medicine (1982)* 23(6): 559–566.

Riles, Annelise, ed. 2006. *Documents: Artifacts of Modern Knowledge*. Michigan, OH: University of Michigan Press.

Savransky, Martin and Marsha Rosengarten. 2015. Situating Efficacy: HIV and Ebola RCTs and the Care of Biomedical Abstractions. 'Situating Efficacy', Symposium at the Brocher Foundation, Geneva, 16–17 February.

Smith, Jeremy N. 2013. The New Book of Life. Available at jeremysmith.com. http://www.jeremynsmith.com/Jeremy_N._Smith/Publications_files/NewBookofLife_1.pdf.

Smith, J. 2015. *Epic Measures: One Doctor. Seven Billion Patients.* New York: HarperCollins.

Smith, R. 1995. The WHO: Change or Die. *British Medical Journal* 310(6979): 543–544.

Specter, M. 2005. What Money Can Buy. *The New Yorker*, 24 October. Available at http://www.newyorker.com/archive/2005/10/24/051024fa_fact_specter.

Star, S. 1990. Power, Technology and the Phenomenology of Conventions: On Being Allergic to Onions. *The Sociological Review* 38(S1): 26–56.

Storeng, Katerini T. and Dominique P. Béhague. 2014. 'Playing the Numbers Game': Evidence-based Advocacy and the Technocratic Narrowing of the Safe Motherhood Initiative. *Medical Anthropology Quarterly*. doi:10.1111/maq.12072.

Strathern, M. 1991. *Partial Connections*. Savage, MD: Rowman & Littlefield.

Strathern, M. 2000. *Audit Cultures: Anthropological Studies in Accountability, Ethics and the Academy*. Abingdon, Oxon: Routledge.

Subramanian, M. 1992a. *Note for the Record. 1993 World Development Report. May 19 1992.* [Archival Source] WHO Archives. Geneva: World Health Organization.

Subramanian, M. 1992b. *Notes for the Record. WHO Working Group for WDR 1993. Summary of Meetings on 18 and 26 March 1992.* [Archival Source] WHO Archives. Geneva: World Health Organization.

The Lancet. 1997. Editorial, From What Will We Die in 2020? *The Lancet* 349(9061): 1263.

The Lancet. 2012. The Global Burden of Disease 2010. Elsevier Digital. Available at http://www.elsevierdigital.com/The-Lancet/GBD/.

Timmermans, Stefan and Marc Berg. 1997. Standardization in Action: Achieving Local Universality through Medical Protocols. *Social Studies of Science* 27(2): 273–305.

Wahlberg, Ayo and Nikolas Rose. 2015. The Governmentalization of Living: Calculating Global Health. *Economy and Society* 44(1): 60–90.

Walt, Gill and Anne Mills. 2001. World Health Report 2000: Responses to Murray and Frenk. *The Lancet* 357(9269): 1702–1703.

WDR. 1993. *World Development Report 1993?: Investing in Health*. Washington, DC: World Bank. Available at https://openknowledge.worldbank.org/handle/10986/5976.

WHA. 1998. WHA51.7: Health-for-All Policy for the Twenty-first Century. World Health Organization, 22 June 2014. Available at http://legacy.library.ucsf.edu/documentStore/g/w/o/gwo93a99/Sgwo93a99.pdf.

White, Kerr L. 2007. Health Services Research and Epidemiology. In *The Development of Modern Epidemiology*, edited by Walter W. Holland, Jørn Olsen and Charles du V. Florey, pp. 183–169. Oxford: Oxford University Press. Available at http://www.oxfordscholarship.com/view/10.1093/acprof:oso/9780198569541.001.0001/acprof-9780198569541.

WHO. 1946. WHO Constitution. World Health Organization. Available at http://whqlibdoc.who.int/hist/official_records/constitution.pdf.

WHO. 1963. Second Report on the World Health Situation 1957–1960. Available at http://apps.who.int/iris/bitstream/10665/85752/1/Official_record122_eng.pdf.

WHO. 1971. Statistical Indicators for the Planning and Evaluation of Public Health Programmes. World Health Organization. Available at http://whqlibdoc.who.int/trs/WHO_TRS_472.pdf.

WHO. 1974. Fifth Report on the World Health Situation. Available at http://apps.who.int//iris/handle/10665/146261.

WHO. 1980. Sixth Report on the World Health Situation: Part 1, Global Analysis, Part 2, Review by Country and Area. Available at http://apps.who.int//iris/handle/10665/44199.

WHO. 1981a. Development of Indicators for Monitoring Process towards Health for All. World Health Organization. Available at http://apps.who.int/iris/bitstream/10665/40672/1/9241800046.pdf?ua=1.

WHO. 1981b. Global Strategy for Health for All by the Year 2000. World Health Organization. Available at http://whqlibdoc.who.int/publications/9241800038.pdf.

WHO. 1993. Report of the Executive Board Working Response to Global Change. World Health Organization. Available at http://hist.library.paho.org/English/GOV/CD/15660.pdf.

WHO. 1995. WHO Response to Global Change. World Health Organization. Available at http://apps.who.int/iris/bitstream/10665/63144/1/PPE_95.4.pdf?ua=1.

WHO. 1996. Summary: Investing in Health Research and Development. World Health Organization. Available at http://whqlibdoc.who.int/hq/1996/TDR_GEN_96.2.pdf.

WHO. 1997. EB101/24 – Programme Budgeting and Priority-Setting. World Health Organization. Available at http://apps.who.int/iris/bitstream/10665/79486/1/eb10124.pdf.

WHO. 1999. WHO | The World Health Report 1999 – Making a Difference. WHO. Available at http://www.who.int/whr/1999/en/.

WHO. 2000. The World Health Report 2000 – Health Systems: Improving Performance. World Health Organization. Available at http://www.who.int/whr/2000/en/.

WHO. 2001. Health Systems Performance Assessment: Report by the Secretariat. World Health Organization. Available at http://apps.who.int//iris/handle/10665/78649.

Yamey, Gavin. 2002. Who In 2002: Have The Latest Reforms Reversed Who's Decline? *British Medical Journal* 325(7372): 1107–1112.

Part III

When solutions make problems

9 More than one world, more than one health

Re-configuring inter-species health

Stephen Hinchliffe

Introduction

For Andrew Lakoff, global health is a 'contested ethical, political, and technical zone whose contours are still under construction' (Lakoff, 2010: 60). More concretely, those contours have undoubtedly been sketched if not fully fashioned around specific objects of concern: emerging infectious diseases, and relating to these, dynamic and often zoonotic pathogens. The assemblage of state and non-state global surveillance networks, the boosting of Cold War-era outbreak investigation capability and martial efforts to contain outbreaks have all contributed to a regulatory regime that Lakoff calls *global health security*. In contradistinction to *humanitarian biomedicine*, this regime of global health is focused on preparedness for the emergence of hitherto unknown communicable diseases, their early detection and the mobilisation of containment procedures (for a critical reading see King, 2002). With a focus on emergence within informal edge landscapes and at interfaces including forest margins, peri-urban zones and human-animal interactions, and the transmission of emergent pathogens to the Global North, this is a tale of scientific intelligence, vigilance and geopolitical pre-emption on behalf of a 'public' that is clearly less than global. Global health in this sense belies a geography of demarcation and regulation of movement rather than an attempt to address the systematic production of inequality and risk.

In recent years, this mix of concerns and materials has been joined by the concept of 'One Health', at root an attempt to marry together clinical, veterinarian and ecological expertise in order to address the shared health fortunes of people, nonhumans (largely but not only food animals) and environments. The contours of One Health are, I will argue, similarly shaped by a focus on emerging infectious diseases, and the result is a tendency to attempt to format the lives of food animals in particular ways that conform to global health security. That this vision of One Health and global health security may in fact be counterproductive is a key question for this chapter.

The chapter uses insights from Science and Technology Studies, Geography and Anthropology along with multi-sited and multi-species qualitative fieldwork on animal livestock and zoonotic influenzas in the UK, to highlight the importance of practical engagements that are concerned with making health. After an introduction to One Health, I argue that there is a tendency to focus on contamination and transmission of pathogens rather than the socio-economic configuration of disease and health, and this tendency conforms to or performs what sociologist John Law calls a one world metaphysics. Following this, three related field cases are used to demonstrate that health is dependent on a patchwork of practices, and is configured in practice by skilled people, animals, micro-organisms and their social relations. From surveillance for influenza viruses to tending animals, good health it turns out is dependent on an ability to construct common sense from a complex of signs, responses and actions. It takes, in other words, more than one world to make healthy outcomes. In light of this, the chapter aims to, first, loosen any association between One Health and a one world-ist metaphysics, and, second, to radicalise the interdisciplinary foundations of One Health by both widening the scope of disciplinarity as well as attending to how different knowledges are brought together. A new common sense is offered, one that emphasises the ability to produce health through the practical articulation of more than one world. It is an articulation that counters some of the uniformity, even imperial aspects, of global health security.

Common sense and its exclusions

While not new, a unified and holistic approach to health took shape in 2004 at a New York meeting hosted by a US conservation organisation (the Wildlife Conservation Society). At the meeting the 12 'Manhattan Principles' defining cross-sectoral and integrated approaches to health were adopted and, indeed, branded as 'One World One Health' (OWOH). The concept immediately gained a foothold in global human and animal health-related institutions. OWOH provided a space for conceptual agreement (it was and is 'common sense' after all) and a chance to interrogate and overcome institutional, disciplinary and other barriers to its realisation. Nevertheless, common sense is rarely a simple, let alone coherent, matter. Common sense is always a mixed blessing (Gramsci, 1971). On the one hand, it is based on popular understanding, is democratic, and can provide the seeds for new practices. On the other hand, common sense is also often embedded within forms of consent to established and often rather staid understandings of the world in which we live. It is with the less progressive forms of common sense with respect to the One Health concept that this chapter is primarily concerned.

The OWOH concept was most readily taken up within or at the edges of national and global animal and public health bodies where practitioners could see the advantages of working on health and disease problems in ways that defied established disciplinary and institutional boundaries (FAO, OIE et al. 2010). Indeed, if the OWOH concept did anything, it helped its champions seek funding for and promote interdisciplinary solutions to long-standing epistemic and political tensions that existed within and between public health, animal health and agriculturally focused organisations. International agencies, including the World Health Organisation (WHO), the World Organisation for Animal Health (OIE) and the Food and Agricultural Organisation (FAO), have traditionally tended to act within their medical/health, veterinary/trade and agriculture/development domains respectively. As Chien (2012) explains, during the first major highly pathogenic Avian Influenza (H5N1) scares at the turn of the century, the WHO prioritised pandemic preparedness, the OIE concentrated on ensuring virus eradication in poultry while the FAO focused initially on the need to reduce potential disease transmission in backyard farms between wild and domestic birds and then between people and their poultry. Tensions though started to mount as disagreements on poultry culling policy revealed differences in terms of priorities and means of disease control. These tensions lay as much within organisations as between them, but in short the favoured option within the WHO of the widespread culling of potentially infected flocks encountered resistance within the FAO and OIE as economists and others questioned the effectiveness of the culls as well as their consequences in terms of livelihoods, food security and ultimately human health. In this sense it was clear that more joined-up approaches to shared matters of concern were necessary.

This analysis is taken further by Scoones and Forster (2011). As well as noting the differences between the institutions, they highlight the similarities and the collective sanctioning of some simple and reductionist accounts or narratives of disease. In doing so, they start to identify a potential problem with seeking unity across disciplines and domains. They refer to three 'outbreak narratives' (Wald, 2008) that existed within international health-related institutions. Each narrative had, they argue, overlapping yet relatively distinct matters of concern. The first was centred on animal health. In this case, Avian Influenza (AI) was a disease of birds, affecting the poultry industry and livelihoods. The response was one of making production more secure, restructuring the industry, particularly in the Global South where initially at least the response to AI targeted backyard production, informal exchange and live bird markets (Hinchliffe and Bingham, 2008). Second, there is the public health narrative, which related to the transmission of AI to and between people. The response here was based on the provision of antivirals, the development of vaccines and behaviour change. Third, there was pandemic preparedness, focusing on 'civil contingency planning, business continuity approaches and containment strategies' (Scoones and Forster, 2011: 21) with the broadest array of actors involved in a scenario-based attunement of government, police, health providers, business, schools, civil society and so on in the development of a readiness to act.

Despite their differences and competition for attention and resources (between and within organisations), each of these narratives shared a single set of core values. Not only did they all assume the compelling outbreak narrative whereby the recognition of human/nonhuman animal interdependence and shared pathogens is succeeded by human mastery, but they also relate to a particular version of disease – one which emphasises what Rosenberg (1992) called 'contamination'. The latter takes contact as its issue of concern and focuses attention on preventing disease transmission (or at least being prepared for any eventual transmission events). Rosenberg contrasted this to a 'configuration' approach to disease, where the focus is less on pathogens and their unregulated movements and rather on the context and therefore the pathogenicity of the disease (see also Farmer, 2004; Leach *et al.*, 2010). It is configuration, Scoones and Forster argue, that has been most readily erased from twentieth- and twenty-first-century disease narratives and associated management regimes, and has been regularly downplayed in responses to Avian Influenza. Vulnerabilities, differentials in social and ecological resilience, accountabilities, risk geographies and abilities to dissimulate are all conditional upon livelihoods, uneven access to political and other resources, and make any response that is solely based on outbreaks and contamination to be partial at best and missing the point at worst.

In contrast, ethnographic work emphasises the ways in which local political resources, economics and social relations configure Avian Influenzas and render them more or less tractable problems. Forster's (2011) ethnography of Avian Influenza in Indonesia highlights the ways in which AI resists being managed through top-down implementation of anti-contamination technologies (like new, centralised market buildings designed to replace informal wet markets). Rather, the disease is configured within informal social and market relations between farmers and market intermediaries (those who often travel on motorcycles collecting poultry from small farmers and so pool risk), between consumers and birds (with many consumers preferring freshly killed birds and therefore live bird markets as a guarantee of their provenance and flavour), and between various risk categories (where Avian Influenza is regarded by farmers as just one among many other, and often more pressing, risks in lives that already exist on the margins). Likewise, Porter's (2013) ethnography of bird flu in Vietnam, and Lowe's (2010) study of the HPAI viral cloud in Indonesia highlight a similar range of entanglements between people, birds and viruses. The conclusion is that Avian Influenza is a socio-economic disease – riddled with all manner of market, social and cultural relations.

To be clear, there is evidence that seasonal and emergency transmission controls can contribute to the reductions of disease burden (for example, periodic closures of live bird markets have seemingly reduced highly pathological H5N1 in Hong Kong (Peiris *et al.*, 2007) and low pathological H7N9 Avian Influenza in China (Yu *et al.*, 2014)). And yet, once disease is framed as predominantly a matter of contamination, we risk missing all manner of key issues for animal and public health.

The point to carry forward is that a one world approach can promulgate a 'common sense' of transmission and contamination as the main issues for disease control. This common sense may miss the vital importance of social conditions and downplay the role of context or, more epidemiologically speaking, the intricate relations between host, pathogens and environment (which includes of course the complex of cultural and social relations) in contributing to disease. To develop the point further and to start to explain the tendency for social relations to be lost from view in One Health, I now look at the 'one world-ist' approach more generally before returning to the socio-economic nature of disease and the multiple dynamics of health later in the chapter.

One world-ism

The late cultural geographer Denis Cosgrove wrote of the imagery and the implicit geographical imagination of the Apollo space missions in the 1960s and 1970s (Cosgrove, 1994). A one-world and whole-earth textual inscription of the Apollo space photographs was linked, in Cosgrove's argument, to a mastering gaze and an imperial, specifically Christian and US geopolitical project, all of which continued to configure a Western geographical imagination.

'One World One Health' arguably shares a similar geographical frame – a singular space or global village, a small world-ism, with dense interconnections. These interconnections, frequently depicted in the maps where flight paths and transmission routes perform a world of contagion, suggest a particular version of disease risk and its mitigation. Indeed, in positing the dense links between people, wild and domestic animals and ecosystems, the image is of a single, bio-communicable planet, with WHO response structures at its centre (Briggs, 2005). A chicken can splutter in Indonesia and a cytokine storm can be triggered in a hospital bed in the UK. The viral storm is both symptom of and contributor to a contagious event whose catastrophic potential is well known. As Braun (2007), Cooper (2008) and others have outlined, there is a geopolitics to this version of one world-ism that can be just as pernicious as the one traced by Cosgrove. For as preventing, containing and preparing for transmission become the key dimensions of disease control, barrier techniques and hygiene are extended across social and agricultural practices (the latter under the rubric of 'disease-free agriculture', an extension that is often capital intensive and a possible threat to all manner of established agro-ecological practice let alone livelihoods). The extension of a global, modern agriculture from the core to a periphery, in the form of disease-free zones and Sanitary and Phyto-Sanitary (SPS) agreements of the World Trade Organisation (WTO), performs a single, biosecure planet. The irony may be that in the pursuit of one world, two worlds are created – a world of self-controlling, virtuous economic actors and a residual (Global South) of inter-species intimacy and contingency.

This one world-ism, as Law (2011) neatly captures it, entails some of the following ontological commitments. First, this is a world of surfaces, volumes and collisions. It is a world made sense of through a particular (Euclidean) geometry. It is a world of objects rather than entangled things, where disease and health are often conceived of as separate spaces, with well-defined objects and properties (pathogens and immune responses), and where one health implies a spatial segregation of forms of 'good' and 'bad' life. Second, this is a world wherein the conditions for knowing that world are systematically effaced in every telling. One world requires no account of the knowledge that makes it possible; it simply is. This is naturalism, or a version of realism, an account of how things are, with any deviation from that real being reduced to ideology, to myth, to poor knowledge. Moreover, this reality is destiny, it is the way things will be – there is no room for politics other than in the shape of presumably short-lived arguments over ways of seeing, or epistemological debates, which are resolved soon enough through recourse to the one world that supplies all the evidence one needs. Third and finally, despite its claim to universalism, this is a world that is made in the Global North, is embedded and naturalised in northern knowledge practices, and exported to other domains through a mixture of the exceptionalism of Western science and a triumphalism of the associated modernism.

Contrast this to a world that is continually made and remade in part through stories we tell about it. Or as Mol (2002) neatly captured it, a world made in various, sometimes overlapping but rarely coherent practices. That is, if we believe that things are made through their relations, or change as they relate to one another – something that doesn't reduce things to one another but simply gives them a more complex history and geography – then if things are practised differently and in different spaces, it follows that there will be more than one thing. Or, better, it follows that the same thing may take on different qualities as it is performed in various ways, and those qualities may exist in tension with one another. The latter suggests that making health is not so much a matter of making one world, but a matter of patching together different realities (Mol and Law, 1994). Here, reality is not so much destiny as a set of sometimes competing, always co-incident, co-productions out of which a more or less settled programme of action may emerge. In developing this more or less coherent way of proceeding, there is no pre-given destiny. Rather there are contingencies, borne out of a heterogeneous world.

In practice, then, there is more than one world, and likewise more than one health. The result is a continuous struggle to produce health in conditions that are rarely of our choosing through a set of non-coherent procedures and practices. Before exploring this empirically, there are two implications which together underline why this approach matters. First, it is crucial that we demonstrate how health is patched together in practices that take account of local conditions (where local refers to the specific mix of materials, knowledges and elsewheres that make a peculiar and particular situation or place). Missing this heterogeneity of practices is to miss the vital means through which health is made. As Law more powerfully and politically puts it, 'one-world metaphysics are catastrophic. . . . They reduce difference. They evacuate reality from non-dominant reals' (Law, 2011: 9). It is the non-dominant reals or the endangered practices within an ecology of practices (Stengers, 2010) that need to be accentuated in health practices. Second, I seek to do this 'at home', within the so-called core of one world-ism. I do so not only to demonstrate that the so-called modern is always and already contingent upon multiple realities, making any export of practices itself a matter for careful translation rather than wholesale extension, but also to demonstrate that the one world story is itself being performed and, in the process, is patching together health in new ways, and with possible deleterious effects. It is part of the analysis then to focus on how this story contributes not to a universe, or even to a pluriverse (or a proliferation of practices) but to a fractiverse, or to put it again in the language of onto-politics (Mol, 1999), to there being more than one world but fewer than many. Again, Law (2011: 2) sums up the political implications:

If we live in a single Northern container-world, within a universe, then we might imagine a liberal way of handling the power-saturated encounters between different kinds of people. But if we live, instead, in a multiple world of different enactments, if we participate in a fractiverse, then there will be, there can be, no overarching logic or liberal institutions to mediate between the different realities. There is no 'overarching'. Instead there are contingent, local and practical engagements.

It is to these contingent, local and practical engagements that I now turn.

Doing animal health and immunity

If one world-ism implies a specific ontology – a world of self-identical objects, with collisions and movements across pre-constituted space or territory – then a One World One Health programme, if it follows suit, is dominated by a particular version of health and disease. Indeed, in the biosecurity strand of responding to emerging and re-emerging infectious disease, one world-ism is alive and well in what I have already characterised as a system of extension wherein barriers to transmission and contamination become the main technology through which health is secured. These barriers are of course semi-porous. Under World Trade Organisation (WTO) rules they need to allow the circulation of goods while selecting out the bads. This is a logic of security, whose result is a material translation of bodily contact, movement and communication into the more regular and regulated exchange, circulation and commerce (Mitropoulos, 2012). As a result, mobility is not so much halted as sanitised or tidied up.

The purpose of the remainder of this chapter is, first, to demonstrate empirically the inability of such practices to meet their own high standards, suggesting that they may even make vulnerable that which they seek to protect. Second, I use empirical engagements with doing animal health in order to highlight how health is made in ways that imply *more* than one world and *more* than one health. Starting from an account of 'viral chatter' (Wolfe, 2011) wherein the locational aspects of disease movements are emphasised, I provide short distillations from three field sites where human/animal health is being practised, effectively drawing together a number of cases in order to emphasise their heterogeneity and practical accomplishments. I conclude with a brief account of how making healthy lives requires attending to the diverse range of practices involved in the doing of health.

Methodologically, this work draws on several years' ethnographic and multi-species fieldwork (undertaken in the UK from 2010 to 2013) involving 70 semi-structured interviews with UK farmers, farm workers, veterinarians, retailers, processors and others; farm visits and observations; fieldwork within an international influenza reference laboratory; and participating in disease surveillance on farms and on wildlife reserves. All interviews were transcribed and these along with field notes were entered into a qualitative database, coded and analysed with the help of software. Sampling was necessarily based on issues of time and access but every effort was used in the research to correct for any bias in terms of differential access (for example, in terms of visiting non-compliant farms and premises) by interviewing and observing people across product chains (so from breeders to retailers) who could share their experience of the whole industry, and by conducting semi-structured interviews with people who were important mediators in the industry (vets, labour organisations and so on). In this way there is confidence in not only generating in-depth accounts of practice but also achieving necessary breadth across the relevant sectors.

The return of configuration

Even within the biological sciences, the distinction between what Rosenberg called dominant 'contamination' and neglected 'configuration' approaches to disease has started to unravel. One source for this has come from virology in the form of 'viral chatter' (Wolfe *et al.*, 2005,2007; Wolfe, 2011). The metaphor of chatter is located first and foremost, the main protagonist admits, in a post 9/11 security logic where online chatter can, controversially, be used to generate and identify signatures of those considered to be a security threat (Wolfe, 2011: 255). But it is also used to capture something of the continuous semiotic and material exchanges that viruses undergo or undertake when in 'conversation' with potential hosts. Most chatter leads nowhere, of course, but the self-styled 'virus hunters' go on to suggest that high rates of chatter increase both viral diversity and the probability of transmission of a virus that can replicate. So, for example, those diseases that manage to cross from animals to people do not simply just happen as a result of contact or viral contamination; they involve repeated crossings, an ongoing conversation – a repetitive material semiotics, or a working-out of a new reality. Contagion, then, is more than contact and viruses don't simply diffuse across space, or extend across a plane through simple transmission. They are configured in relation. Anthropologists Brown and Kelly (2014) go on to read viral chatter as a means of emphasising that disease risk is not located – it is locational – arising from the particular mix of social, biotic and material conditions. Contagion, then, is made in intensive relations where repetition and difference count as much as touching. It is, in that sense, about configuration as much as it is about contamination.

Nevertheless, a geography of point location and contact, rather than the repetition and difference of contagion, is embodied and reproduced in biosecurity programmes (or the protection of production systems from disease). A version of immunity is built from two main investments: a contractual economy of disease-free agriculture (replete with technologies honed in the retail and food safety sector) and scanning surveillance or early warning of viral presence. I will now touch on three case studies that illustrate these approaches and their limitations.

Contract and contagion in chickens

In the UK, poultry farms are contracted to produce chickens for meat (broilers) for five main processors who in turn are contracted to supply the retailers, notably the big supermarket chains. As participants in the chain suggest, this purportedly allows for logistical and management control of the production process, if not from farm to fork then certainly from breeding to hatching to raising, to processing and to supermarket shelves.

> Whichever way you do it, [by owning farms or contracting the growing], you make sure you have full control to make changes on farms. . . . Biosecurity is more straightforward with *your* management structure.
>
> (Major UK poultry processor, interview 2011, emphasis in original)

> [The retailer] Tesco's [a UK major supermarket chain] probably knows more about the farms than the integrators know about the farms. They will have a file on every farm supplying them, they'll know their mortality, their records, they'll know antibiotics used – because they're absolutely petrified of having anybody saying they've got any problem after eating their food because the financial effect is so great on them.
>
> (Poultry vet, interview 2011)

While protagonists emphasise the security and food safety aspects of a contractual and/or integrated environment where there is managerial control, these relations are also and primarily a means to manage and distribute financial risk. In doing so, the contractual environment exerts upward pressure on everything apart from labour – so that stocking rates, throughput, growth rates, densities and application of logistics are all scaled up, whereas labour is scaled down. Commercial farms range from 20,000 to 300,000 poultry, with each farm usually employing only one or two workers. The high-volume, low-unit margin structure results in a compressed life for chickens, as they are managed from hatchery to harvesting within tightly regulated houses and with minimal human contact in order to reduce disease risk. The chickens are like 'racehorses', one industry vet suggested in interview, primed in this case to reach the table as quickly and cheaply as possible. The result is a bird that lives at a 'biological threshold', experiencing tissue growth at rates unimaginable only a few decades ago. While ostensibly contained and biosecure, the birds are arguably immuno-compromised as a result of accelerated growth rates and continuous throughput of feed (Humphrey, 2006; Humphrey *et al.*, 2007).

However, the trade-offs between margin, volumes, growth rates and the susceptibility of birds and people to ill-health temporarily unfold at the points of thinning and harvesting, when additional, casualised labour is needed to catch and move chickens to the processing plant. Thinning of poultry houses is required in an industry where tight margins impose the need to stock houses to their capacity, and in such a way that maximises throughput and meat production without violating animal welfare regulations. So a standard commercial poultry farm will comprise around ten sheds, with each shed stocked with 30,000 one-day-old chicks. The flocks are then thinned at approximately four to five weeks when the birds have grown to an extent that is set to exceed statutory stocking rates.

Thinning involves the removal of around 15 to 25 per cent of the stock for slaughter (the exact number is determined by the processor and by growth rates), with the remaining birds kept for another week to put on more body mass (and possibly to incubate any diseases related to the thin) and to be harvested at full weight. At the thin and the harvest, birds that are hitherto used to a regulated diurnal regime and continuous feed are denied food and sleep for 24 hours to make them docile. They are then caught by a catching team that moves from farm to farm on a subcontracted, casual employee basis with little or no access to sickness benefits and working under tight time regimes in order to meet factory capacity at the processing plant. Here the socio-economy of the margin combines with the socio-biology of labour and poultry to produce the necessary locational elements for viral chatter. As stressed guts are flooded with noradrenalin, and the precarious human and chicken bodies meet skin to skin, the 'immunity' conferred by walls and doors seems somewhat beside the point. So, even when highly regulated, the tidying up of mobility into exchange, circulation and commerce is always far from perfect. Contact, movement (even in and of the gut), and communication (chatter) reappear in this heavily contracted and therefore 'drawn together' or intensely compressed network of production. Transmission is in this sense only part of the problem, as the intense configuration of the poultry economy and socio-biology adds in new disease risks.

The point here is to emphasise that One World One Health cannot afford to accede to a model of disease whereby transmission is the only issue for attention. Quite clearly, even in the core of modernised farming practice, health is dependent upon more than reduced transmission and regulatory fixes. Health is socioeconomic and any health programme needs to address how disease risks are configured in particular socio-economic and cultural settings.

Surveillance for influenza

If modernised poultry production is hardly immune to infection, then a second line of defence is the early warning through a programme of scanning surveillance for newly emerging or re-emerging microbiological threats. But there are several reasons that make this less straightforward than it sounds.

First, surveying for microbes is rarely a matter of the presence or absence of known viruses (Hinchliffe and Lavau, 2013). Poultry surveys, for example, generally employ haemagglutinin inhibition (HI) tests of blood samples in order to trace previous infections such as antibodies within the blood of sampled birds that are produced in response to predetermined antigen (HA or haemagglutinin) proteins on the coats of viral particles. These tests are, however, dependent on responsive and clear immune responses in host birds, something that is not always easily assumed in intensive poultry houses. Responses and antibody production may be subdued or, conversely, 'noisy' as a result of maternally conferred immunity, co-infections and any previous vaccinations. It is also common for serological tests to produce positive results but for no live virus to be detected in the sample (so-called cryptic infections), suggesting either that infections have passed through or that the antibodies are being produced in response to a complex of conditions and microbial challenges. Meanwhile, the tests themselves need to be continually balanced as they may be over-sensitive, producing false positives, or conversely not sensitive enough, being overly specific to a suite of pathogen strains and therefore likely to miss any dangerous shifts or drifts in the virus and in immune responses. The complexity of this disease ecology and the attendant knowledge practices makes scanning surveillance less a matter of detecting known enemies and more a procedure of piecing together evidence from a variety of tests, learning to respond with various epistemic objects including HA proteins, viruses, red blood cells as well as population data and disease models, in order to build up a picture of viral circulations.

Second, surveillance is expensive and tends in most cases to be passive, proceeding after symptoms have been reported in domestic and/or wildlife flocks and herds. Yet, in the case of zoonotic influenza diseases, it is increasingly apparent that infections can often be asymptomatic or at least are expressed through a variety of often minor clinical symptoms. This inconsistency in terms of expression of symptoms for influenza virus lineages and sub-lineages and variations in the locations of virus attachment and therefore symptoms across different avian and mammal species groups makes disease surveillance for a segmented and highly mutable virus into a continuous challenge. The possibility for viruses that are dangerous to people circulating undetected in large domestic animal populations is therefore large. H7N9, a new 'Avian' Influenza that claimed over 100 human lives in China in the spring of 2013, is, for example, defined as low pathogenic in chicken and would not necessarily be picked up in a passive animal health surveillance system. Active surveillance, with randomised or risk-based sampling of apparently healthy animals, may be part of the answer. However, an industry with already tight margins and state-led reductions in public spending means that, apart from some key research programmes, maintaining let alone expanding the surveillance of a large and growing standing biomass of flu-susceptible life is difficult. In this context there are calls for smart surveillance (Daszak, 2009), or a focusing of scarce resources at key risk sites. However, being smart isn't simply a matter of directing scarce resources at specific at-risk loca-tions; it may also involve an acceptance of the systematic production of risks which are 'locational'. In this sense it should aim to draw together existing data in ways that can interpret mixed signals, understand indeterminacies in scientific practice (Fish *et al.*, 2011) and crucially develop a transdisciplinary approach to disease knowledge from veterinarians, medics, farmers, stock-people, ornitholo-gists and so on.

This need for an array of different knowledge practices and objects of concern – from the organism to the virus, to haemagglutinin proteins and reagents, and from populations to clinical signs in individual birds – suggests a requirement for an ontology of disease that is multiple rather than universal, accepting and care-fully combining the signals of health and disease. A transdisciplinary approach utilising health trend and anomaly data, for example, combines a broad set of knowledges in order to provide early warnings that may otherwise be missed.

This non-pathogen specific surveillance relies on 'producers, animal health technicians, and veterinarians [as well as slaughter personnel and laboratory scientists] that directly observe animals on an ongoing basis' (Scott *et al.*, 2012) to participate in disease surveillance. System specificity emerges in this case not through pathogen specificity but through the multiple reading and corroboration of often subtle signs within a variety of spaces and settings. It involves piecing together several practices and practitioners, each with different obligations, traditions and embedded uncertainties. Health is more than locating disease threats or contaminants; it is understanding the ecologies and configurations of viruses, hosts, responsive bodies, reagents and the stresses of production systems.

The general point is that not only is a collective approach to health interdisciplinary (something the OWOH concept emphasises); it transgresses disciplines and requires numerous objects, skills and the careful piecing together of the indications of that which makes health possible. In other words, it requires a multiple rather than single approach to disease, one that cannot be reduced to simple objects that need to be regulated and monitored but is rather the careful and highly skilled bringing together of numerous engagements with health and disease in order to provide a suitable diagnosis and guide healthy practices.

Keeping pigs safe

This requirement to assemble together those who observe and work with animals and microbes on a daily basis is taken further in my final case of health practices with pigs. Pigs have a 'potentially increased permeability to infection with influenza viruses of avian or human origin' (Brown and Done, 2013: 8) and act as mixing vessels for flus (Smith *et al.*, 2009). Contemporary long-distance movements of pigs, people and pig products mean that these influenzas can move rapidly. The 2009 pandemic swine flu (H1N1) strain, for example, moved quickly from its reported site of zoonosis in Mexico, to become a global pandemic in humans, and is now established and almost certainly endemic in global pig populations as a result of reverse zoonosis and highly efficient pig-to-pig transmission. This rapidity and flux is well known, but building up a detailed picture is difficult. Influenza surveillance and understanding in pigs is fraught with a series of challenges. Some of the complexities include: the co-circulation of highly segmented influenza A viruses that are subject to rapid re-assortments and antigenic drift; complex immune responses which introduce uncertainties into serological tests; and an industry that may be reluctant to look for and publish a disease burden. This complexity means that serology panels need to be regularly revalidated in order to confirm their suitability, and results of tests need to be examined across herds or populations 'to gain qualitatively correct interpretations' (Brown and Done, 2013: 9). In this sense, swine and avian influenzas are anything but self-same objects colliding with healthy bodies. Rather they are intricate and continuously changing knots of animals, people, viruses and economies, with which it is difficult to keep pace.

This picture of complexity and risk is countered within the industry by claims to have the highest levels of biosecurity. In the UK's commercial pig sector, and in the main, a system of closed herds is operated. In this, replacement stock is provided by companies who use a breeding pyramid of geographically separated nuclei, multiplier and commercial stock to either plan and deliver the genetics of a herd using artificial insemination or to send replacement gilts (young females) onto farms from secure or disease-free units. Ninety-eight per cent of UK pigs for slaughter are finished indoors (BPEX, 2013) in highly regulated conditions in an industry that has consolidated in the last decades, roughly following a US model of increasing the size and reducing the number of holdings (with most production now on 1400 or so farms with average herds of 500) (House of Commons, 2009). Breeding companies make use of an international network of remote nuclei and multiplier units to produce biosecure pigs, which are often termed, in the breeding industry, as disease-free or high health. And yet, farmers and field vets quickly translate these terms in practice (see Hinchliffe and Ward, 2014). Disease-free, for example, is soon translated by vets to 'specific pathogen-free', while vets and farmers use a variety of means to make sure that the naïve pigs entering or being born on the farm *gain* pathogens that are locally circulating in order that the pigs develop immunity and do not constitute a sero-negative sub-population which could accelerate viral circulation. Indeed, the first thing that happens to new arrivals on a pig unit is isolation (where infrastructure allows) to make sure incoming pigs are not sick pigs, followed by acclimatisation, and the latter often sees pristine, biosecure bodies covered in pig muck (from the farm) in order to make them, and the farm, safe. In this sense health again becomes not so much a single world in need of security, but the translation of contact, movement and communication into the more regular and regulated exchange, circulation and commerce. Indeed, contact, movement and communication are involved in the practices of making life safe. Likewise, as is the case for disease surveillance and understanding, farming practice is not so much a matter of a single world or universe of self-identical objects, which collide and cause effects, but a complex of objects that can both attack *and* condition life (Napier, 2012). Farming pigs safely is likewise not only about establishing boundaries and excluding microbes, of halting transmission, but requires an approach to health that patches together or manages (in the sense of caring for and continuously monitoring and adjusting) life. Indeed, it may well be that the pursuit of a single world of disease-free farming could endanger the very localised and contingent practices that make safe life a possibility (Hinchliffe and Ward, 2014). Hypertrophic security, as is well known, often produces the conditions of possibility for new dangers. And as the critique of one world-ism suggests, this form of one world-ism can reduce biological and social difference rather than manage its role in conditioning life and making health possible.

Conclusions

A one world-ist ontology, to repeat Law's characterisation, involves a world of objects and collisions, of single truths and of Western triumphalism. In turn, there is a tendency to prioritise certain understandings or enactments of disease and

global health security, emphasising contamination over configuration, and a normative programme of extending controlled forms of agricultural practice and surveillance. In passing I note that this cannot help but produce two worlds divided along
the lines of the virtuous and the pathological. And yet, as the empirical engagements have demonstrated, even in the so-called core of this one world-ist world,
life is pathological. That is, the objects of disease are never straightforward, virtu-
osity and regulation never quite eliminate contingency and movement, and farming
well requires practices that engage with rather than eliminate biological difference.
So, sick birds and HPAI risks are not solely found in backyard or unregulated
systems. The configurations of intense contractual markets can produce the conditions for viral chatter. In this account, disease objects become so entangled with the
bio-social and technological approaches to farming that new kinds of risk and
disease object can emerge. Such objects are slippery, difficult to monitor and
require a pooling of not only veterinary and medical expertise but also draw upon
a range of practitioners, scientific, lay, professional and amateur, in order to identify
the locational aspects of disease risk. Finally, the patching together of health, on
farms and in other settings, suggests that disease and health are not, in practice,
regarded as things that can be divided into separate spheres. Pig keepers and their
vets understand that health is something of an achievement, a patching together or
reconfiguring of good husbandry practices, promoting immune responses, vaccinations, sourcing and matching stock and so on.

   To be clear, nothing I have said here disqualifies the One Health intention of
focusing on the synergies and mutual advantages of improving human, animal
and environmental health. The common sense with which I started holds, as does
the requirement to critique any version of global health that is narrowly premised
on human communities. Clearly, health is a multi-species matter. Likewise, the
will to develop interdisciplinary modes of working across previously separate
domains of health is, if anything, amplified in the accounts I have given here. In
engaging with some of the practices involved in doing health, I have highlighted
the need to uncouple a one world-ist metaphysics from this aspect of One Health,
especially when such a metaphysics elevates contamination, simple objects and
spatial divisions over attending to the various configurations, complex things and
relations that make health and disease. I have suggested that working towards
shared health across species lines and locational specificities requires a recognition of the multiple dimensions of health. This is not to say that health is culturally
relative, but it is to recognise and value the continuous work that is carried out on
farms, in laboratories and elsewhere in order to produce healthy outcomes. This
requires a new common sense, and a finer grained approach towards global health.
It is one that brings together and interrogates rather than romanticises the various
knowledge practices that make health possible across these domains. It also
suggests, perhaps, that the physical model underpinning a one-world-ist approach
where objects collide and cause effects is replaced with a more chemical model.
Here, objects transform as they undertake new relations and form compound
things that alter as they move. It is this dynamism and polymorphism that underpins a sense of more than one health, more than one world.

References

BPEX (2013). British Pig Executive Website. Available at http://www.bpex.org.uk/prices-facts-figures/industry-structure/UKpigbreedingherd.aspx.

Braun, B. (2007). Biopolitics and the molecularization of life. *Cultural Geographies* 14, 6–28.

Briggs, C.L. (2005). Communicability, racial discourse, and disease. *Annual Review of Anthropology* 34, 269–291.

Brown, H. and A.H. Kelly (2014). Material proximities and hotspots: Towards an anthropology of Viral Haemorrhagic Fevers. *Medical Anthropology Quarterly*, doi: 10.1111/maq.12092.

Brown, I.H. and S.H. Done (2013). Current risks and developments with influenza in UK swine populations. *The Pig Journal* 68, 8–11.

Chien, Y-J. (2012). How did international agencies perceive the avian influenza problem? The adoption and manufacture of the 'One World, One Health' framework. *Sociology of Health and Illness* 35(2): 213–226.

Cooper, M. (2008). *Life as Surplus: Biotechnology and Capitalism in the Neoliberal Order*. Seattle: University of Washington Press.

Cosgrove, D. (1994). Contested global visions: One-world, whole-earth, and the Apollo space photographs. *Annals of the Association of American Geographers* 84, 270–294.

Daszak, P. (2009). A call for smart surveillance: A lesson learned from H1N1. *EcoHealth* 6, 1–2.

FAO, OIE and WHO (2010). The FAO–OIE–WHO collaboration: Sharing responsibilities and coordinating global activities to address health risks at the anima–human–ecosystems interfaces: A Tripartite Concept Note. Available at http://www.who.int/influenza/resources/documents/tripartite_concept_note_hanoi_042011_en.pdf. O. FAO, WHO. Rome, Paris, Geneva.

Farmer, P. (2004). *Pathologies of Power*. Berkeley: University of California Press.

Fish, R., Z. Austin, R. Christley, P.M. Haygarth, L. Heathwaite, S. Latham, W. Medd, M. Mort, D.M. Oliver, R. Pickup, J.M. Wastling. and B. Wynne. (2011). Uncertainties in the governance of animal disease: An interdisciplinary framework for analysis. *Philosophical Transactions of the Royal Society B* 366, 2023–2034.

Forster, P. (2011). Risk, modernity and the H5N1 virus in action in Indonesia: A multi-sited study of the threats of avian and human pandemic influenza. Ph.D., University of Sussex.

Gibbs, E.P.J. (2014). The evolution of One Health: A decade of progress and challenges for the future. *Veterinary Record* 174, 85–91

Godley, A. and B. Williams (2008). The chicken, the factory farm and the supermarket: The emergence of the modern poultry industry in Britain. In *Food Chains: Provisioning, from Farmyard to Shopping Cart*, ed. W. Belasco and R. Horowitz. Philadelphia: University of Pennsylvania Press, pp. 47–61.

Godley, A. and B. Williams (2009). Democratizing luxury and the contentious 'invention of the technological chicken' in Britain. *Business History Review* 83(summer), 267–290.

Gramsci, A. (1971). *Selections from the Prison Notebooks*. London: Lawrence and Wishart.

Hinchliffe, S. (2013). The insecurity of biosecurity: Re-making emerging infectious diseases. In *Biosecurity: The Socio-politics of Invasive Species and Infectious Diseases*. In A. Dobson, K. Barker and S. Taylor. London: Earthscan/Routledge, pp. 199–213.

Hinchliffe, S., J. Allen, S. Lavau, N. Bingham and S. Carter, (2013). Biosecurity and the topologies of infected life: From borderlines to borderlands. *Transactions of the Institute of British Geographers* 38(4), 531–543.

Hinchliffe, S. and N. Bingham (2008). Securing life – the emerging practices of biosecurity. *Environment and Planning A* 40, 1534–1551.

Hinchliffe, S., N. Bingham, J. Allen and S. Carter (2016). *Pathological Lives: Disease, Space and Biopolitics*. London: Wiley Blackwell.

Hinchliffe, S. and S. Lavau (2013). Differentiated circuits: The ecologies of knowing and securing life. *Environment and Planning D: Society and Space* 31, 259–274.

Hinchliffe, S. and K. J. Ward (2014). Geographies of folded life: How immunity reframes biosecurity. *Geoforum* 53, 136–144.

House of Commons (2009). The English pig industry: First report of Session 2008–9. House of Commons – Environment, Food and Rural Affairs Committee. London.

Humphrey, T.J. (2006). Are happy chickens safer chickens? Poultry welfare and disease susceptibility. *British Poultry Science* 47, 379–391.

Humphrey, T. J., S. O'Brien and M. Madsen (2007). Campylobacters as zoonotic pathogens: A food production perspective. *International Journal of Food Microbiology* 117, 237–257.

Kelly, A., B. Osburn and S. Salman (2014). Veterinary medicine's increasing role in global health. *The Lancet Global Health* 2, 379–380.

King, N.B. (2002). Security, disease, commerce: Ideologies of postcolonial global health. *Social Studies of Science* 32(5–6), 763–789.

Lakoff, A. (2010). Two regimes of global health. *Humanity: An International Journal of Human Rights, Humanitarianism, and Development* 1(1), 59–79.

Law, J. (2011). What's wrong with a one-world world? Available at http://www. heterogeneities.net/publications/Law2011WhatsWrongWithAOneWorldWorld.pdf.

Leach, M., I. Scoones and A. Stirling (2010). Governing epidemics in an age of complexity: Narratives, politics and pathways to sustainability. *Global Environmental Change* 20, 369–377.

Lowe, C. (2010). Viral clouds: Becoming H5N1 in Indonesia. *Cultural Antrhopology* 25(4): 625–649.

Mitropoulos, A. (2012). *Contract & Contagion: From Biopolitics to Oikonomia*. New York: Minor Compositions.

Mol, A. (1999). Ontological politics, a word and some questions. In *Actor Network Theory and After*, ed. J. Law and J. Hassard. Oxford and Keele: Blackwell/Sociological Review, pp. 74–89.

Mol, A. (2002). *The Body Multiple: Ontology in Medical Practice*. Durham, NC: Duke University Press.

Mol, A. and J. Law (1994). Regions, networks and fluids: Anaemia and social topology. *Social Studies of Science* 24, 641–671.

Napier, A.D. (2012). Non-self help: How immunology might reframe the enlightenment. *Cultural Anthropology* 27(1), 122–137.

Peiris, J.S.M., M.D. de Jong and Y. Guan (2007). Avian Influenza Virus (H5N1): A threat to human health. *Clinical Microbiology Reviews* 20(2), 243–267.

Porter, N. (2013). Bird flu biopower: Strategies for multi-species coexistence in Vietnam. *American Ethnologist* 40(1), 132–148.

Rosenberg, C.E. (1992). *Explaining Epidemics: And Other Studies in the History of Medicine*. Cambridge: Cambridge University Press.

Scoones, I. and P. Forster (2011). Unpacking the international responses to Avian Influenza: Science, policy and politics. In *Avian Influenza*, ed. I. Scoones. London: Earthscan, pp. 19–64.

Scott, A.E., K.W. Forsythe and C.L. Johnson (2012). National animal health surveillance: Return on investment. *Preventive Veterinary Medicine* 105, 265–270.

Shukin, N. (2009). *Animal Capital: Rendering Life in Biopolitical Times*. Minneapolis: University of Minnesota Press.

Smith, G.J.D., D. Vijaykrishna, J. Bahl, S. Lycett, M. Worobey, O. Pybus, S.K. Ma, C.L. Cheung, J. Raghwani, S. Bhatt, J.S.M. Peiris, Y. Guan and A. Rambaut (2009). Origins and evolutionary genomics of the 2009 swine-origin H1N1 influenza A epidemic. *Nature* 459, 1122–1126.

Stengers, I. (2010). Including nonhumans in political theory: Opening Pandora's box? In *Political Matter: Technoscience, Democracy, and Public Life*, ed. B. Braun and S. Whatmore. Minneapolis: University of Minnestoa Press, pp. 3–33.

Wald, P. (2008). *Contagious: Cultures, Carriers, and the Outbreak Narrative*. Durham, NC: Duke University Press.

Wolfe, N. (2011). *The Viral Storm*. London: Penguin.

Wolfe, N., P. Daszak, A.M. Kilpatrick and D.S. Burke (2005). Bushmeat hunting, deforestation, and prediction of zoonotic disease emergence. *Emerging Infectious Diseases* 11(12), 1822–1827.

Wolfe, N., C.P. Dunavan and J. Diamond (2007). Origins of major human infectious diseases. *Nature* 447, 279–283.

Yu, H., J.T. Wu, B.J. Cowling, Q. Liao, V.J. Fang, S. Zhou, P. Wu, H. Zhou, E.H.Y. Lau, D. Guo, M.Y. Ni, Z. Peng, L. Feng, H. Luo, Q. Li, Z. Feng, D.W.Y.Yu Wang and G.M. Leung (2014). Effect of closure of live poultry markets on poultry-to-person transmission of avian influenza A H7N9 virus: An ecological study. *The Lancet* 383(9196), 541–548.

10 The needs of the 'other' global health

The case of Remote Area Medical

Paul Jackson and Caitlin Henry

> They may be poor, but that does not mean they don't work and in many cases work 7 days a week. They just can't make enough to support their family in all directions. You see, they may be able to put food on the table and pay their electric bills, but they can't do that AND pay for all the doctor's co-pays and high deductibles or pay for the dentist when they need a filling. They are always just one pay check from losing it all and falling yet more and more behind. 'That kind of stress can weigh on a person – you know,' says one man attending a RAM clinic. 'It's every day, all the time. One simple flat tire on my truck could mean the difference of buying groceries. Life right now makes you face hard choices that no one wants to make. The kind of choices like which child gets to go to the dentist or the fear of someone needing a pair of glasses. We just can't afford it. And if it means me as a dad or my kids getting care, it will be my kids every time. What does that mean for me? I am last. I hardly get the care I need. I can't give the time away from work and can't afford to help my kids and myself too.' (*sic*)
>
> —'Stop the Suffering in Appalachia', *Remote Area Medical Magazine* (2014a)

New York City, Thanksgiving weekend, 2014, 7000 people were estimated to attend a free health clinic put on by the organisation Remote Area Medical (RAM). This pop-up clinic of dental, vision and medical care was to be held at the Javits Center that usually hosts technology expos and clothing trade shows, blocks away from Times Square.[1] The New York Governor's office shut down the clinic because doctors were not allowed to cross state lines to practise medicine, even if they are not being financially reimbursed for the work. New York City – one of the richest cities in the world and recently scared by doctors and nurses coming back from West Africa's Ebola epidemic – could not give away free healthcare, despite the overwhelming demand. This geography of need indicates the persistence of health inequality in the USA, echoed in the testimonial above. Despite recent developments of the Affordable Care Act (ACA), essential healthcare services still fall on a wide variety of community clinics, non-profits, street health and non-governmental organisations. How then can we understand this situation where the USA is both known for being a major player in global health and at the same time is known for massive health inequality?

Global health lacks a precise definition. The anthropologist Arthur Kleinman (2010: 1518) says, 'Global health . . . is more a bunch of problems than a discipline.' Rather than attempting to understand global health as a single entity, we ask what work the modifier "global" does when applied to health. Does it signal market integration, neoliberalism and proposals of a flat world? Does it lead to thinking of the spaces of logistics, pharmaceutical commodity chains, or NGOs deploying people and resources? The meaning and spatial imagination of global health is widely debated outside the discipline of geography (see overviews by Brown *et al.*, 2006; Bozorgmehr, 2010; Lakoff, 2010). We suggest that geographers can contribute to defining global health through careful attention to specific locations and cases, supported by the discipline's extensive interrogation of how geographies are both produced and uneven (Smith, 1984; Harvey, 2006). Geographical difference has long been a crucial debate in understanding the world, to the point that the global scale has been taken apart as too limiting (Marston *et al.*, 2005). In addition, the geographies of health and inequality are currently being 'revised and reterritorialised' according to Matt Sparke (2009: 132) through neoliberalism and recent austerity regimes.

In response, we take a page from Paul Farmer (1999, 2005, 2006) and other medical anthropologists (Nguyen, 2010; Scheper-Hughes, 1993; Biehl and Petryna, 2013b; Petryna, 2002) who have long paid close attention to the lived experience of global health inequalities. Through the case of RAM, this chapter will show how the spatial imagination of global health obscures the urgent need for care work within the USA in places that Meyers and Hunt (2014) call the 'other global South'. We will discuss how to interrogate these 'other' global health geographies, and return to the social justice roots of primary healthcare of the 1970s (Cueto, 2004). Focusing on the 'other' global health inverts the development paradigm which implicitly assumes that assistance comes from the Global North and is given to the Global South. We propose that this 'other' global health emphasises a relational geography of need and care that is fundamentally uneven. A grounded, embodied and material definition of health, built upon a foundation of material resources and workers, highlights the differences *between* New York City and Freetown, as well as *within* them. We focus on care work and access to resources in our analysis because, as Farmer (2014) summed up while visiting Liberia during the recent Ebola epidemic, 'Without staff, stuff, space and systems, nothing can be done'. Through an analysis of the work of Remote Area Medical, this chapter attempts to rethink the 'global' of global health by considering other uneven geographies of care work and the politics of health access in the USA. When we put the patients and the volunteer work of RAM at the centre of global health, this opens up the question of need and necessity that transforms health into a particular articulation of social reproduction. Accordingly, envisioning health as social reproduction requires an analysis of labour and an overt politicisation of care.

Introducing RAM and rethinking remote geographies

The extreme unevenness of healthcare provision and access within the USA prompted the founder of RAM to rethink his own practice of *doing* global health.

RAM began in the mid-1980s as a volunteer airborne medical relief corps that provided services to the Global South, specifically communities in Guyana, Haiti, Dominican Republic, Honduras, Guatemala, East Africa, India, Nepal and others (Brock and Wilson, 2011). Stan Brock – a nature lover who co-hosted the television show *Mutual of Omaha's Wild Kingdom* in the 1970s – founded RAM after experiencing the isolation from medical care of the Wapishana indigenous people in Guyana. Since then RAM has expanded, as Brock explains, to provide care 'to thousands around the world in similar conditions. In other words, there are Wapishanas everywhere.' Based in Knoxville, Tennessee, RAM go where they are invited. In the early 1990s they began to receive invitations from neighbouring counties after getting local press coverage for their international work. As word spread, the demand for their services began to overwhelm their occasional clinics. Consequentially, RAM's mission includes regular monthly clinics in the USA, surpassing 60 per cent of their 'expeditions' (Brock and Wilson, 2011; Whitney, 2009; Goodman, 2009; Remote Area Medical, 2015). Initially focused on rural Appalachia, RAM could no longer ignore the medical 'isolation' of large segments of the population across the entire country. For RAM, North/South binaries and international development narratives did not constrict what isolation from health meant.

We argue that with this geographic shift back to the USA, RAM effectively changed the definition of 'remote'. Here, then, *remote becomes relational* and is no longer limited to physical distance between two positions (in the tradition of the core–periphery paradigm of international development). Rather than a static geography, remote should be seen as a fluctuating relationship of support from care workers and access to resources, including livelihoods, food, water and other necessities for survival. Remote here means proximity and access to capital, both physically and socially. Thus, many residents of New York City, the centre of global capital, can find themselves remote from health, even if they can see a hospital from their front stoop. These residents become isolated from health services through such factors as finances, employment, housing and navigating government bureaucracy. For RAM, the definition of isolation and remoteness is rooted in human suffering, pain and need. This stretches our understanding of space and distance, and highlights the stark segregation that exists even in wealthy cities. Patients and the volunteers of RAM experience a form of 'global health' through intimate and embodied relationships of care work (Pratt and Rosner, 2012; Mountz and Hyndman, 2006). Remote thus refers to attainability rather than simply proximity, making inherently political the spatial analyses of health-care access.

We propose situating health in care work, the suffering of bodies and structural inequalities. While the meaning of health has long been debated, especially within the subdisciplines of health and medical geography (Brown *et al.*, 2009; Dyck, 2003; Greenhough, 2011; Kearns and Moon, 2002; Sparke, 2014), others have argued that health, as a term, is increasingly a conceptual block, something to be worked against (Metzl and Kirkland, 2010). To bypass this obstruction the philospher and historian of science Georges Canguilhem in *The Normal and The*

Pathological helps by reversing the category of health. Canguilhem (1989: 148; see also Philo, 2007) writes, 'Health is a set of securities and assurances . . . securities in the present, assurances for the future. . . . To be in good health means being able to fall sick and recover, it is a biological luxury.' This reversal suggests that health is not some a priori pure state of bodily integrity. Disease is not introduced into purity; rather, disease reduces one's tolerance to ongoing environmental and biological processes. From this perspective, then, disease can be framed as the whittling away of structures of biological and social support. Translated into the language of RAM: disease is suffering. A life of luxury (or health) is the absolute reduction of suffering supported by either privilege or collective social formations (such as national healthcare, insurance or political mobilisation). Global health's fixation on places such as Liberia as 'pathological' implies that the USA is 'normal', and this hinders explanations about how these geographies are produced and where people in need are located. Accordingly, the Global North is not inherently healthy and countries in the Global South are not inherently sick or 'failed' health states. Instead, privileges accrue for some while support is diminished for others, or impeded through histories of capitalism, colonialism, imperialism, racism and patriarchy. To counter this diminishment, Jenna Loyd gives a very particular formulation of health in her book *Health Rights are Civil Rights*. She envisions health as 'individual *and* collective bodily self-determination' (Loyd, 2014: 2, emphasis added). This version also avoids the 'normal and pathological' binary that limits the imaginations of doctors, experts and policy makers. Health must be a necessarily political definition for Loyd, even prefiguratively political. Combining individual politics with collective social formations, Loyd crucially focuses on bodies – both singular and collective – through everyday politics and everyday life. Put together, health is not about achieving a position of privilege (luxury), but depends on politics, advocacy and social justice (self-determination). Finally, a political health project does not stop at the body or a medical procedure, but starts, in the words of RAM, to 'generate a people's movement' for 'community transformation'.

This formulation of heath contextualises RAM's work of delivering assistance to those in need. RAM's motto is 'Stop Pain, End Suffering'. By starting with pain and suffering, RAM recasts health as a lived experience rather than producing pure bodies by way of technological and pharmaceutical fixes. RAM shifts the debate away from defining what health *is* to think about what health *work does*: the work of stopping and ending. Our emphasis on health work is echoed by recent calls in geography (Connell and Walton-Roberts, 2015; Andrews and Evans, 2008); yet we follow RAM by putting suffering before the medical profession. Similarly, anthropologists Biehl and Petryna in their introduction to *When People Come First* (2013a: 4) suggest that 'disease is never just one thing, technology delivery does not translate into patient care' and ask a question relevant to RAM's work: 'By what trajectories and means do the people who desperately need care access it (or fail to access it)?' To help answer this question, we suggest thinking of global health along a spectrum. The right side of the spectrum is dominated by magic bullets (drug development, biomedical research, logistics, management consultants) and the left side builds upon collective self-determination (political organising, care work and the everyday struggles of survival). We suggest that global health needs to lean more to the left, and pay attention to the workers and patients in the multiple geographies where suffering exists.

Global health or uneven burdens?

According to Brown and colleagues' history (2006: 63), global health emerged in the 1990s as a discourse that evoked intergovernmental affairs, international relations and universal rights, while at the same time the term was dismissed as 'meaningless jargon' by some leaders in the field. Global health combines contradictory programmes and abandoned paradigms (such as tropical medicine, primary health-care and international health) that was guided for a time by the World Health Organisation (Brown *et al.*, 2006; see also Garret, 2013); however, there is currently no single coordinating agency. Global health is now a patchwork of international agencies and organisations ill-fitted for dealing with global health concerns. The name is misleading, since, as we argue, the global does not mean healing the entire global population. For critics, global health was a re-articulation of the colonial efforts of the International Sanitary Conferences of the nineteenth century (Brown, 2011; see also Arnold, 1993) that locked in the relationship of knowledge and resources moving from Global North to South in order to reduce the global burden of disease, most recently HIV/AIDS, malaria and tuberculosis (Ingram, 2009; Koplan et al., 2009). Therefore global health cannot be disentangled from colonialism and imperialism, and any new formulation and geopolitical encounter is read through that history. For Lakoff (2010: 59), there are 'two contemporary regimes for envisioning and intervening in the field of global health: global health security and humanitarian biomedicine . . . [and] each envision a form of social life that requires the fulfilment of an innovative technological project'. This technological project has been profoundly shaped by philanthro-capitalism (McGoey, 2012, 2014; McGoey *et al.*, 2011), as the Bill and Melinda Gates Foundation dominates the landscapes of funding and drug development. Global health is locked into biomedical and geopolitical registers. Expertise fixates upon how diseases affect multiple countries and solutions arise from biomedical innovations (Koplan *et al.*, 2009; Bozorgmehr, 2010). While global health cannot exist outside markets and states, we chose to look elsewhere, away from the global health complex and its blind obsession over pharmaceutical solutions. The danger is in taking these global health geographies and solutions for granted, and conceding our imaginations to the likes of Bill Gates who envision entrepreneurs as the true healers.

In response, we suggest focusing on the care work happening in 'other' places. In critiquing global health's fixation on the Global South, Meyers and Hunt (2014) propose that there is the 'other global South' found in disinvested communities like Detroit with abandoned hospitals and suffering people. They do not suggest that we must compare and contrast the needs of places like Detroit and Dhaka since that hinders our understanding of who is included and excluded from global health. We support Meyer and Hunt's critiques of global health's overdetermined development paradigm; however, why re-inscribe this North–South geographic binary? We suggest dropping the 'South' and instead we ask: Where are all the 'other' spaces of global health? This refocuses attention on more spatially variegated questions about who is injured and where they are suffering. Meyers and Hunt (2014: 1921) explain:

> Illness is but one injury. If entangled with other forms or situations of lack and insult, injury may be hard to quantify but even harder to ignore. . . . a focus on specific forms of harm and their consequences is a valuable analytic starting point for broadening discussions and practices of global health.

Suffering, injury and pain are also where RAM start their work. Each individual injury requires collective responses. The point is that injuries are unevenly produced and the burdens of care are unevenly carried. To declare that there are pockets of the 'third world' in the USA is an important rhetorical manoeuvre; however, the harder work is to care for those inflicted by the consequences of the structural inequities that produce these 'other' spaces. Franz Fanon says that '[in medicine] there is always an opposition of exclusive worlds, a contradictory inter-action of different techniques, a vehement confrontation of values' (in Meyers and Hunt, 2014: 1922). The remoteness of the 'other' global health means getting *close* to the inherent contradictions in care work's embodied interactions. The political point is to dismantle these asymmetries and processes of exclusion, not merely plot the geographic coordinates of the wretched places of the earth.

Our argument here is not to suggest that global health institutions, in particular funding and projects emerging from the USA, only engage with domestic health problems. We believe that it is more productive to start by examining, following Chouinard (2013), how injury, impairment and disability is produced and embodied in the context of a global capitalist order. She suggests that there is 'a particular corporeal class order' that constructs 'able' bodies as normal, exalted and valued, and disabled bodies as abnormal, abject and devalued. RAM's work in the USA demonstrates how this 'corporeal class system that orders and regulates bodies' is international in scope, yet 'geographically uneven in its outcomes' (Chouinard, 2013: 342). These uneven burdens weigh more heavily on bodies in the Global South and the 'other Global South', along with those who take care of them.

David Harvey's work is helpful in focusing on how these burdens and privileges are unevenly produced. Indeed, as he writes,

> [T]he uneven geographical development of social infrastructures is, in the final analysis, reproduced through the circulation of capital. . . . The social geography which evolves is not, however, a mere mirror reflection of capital's needs, but the locus of powerful and potentially disruptive contradictions.
>
> (Harvey, 2006: 401)

The vast array of global health institutions – from the WHO to the Gates Foundation to RAM – illustrate how these social infrastructures of health do not work as a coherent whole but attempt to mitigate the consequences of uneven development. Contradictions can therefore be pulled apart in the differences: between private health and public health; paid and unpaid care work; that injury and illness exists surrounded by wealth. For example, while RAM has a similar mission to MSF, RAM's temporary and pop-up clinic delivery system does not even provide basic needs (food, water, shelter) nor, according to Redfield's (2013: 18) notion of minimal biopolitics, does it provide 'contemporary functions of governing, if on a minimal, immediate scale'. Global health then is not something to be optimised and perfected; instead it is a particular geographic formulation among many that embodies the contradictions of capital at this particular time.

These contradictions are not new. In the late 1960s and 1970s, politics, social justice and calls for structural transformation through health rose to the surface within international organisations like the WHO. According to Cueto's history, primary healthcare emerged as a response to the overemphasis in the 1950s on: vertical international health programmes; elitism within the medical profession; and the obsession with disease-oriented technologies (Cueto, 2004, 2005). Promoted by many of the decolonising nations of that era, primary healthcare was grounded in social justice and calls for 'Healthcare for All by 2000'. As Cueto (2004: 1871) says, 'In its more radical version, primary health care was an adjunct to social revolution'. However, almost immediately this international movement was eroded and supplanted with a turn to 'selective' primary healthcare that focused on metrics and deliverables (what WHO official Kenneth Newell called a 'counter-revolution'). Primary health care became mired in the struggle of two competing visions of how to achieve health: utopian versus pragmatic. In the Global South, primary healthcare continues through organisations like Partners in Health (Farmer *et al.*, 2006) while in the Global North it is about optimising services and access in the health sector (Crooks and Andrews, 2009) or invoked for calls for increased funding for community clinics (Brock, 2014). The dismantlement of a justice-based primary healthcare coincided with the rise of neoliberalism of the 1980s and the rollback of state services, along with deindustrialisation throughout the USA. Stan Brock and RAM, it may be argued, is a continuation of that original social justice-based primary healthcare movement. As the global utopian dreams began falling apart, he put a dentist's chair in the back of his pick-up truck and began to do the work, quietly and without fanfare. Rather than focusing on funding or metrics, Brock focused on where people were in pain and needed glasses. Although not necessarily a model of efficiency or efficacy, we argue that Brock's efforts represent a rethinking of global health centred on need. He asked the geographic question: Where is the need? We follow Brock to focus on social reproduction and put care work as the foundation of the 'other' global health: a return to those utopian roots of the primary healthcare lineage.

The case of RAM

Stan Brock's oft-repeated origin story of RAM is grounded in a rethinking of time and space, along with a reckoning with distance. As he tells it, Brock was in

Guyana in the 1950s working with the Wapishana community on large cattle operations (he says he 'became a cowboy in a place where all the cowboys were Indians'). He was injured and was told that the nearest doctor was 26 days away on foot. Later, when telling this story to the astronaut Ed Mitchell, the astronaut's response was: 'Gosh, I was on the moon and I was only three days away from the nearest doctor.'[2] This contradiction drove Brock to bring doctors 'closer' to those in need. For Brock, the distance of the 26-day walk in Guyana hid more than it revealed. That Guyana was effectively more remote than the moon in terms of access to healthcare demonstrates how distance is not merely a geographic category but is also reconfigured through investment, funding and priorities. The body of an astronaut marshals more attention and support than a single mother in Appalachia. RAM does not focus on epidemics, bed nets or clean water, but on bodies suffering or in pain. Accordingly, their primary services are general medical services; dental (cleanings, fillings, extractions); vision (dilated eye examinations, testing for glaucoma, testing for diabetic retinopathy, glasses made on site); prevention (breast examinations, diabetes screening, physicals, women's health); and education (resources and information provided throughout service areas). RAM's work is therefore more akin to triage than to public health or health promotion.

Remoteness has taken on a new meaning over the past 30 years, as speed of travel and logistical infrastructures have only increased the time–space compression. This myth of a 'small world' of immediate connections has led to the assumption that nothing is remote anymore. However, new technological developments have not completely annihilated the spaces of injury or sickness. RAM has actually witnessed a growing demand for their services by large segments of the US population. Starting with a pick-up truck and one dentist's chair driving around the Amazon, RAM has expanded slowly with more equipment and more volunteers. Using similar methods of setting up mobile clinics in remote areas in foreign countries, RAM creates temporary spaces of care in stadiums, conventions centres, schools and airports throughout the USA. With more than 600 'expeditions' after 30 years of work, RAM remains a charitable, no-cost and all-volunteer organisation. RAM has also received very little corporate support; by 2009 they only had one or two corporate donors. Brock says he would love fuel donations from an oil company because that is their biggest cost (Goodman, 2009).

Brock sets the tone of RAM and his presence is fairly incongruous: an elderly, yet fit, charismatic British man in a beige flight suit who is 'on expedition' in the rural mountains of Appalachia. Brock, now in his late seventies, 'has no money and no possessions and subsists mainly on the oatmeal and fruit given to him by friends. He often sleeps on the floor' (Whitney, 2009). The other senior members of RAM also wear flight suits that give a military tenor to their calling as a 'Volunteer Corps'. Yet RAM is merely the spark around which gather a wide-ranging assortment of local volunteers, including doctors, nurses, church groups, Lions Clubs, dental/medical schools and state-level service providers, along with individual volunteers throughout the region who have heard about these clinics and want to help in any way they can. RAM is not religious, yet many who volunteer embody Christianity through prayer, and the call to be a Good Samaritan. RAM has started to become media savvy; however, this may not be by design but rather as a response to the intermittent national media attention their work has received. While RAM wants to run more clinics, there is no indication that they want to 'scale up' their organisation. By focusing on suffering, RAM's care work remains horizontal, diffuse and localised. The pop-up nature of their clinics relies almost entirely on volunteer labour that divides the care work according to tasks: parking and camping provision, intake and data collection, emergency and specialised medical services, cooking for the volunteers, and even basic patient navigation around the chaotic clinics. The volunteers do the same task all day long (either pulling teeth, entering data or helping patients find their queues). Secondary volunteer services are also pop-up, but are entirely dependent on specific volunteers that might give away free clothing, massages or counselling, along with lunches and snacks for those waiting in line. RAM relies on volunteers to provide 'no-cost healthcare'; however, the price comes in the form of disarray, inherent to an organisation that flies by the seat of its pants. While chaotic and the work repetitive, volunteers witness lines upon lines of suffering patients over the entire weekend, along with many more who are turned away.

At each clinic, many attendees drive long distances and wait for days for the chance to receive basic health services. RAM is not the only free health clinic in the USA. A 2010 survey found 1007 clinics that serve and do not charge 1.8 million people, accounting for 3.5 million medical and dental visits. Of that number, 58.7 per cent receive no government funding (Darnell, 2010). What distinguishes RAM is their practice of setting up temporary clinics. Both the care workers and the patients require mobility. Need and service provision, therefore, are not anchored in place. Rather, these pop-up clinics are simultaneously spatially specific while also dynamic, fluid and moveable. RAM seizes on this aspect of their work saying:

> The healthcare crisis in America has reached a point where people are becoming 'weekend refugees' to simply get basic medical attention. At any given RAM Clinic you will find those so desperate that they sleep for days in their car with their entire family in all kinds of conditions to find help.
>
> (Remote Area Medical, 2014b: 36)

By reframing their patients as geopolitically displaced populations due to war and famine, RAM's implicit political critique turns the USA into a 'failed state', but only for some.

We are suggesting that putting the patients and volunteers of RAM at the centre of global health questions how health gaps between populations become naturalised and how vulnerability for some becomes subsumed into a universal condition. The 'other' global health disrupts the North–South binaries and imaginations that dictate the terrain of care provision. Brown and Moon (2012) have questioned the call around 'closing the gap' in global health, along with the struggle to create a bridge across health disparities. However, we emphasise how these gaps are *produced* for particular people in particular places through remoteness. Gaps are not merely inequitable or inefficient access to resources, but how people and communities become displaced, dispossessed and distanced from necessary care. For those waiting in line for days at a RAM clinic, pulling a rotten tooth does not make the gap disappear because health gaps are deeply intertwined with job and care gaps, to say nothing of class, gender and race. RAM attendees are vulnerable, but this precariousness is particular to each person. While the head of the WHO claims that 'vulnerability is universal', Brown (2011) shows how this understanding of vulnerability is confined to a longer history of fears of pandemics. This version of vulnerability fixates on the speed of disease transmission and predictions of the 'coming plague'. To counter this fixation on the speed of outbreaks, we suggest focusing on how slow violence (Nixon, 2011) and slow death (Berlant, 2007) contribute to isolation. In the 'other' global health that starts from suffering and injury, vulnerability shifts from nebulous prediction to lived experience. For RAM attendees, a vulnerable life changes when a person loses their job or receives a set of free eyeglasses.

Supplies and demands: health, care and social reproduction

The different ways in which people and communities are made remote – geographically, but also socially and economically – are glossed over by global health's development and geopolitical paradigms. People become remote in terms of their distance from capital, along with the power, agency and health that privilege affords. Everyday suffering becomes invisible when analyses of global health become stuck at the scale of the nation state and focused on geopolitical relations. In other words, the development paradigm of global health obscures need. Care, by contrast, is necessarily grounded in the interactions among people. Care must happen with or on bodies in need, at the scale of the body. Workers and patients can move, but the need is situated in the body and bodies become isolated. However, these are not permanent designations. Care and need constitute a dynamic geography of remoteness and proximity to capital. So, while suffering embodies isolation, care work brings the remoteness of pain 'closer' to collective social formations based on redistributed surpluses of labour and capital. The defining questions of the 'other' global health are: Who does the work of care, and how is the care organised?

Health needs and care deficits

The growing demand for RAM's services illustrates the care deficits that punctuate the uneven geographies of the USA. A care deficit refers to the lack of care provisioning available in a society (Raghuram, 2012; Hochschild, 2000). This includes both paid and unpaid care workers – from parents to domestic workers to nurses and doctors. Structures of caring, such as a healthcare system, may be inadequate for meeting the health needs of the population; thus emerges a structural care deficit that can be national and global (Aiken, 2007; Raghuram et al., 2009; Ross *et al.*, 2005). As the US population ages, more people will need long-term and end-of-life care, yet the system is too small, under-resourced and under-staffed to meet the growing health needs in the coming decades (Guo and Castillo, 2012; Poo, 2015). The healthcare system overall is in deficit, with large and small pockets across the country deep in the red. Volunteer groups like RAM attempt to push this deficit into the black. Global health does little to help us understand this shifting labour geography and how it is produced.

Care deficits and deficits of care workers are connected. If there are no workers to provide care, along with no institutions or structures, then the work of providing health becomes difficult or, in our words, increasingly remote. Therefore, when we consider need, we must not only consider injury and sickness but also the needs of healthcare workers. Nursing scholar Mireille Kingma (2006) problematises the ways deficits or shortages of healthcare workers are circum-scribed by the discipline of economics. Labour shortages should not be limited by the simple economic logic of supply and demand. Instead, Kingma shows that need:

> is a subjective judgment about the ideal amount of a product or service that should be available regardless of the price . . . those who finance health care . . . insist that there is no shortage in terms of demand, whereas in fact there is a shortage when one considers need.
>
> (Kingma, 2006: 29)

Kingma's definition of shortage determined by need analyses care work from a position akin to the 'other' global health and the work of RAM: start with injury and suffering rather than regional, national or global demand based on HR depart-ments' labour projections. Kingma's approach to labour considers more than workers because it incorporates patients' (and society's) *need* for care and health. Understanding the relationality between caregiver and care recipient is thus a more collective understanding of health. Applied to our case, RAM seeks out the geographies of need and brings the care work to where they are needed. This formulation opens up the rich possibilities of collective solidarity that pays close attention to the 'global intimate' relations of care work on suffering bodies (Pratt and Rosner, 2012; Mountz and Hyndman, 2006).

The 'other' global health should not concede to capital or economic rationales on how to define need. Orzeck (2007: 511) reminds us of capital's constant attempts to manipulate needs and at the same time fulfil them. Yet, bodies resist this constant manipulation. She explains that 'needs may be remarkably elastic, they may vary enormously through time and across space, but our bodies can never get used to certain types of privation and exposure'. Thus, even though funders, financiers and philanthro-capitalists may attempt to inflate demands or minimise needs, our individual and collective bodies have innate limits. If we see health as a privilege (or a surplus), then the collective project is to determine where needs exist and support those who do the work.

When attention shifts away from economic definitions of supply and demand and towards collective needs, new 'remote' areas come into view. Each pop-up RAM clinic illustrates this need, in the words of Stan Brock:

> They cannot afford healthcare. This leads some of our American families, with their children, to sleep in tents and cars, often for over 24 hours, waiting for a RAM event to open its door. Blindfolded, you can stick a pin on a map of America and wherever it lands, you will find hundreds, if not thousands of sick hurting people in need of care that they cannot obtain.[3]

By their own numbers, RAM cared for more than 27,500 people in 2014 with the labour of 7400 volunteers, with an estimated total value of US$9 million in free care. RAM's work for the 'other' global health is for those who have no choice. It is care work for surplus populations: the unemployed, the marginal, those without visas, people who are not eligible for the benefits of the Affordable Care Act. RAM cares for the precarious worker, the temp and the unemployed, the discouraged, those with chronic pain, those on disability, even those full-time workers who cannot afford to pay the dentist. Nowadays, it is not just the factory that wears down the body, but the ongoing neglect of everyday life. These clinics are a version of Biehl's (2005: 137) *Vita*, a space of social abandonment and a social destiny in landscapes where 'social death and selective life extension coexist'. And yet this is not a story of abandonment because volunteers give their time and do the work, facing those people against whom capital and the state has turned its back. RAM's pop-up clinics throw into sharp relief the demands of the suffering in the USA and the volunteers who supply the care. Pulling teeth in the middle of a NASCAR racetrack reveals the incongruous state of the healthcare system in the USA.

RAM's clinics illustrate how care deficits happen even in very healthy 'rich' places. The US healthcare system is rich in terms of technology, knowledge and research funding. These productive aspects of the system are, for the most part, well supported. From the development of new technologies and pharmaceuticals to elective procedures to health insurance, these aspects of the healthcare system are quite robust, generating billions of dollars annually. While global health is dominated by philanthro-capitalism (McGoey, 2014), the work of the 'other' global health is dismissed, a point that has been repeatedly raised by scholars of social reproduction.

Health and social reproduction

Social reproduction interrogates 'how we live' (Mitchell *et al.*, 2003: 416) and what it takes to reproduce 'ourselves or others according to our and their desires' (Federici, 2012: 99).We suggest building upon the work done by geographers of social reproduction (Bakker and Gill, 2003; Mitchell *et al.*, 2004; Heynen, 2009; Heynen *et al.*, 2011; Roberts, 2008) to contribute to this 'other' global health. Introducing social reproduction into global health raises the important question:

Who does the work? Mitchell *et al*. (2003: 426) say this question has long been overlooked because social reproduction was 'conducted by slaves and their descendants, colonial and postcolonial subjects, children, and women' and that 'the work [was] considered "outside" of production, either unwaged or paid so poorly it cannot serve to reproduce the labourer himself or herself'. This work of feeding, cleaning and caring is vital because it underpins both households and systems of production, while it is undervalued or not valued at all. Therefore in this 'other' global health, volunteers and family members, not entrepreneurs, do the work.

The work of social reproduction involves 'three components: biological reproduction, the reproduction of the labouring population, and provisioning and caring needs' (Strauss, 2013: 182). Health becomes substantiated differently in each of these components, but there are interlocking sites of contestation and collective organising. Biological reproduction requires healthy bodies to carry and deliver babies, as well as healthcare workers to help people deliver those babies. The biological also focuses on the ability of the body to repair and heal in rapidly changing environments that are contoured by poverty, state violence and racialised geographies (Mansfield and Guthman, 2014, Guthman and Mansfield, 2013; Sze, 2007; Bullard, 1990). Reproducing the 'labouring population' requires a healthcare system that can help people lead healthy lives, heal when sick or injured, or assist them at the end of their lives. Finally, provisioning emphasises how the necessities of survival are organised, such as forms of combating hunger (Heynen, 2006) or education over the rights of women's bodies. Each of these components involves a need that care work supplies.

RAM's volunteer labour force is a form of social reproduction. Their work solves immediate health problems rather than waiting for pharmaceutical, technological and biomedical research and development. This healthcare landscape leaves many to live with chronic pain and debility. Most people cannot pull their own teeth, even though many are driven to do so. This social reproduction between caregiver and patient meets everyday needs. While this work can be found in particular aspects of the current healthcare system, across the USA, hospitals are closing (Henry, 2015) and both inner city and rural facilities struggle to fill nurse and physician positions, as communities lose jobs and lack healthcare services. Medicaid – the state-based public insurance option for low-income and disabled persons – varies from state to state, so that the geography of health insurance is increasingly uneven (Whitehouse.gov, 2015). Entire states become politically, economically and socially remote through austerity programmes that undermine welfare, food stamps, public transportation and women's health services.

For the 'other' global health, the work and care workers are part of the individual and collective struggles, successes and manifestations of health. A political approach to health foregrounds the organising work that goes into supplying the needs of the 'other' global health. One of the Foundational Principles of RAM is to 'Generate a People Movement', saying:

> We are strengthened by the dedication of compassionate volunteers – they
> are our heroes. We are driven by people who want to bring needed change to

communities. Remote Area Medical provides those people with the perfect opportunity to witness community transformation. This generates a people movement made up of dynamic and caring people seeking to change their world.

While the volunteer labour of ending pain and suffering takes precedent, the political work of organising a movement follows. Federici (2012: 111) explains: 'What is needed is the reopening of a collective struggle over reproduction, reclaiming control over the material conditions of our reproduction and creating new forms of cooperation around this work outside of the logic of capital and the market.' Social reproduction is an apt lens for this approach because of its emphasis on work and work that *needs* to get done, in this case the labour that goes into providing health services. RAM's strategy is an example of cooperation between volunteers and patients, along with a growing collective struggle to help others in need. Each temporary clinic introduces a dynamic of local politi-cisation that starts to 'generate a people movement'. Remote Area Medical shows that the way to achieve health for individuals depends on collective organising.

Katz's (2001: 711) classic line that 'social reproduction is the fleshy, messy, and indeterminate stuff of everyday life' implies that the 'other' global health should start where bodies and workplaces actually lack clear and defined contracts *and* cures. Since RAM's mandate is not to provide long-term institutional services, the pop-up and nomadic nature of their work provides unique spaces for consciousness-raising while ending suffering. These are not fixed spaces of care, but temporary and fleeting moments. The only constant is the work. RAM is doing the fleshy work through their pop-up clinics of pulling teeth and screening eyes. Care work situates the 'other' global health. RAM emphasises the mundane, everyday health needs that (1) people experience everywhere, and (2) are found-ational to good health, or as Loyd would say, individual and collective bodily self-determination. This approach refuses to exceptionalise health needs and seeks a more grounded analysis of global health justice.

Conclusion: trying to take care of our own

> We try to take care of our own, but if we don't have the means to do that, how are we supposed to?
>
> —RAM clinic attendee in Bristol, Tennessee
> (Reichert and Zaman, 2013)

When the category of 'our own' is scaled up and applied to general human suffering, the problem of global health becomes 'How can we take care of our own with limited resources?' RAM's answers are not further research and new drug development, but supporting care work to ease bodies in pain. To ground the geographies of 'other' global health, we suggest building upon the contribu-tions of geographers of social reproduction to focus on how bodies are suffering and who does the work in caring for them. Orzeck (2007: 499) working with Harvey argues that 'the body, for Marx, is porous: the dialectical product of worlds without and within'; as a result then, 'if the body reflects the world it must have a mechanism for absorbing that world'. The bodies of RAM clinic patients reflect the state of healthcare in the USA. They absorb structural inequalities through chronic pain and rotting teeth. The hope of getting a job blurs with macular degeneration. As a discussion of health cannot avoid the body, Orzeck states (2007: 503): 'Different types of labour transform the body in different ways. Workers lose limbs, digits, fingernails, eyes; they develop repetitive strain injuries, respiratory diseases, skin diseases, diseases from exposure to asbestos, pesticides, and other hazardous substances.' The chronic lack of care transforms the body yet again for the patients of RAM. Bodies absorb the uneven geographies in specific and varied ways. Yet collective responses of care and social reproduction mediate these worlds without and within – be it in Lagos or rural Kentucky. The point is to understand the dialectical processes that produce bodies and spaces. The 'other' global health must start with the body or the injury, and then expand beyond suffering to understand how each body is surrounded by a whirlpool of social relations, punctuated with eddies of race, class and gender along with waves of unemployment and state violence. As Orzeck continues (2007: 503): 'Income, access to healthcare and education, environmental racism, etc are all, like occupational injury and disease, factors that shape bodies, and frequently in ways that are both deleterious and indelible.' If bodies are shaped by both privilege and inequality, bodies can be shaped yet again by the care work of RAM.

Social reproduction and health are embodied in the relationship between the care worker and the patient. Together they can mutually constitute a collective effort to achieve self-determination. The embodiment of an individual's health, even if direly remote, can make these concerns, somewhat conversely, intimate. It is this perpetual intimacy that makes health political. Health is a matter of proximity and remoteness, or, as Orzeck states, how bodies are open to a range of dangers and privileges. The practice of making health a reality for many in the 'other' global health calls for collective responses. As Butler (2010: 13–15) argues, 'survival is dependent on what we might call a social network of hands'. RAM is those hands for many. To be 'alive' and to be healthy is to be in the hands of *others*. Being dependent, being impinged upon, and organising the social network of hands makes the world a little less remote.

Notes

1   This event was written about by Reichert and Zaman (2014). For an excellent overview of the work RAM do we highly recommend their documentary (Reichert and Zaman, 2013).
2   This original story is told in many places, including in interviews (Whitney, 2009) and the film *Remote Area Medical* (2013).
3   Brock (2014) said this while testifying in front of Congress on the needs for expanded resources to go to primary care in the USA.

References

Aiken, L.H. (2007) US nurse labor market dynamics are key to global nurse sufficiency. *Health Services Research* 42: 1299–1320.

Andrews, G.J. and Evans, J. (2008) Understanding the reproduction of health care: towards geographies in health care work. *Progress in Human Geography* 32: 759–780.

Arnold, D. (1993) *Colonizing the Body: State Medicine and Epidemic Disease in Nineteenth-century India.* Berkeley: University of California Press.

Bakker, I. and Gill, S. (2003) *Power, Production and Social Reproduction.* Basingstoke: Palgrave Macmillan.

Berlant, L. (2007) Slow death (Sovereignty, obesity, lateral agency). *Critical Inquiry* 33: 754–780.

Biehl, J.G. (2005) *Vita: Life in a Zone of Social Abandonment.* Berkeley: University of California Press.

Biehl, J. and Petryna, A. (2013a) Critical global health. In Biehl, J. and Petryna, A. (eds) *When People Come First: Critical Studies in Global Health*, pp. 1–20.

Biehl, J. and Petryna, A. (2013b) *When People Come First: Critical Studies in Global Health.* Princeton, NJ: Princeton University Press.

Bozorgmehr, K. (2010) Rethinking the 'global' in global health: a dialectic approach. *Global Health* 6: 19.

Brock, S. (2014) Addressing primary care access and workforce challenges: voices from the field. The U.S. Senate Committee on Health, Education, Labor & Pensions.

Brock, S. and Wilson, A. (2011) Remote Area Medical®: pioneers of no-cost health care. In R.A. Williams (ed.) *Healthcare Disparities at the Crossroads with Healthcare Reform.* New York: Springer Science & Business Media, pp. 413–420.

Brown, T. (2011) 'Vulnerability is universal': Considering the place of 'security' and 'vulnerability' within contemporary global health discourse. *Social Science and Medicine* 72: 319–326.

Brown, T., McLafferty, S. and Moon, G. (2009) *A Companion to Health and Medical Geography.* New York: John Wiley & Sons.

Brown, T. and Moon, G. (2012) Geography and global health. *The Geographical Journal* 178: 13–17.

Brown, T.M., Cueto, M. and Fee, E. (2006) The World Health Organization and the transition from international to global public health. *American Journal of Public Health* 96: 62–72.

Bullard, R.D. (1990) *Dumping in Dixie : Race, Class, and Environmental Quality.* Boulder, CO: Westview Press.

Butler, J. (2010) *Frames of War: When is Life Grievable?* London and New York: Verso.

Canguilhem, G. (1989) *The Normal and the Pathological.* New York: Zone Books.

Chouinard, V. (2013) Precarious lives in the Global South : on being disabled in Guyana. *Antipode* 46: 340–358.

Connell, J. and Walton-Roberts, M. (2015) What about the workers? The missing geographies of health care. *Progress in Human Geography* 40(2): 158–176.

Crooks, V.A. and Andrews, G.J. (2009) *Primary Health Care: People, Practice, Place.* Farnham: Ashgate Publishing.

Cueto, M. (2004) The origins of primary health care and selective primary health care. *American Journal of Public Health* 94: 1864–1874.

Cueto, M. (2005) The promise of primary health care. *Bulletin of the World Health Organization* 83: 322.

Darnell, J.S. (2010) Free clinics in the United States: a nationwide survey. *Archives of Internal Medicine* 170: 946–953.

Dyck, I. (2003) Feminism and health geography: twin tracks or divergent agendas? *Gender, Place & Culture* 10: 361–368.

Farmer, P. (1999) *Infections and Inequalities: the Modern Plagues.* Berkeley: University of California Press.

Farmer, P. (2005) *Pathologies of Power: Health, Human Rights, and the New War on the Poor.* Berkeley: University of California Press.

Farmer, P. (2006) *Aids and Accusation: Haiti and the Geography of Blame.* Berkeley: University of California Press.

Farmer, P. (2014) Diary. *London Review of Books* 36: 38–39.

Farmer, P.E., Nizeye, B., Stulac, S. and Keshavjee, S. (2006) Structural violence and clinical medicine. *PLoS Med* 3: e449.

Federici, S. (2012) *Revolution at Point Zero: Housework, Reproduction, and Feminist Struggle.* ?PM Press.

Garret, L. (2013) *Existential Challenges to Global Health.* New York: Center on International Cooperation, New York University.

Goodman, A. (2009) Uninsured travel from across US for free healthcare from Relief Group Remote Area Medical. *Democracy Now!* : Available at http://www.democracynow.org/2009/7/22/uninsured_travel_from_across_us_for (accessed 27 September 2016).

Greenhough, B. (2011) Citizenship, care and companionship: approaching geographies of health and bioscience. *Progress in Human Geography* 35: 153–171.

Guo, K.L. and Castillo, R.J. (2012) The US long term care system: development and expansion of naturally occurring retirement communities as an innovative model for aging in place. *Ageing International* 37: 210–227.

Guthman, J. and Mansfield, B. (2013) The implications of environmental epigenetics: a new direction for geographic inquiry on health, space, and nature–society relations. *Progress in Human Geography* 37(4): 486–504.

Harvey, D. (2006) *The Limits to Capital.* New York: Verso.

Henry, C. (2015) Hospital closures: the sociospatial restructuring of labor and health care. *Annals of the Association of American Geographers* 105: 1094–1110.

Heynen, N. (2006) 'But it's alright, Ma, it's life, and life only': radicalism as survival. *Antipode* 38: 916–929.

Heynen, N. (2009) Bending the bars of empire from every ghetto for survival: the Black Panther Party's radical antihunger politics of social reproduction and scale. *Annals of the Association of American Geographers* 99: 406–422.

Heynen, N., Hossler, P. and Herod, A. (2011) Surviving uneven development: social reproduction and the persistence of capitalism. *New Political Economy* 16: 239–245.

Hochschild, A.R. (2000) Global care chains and emotional surplus value. In W. Hutton, A. Giddens and N. Myers (eds) *On the Edge: Living with Global Capitalism.* London: Jonathan Cape.

Ingram, A. (2009) The geopolitics of disease. *Geography Compass* 3: 2084–2097.

Katz, C. (2001) Vagabond capitalism and the necessity of social reproduction. *Antipode* 33: 709–728.

Kearns, R. and Moon, G. (2002) From medical to health geography: novelty, place and theory after a decade of change. *Progress in Human Geography* 26: 605–625.

Kingma, M. (2006) *Nurses on the Move: Migration and the Global Health Care Economy.* New York: Cornell University Press.

Kleinman, A. (2010) Four social theories for global health. *The Lancet* 375: 1518–1519.

Koplan, J.P., Bond, T.C., Merson, M.H., Reddy, K.S., Rodriguez, M.H., Sewankambo, N.K., Wasserheit, J.N. and Board, CoUfGHE (2009) Towards a common definition of global health. *The Lancet* 373: 1993–1995.

Lakoff, A. (2010) Two regimes of global health. *Humanity: An International Journal of Human Rights, Humanitarianism, and Development* 1: 59–79.

Loyd, J.M. (2014) *Health Rights are Civil Rights : Peace and Justice Activism in Los Angeles, 1963–1978.* Minneapolis: University of Minnesota Press.

Mansfield, B. and Guthman, J. (2014) Epigenetic life: biological plasticity, abnormality, and new configurations of race and reproduction. *Cultural Geographies* 22: 3–20.

Marston, S.A., Jones, J.P. and Woodward, K. (2005) Human geography without scale. *Transactions of the Institute of British Geographers* 30: 416–432.

McGoey, L. (2012) Philanthrocapitalism and its critics. *Poetics* 40: 185–199.

McGoey, L. (2014) The philanthropic state: market–state hybrids in the philanthrocapitalist turn. *Third World Quarterly* 35: 109–125.

McGoey, L., Reiss, J. and Wahlberg, A. (2011) The global health complex. *BioSocieties* 6: 106–118.

Metzl, J. and Kirkland, A.R. (2010) *Against Health: How Health Became the New Morality.* New York: New York University Press.

Meyers, T. and Hunt, N.R. (2014) The other global South. *Lancet* 384: 1921–1922.

Mitchell, K., Marston, S.A. and Katz, C. (2003) Introduction: Life's work: an introduction, review and critique. *Antipode* 35: 415–442.

Mitchell, K., Marston, S.A. and Katz, C. (2004) *Life's Work: Geographies of Social Reproduction.* Oxford: Blackwell.

Mountz, A. and Hyndman, J. (2006) Feminist approaches to the global intimate. *Women's Studies Quarterly* 34: 446–463.

Nguyen, V-K. (2010) *The Republic of Therapy: Triage and Sovereignty in West Africa's Time of AIDS.* Durham, NC: Duke University Press.

Nixon, R. (2011) *Slow Violence and the Environmentalism of the Poor.* Cambridge, MA: Harvard University Press.

Orzeck, R. (2007) What does not kill you: historical materialism and the body. *Environment and Planning D: Society and Space* 25: 496–514.

Petryna, A (2002) *Life Exposed: Biological Citizens after Chernobyl.* Princeton, NJ: Princeton University Press.

Philo, C. (2007) A vitally human medical geography? Introducing Georges Canguilhem to geographers. *New Zealand Geographer* 63: 82–96.

Poo, A-J. (2015) *The Age of Dignity: Preparing for the Elder Boom in a Changing America.* New York: TheNew Press.

Pratt, G. and Rosner, V. (2012) *The Global and the Intimate: Feminism in our Time.* New York: Columbia University Press.

Raghuram, P. (2012) Global care, local configurations – challenges to conceptualizations of care. *Global Networks* 12: 155–174.

Raghuram, P., Madge, C. and Noxolo, P. (2009) Rethinking responsibility and care for a postcolonial world. *Geoforum* 40: 5–13.

Redfield, P. (2013) *Life in Crisis: The Ethical Journey of Doctors without Borders.* Berkeley: University of California Press.

Reichert, J. and Zaman, F. (2013) *Remote Area Medical.* Candescent Films, Green Film Company.

Reichert, J. and Zaman, F. (2014) Dear New York City's uninsured: screw you, love Governor Cuomo. *Huffington Post.* Availablee at http://www.huffingtonpost.com/jeff-reichert/dear-new-york-citys-unins_b_6184470.html: Huffington Post.

Remote Area Medical (2014a) Stop the suffering in Appalachia. *Remote Area Medical Magazine*. RAMUSA.org.

Remote Area Medical (2014b) Weekend refugees. *Remote Area Medical Magazine*. RAMUSA.org.

Remote Area Medical (2015) About. Remote Area Medical. https://ramusa.org/about/.

Roberts, A. (2008) Privatizing social reproduction: the primitive accumulation of water in an era of neoliberalism. *Antipode* 40: 535–560.

Ross, S.J., Polsky, D. and Sochalski, J. (2005) Nursing shortages and international nurse migration. *International Nursing Review* 52: 253–262.

Scheper-Hughes, N. (1993) *Death Without Weeping: the Violence of Everyday Life in Brazil*. Berkeley: University of California Press.

Smith, N. (1984) *Uneven Development: Nature, Capital, and the Production of Space*. New York: Blackwell.

Sparke, M. (2009) Unpacking economism and remapping the terrain of global health. In A. Kay and O. Williams (eds) *Global Health Governance: Transformations, Challenges and Opportunities Amidst Globalization*. New York: Palgrave Macmillan, pp. 131–159.

Sparke, M. (2014) Health. In R. Lee, N. Castree, K. Rob, V. Lawson, A. Paasi, S. Radcliffe and C. Withers (eds) *The SAGE Handbook of Progress in Human Geography*. London: Sage Publications.

Strauss, K. (2013) Unfree again: social reproduction, flexible labour markets and the resurgence of gang labour in the UK. *Antipode* 45: 180–197.

Sze, J. (2007) *Noxious New York: The Racial Politics of Urban Health and Environmental Justice*. Boston, MA: MIT Press.

Whitehouse.gov (2015) 22 states are refusing to expand Medicaid. Here's what that means for their residents. Available at https://www.whitehouse.gov/share/medicaid-map.

Whitney, J. (2009) Healthcare on the Moon: Jake Whitney interviews Stan Brock. *Guernica/A Magazine of Art & Politics*. Available at https://www.guernicamag.com/interviews/healthcare_on_the_moon/.

11 Eat your greens, buy some chips

Contesting articulations of food and food security in children's lives

Jane Battersby

Introduction

Food and nutrition have long been viewed as a critical issue for human health and development, but, until quite recently, the 'food problem' was primarily framed as one of malnutrition or hunger and the main concern was ensuring caloric sufficiency. There was, in other words, little or no mention of food in relation to obesity and chronic disease, be it in the international health agenda or the global food security literature (Reubi *et al.*, 2016). This framing has been increasingly challenged over the past few years.

To start with, there has been a growing interest in obesity as a global health problem of late (Haddad *et al.*, 2015). This, however, has yet to be adequately connected to the food security agenda, which drives much of the global policy and programming on food issues. Furthermore, there has been an increased focus on the nutritional aspects of food security, as is evident in the second Sustainable Development Goal: 'end hunger, achieve food security and improved nutrition and promote sustainable agriculture.' But, although nutrition is increasingly considered as part of food security, this understanding of nutrition remains linked to *mal*- or *under*-nutrition.

Such an understanding fails to capture the ways in which food security manifests itself are changing. Indeed, in many parts of the Global South, obesity and diet-related diseases are increasingly prevalent, although at the same time hunger and hunger-related diseases continue to be present (Doak *et al.*, 2005). Despite this having been acknowledged by UN agencies as early as 2003 (WHO/FAO 2003, 8), the global food and nutrition policy agenda has not yet shifted its focus to acknowledge the impacts of the nutrition transition, as defined by Popkin (1999). As Haddad and colleagues (2015, xxiii) note in the new *Global Nutrition Report*:

> In 2014 we reported that out of the proposed 169 SDG targets, nutrition is mentioned in only one; this situation has not changed. New SDG document-ation also shows that overweight and obesity are not mentioned once in the entire document, and none of the three implementation targets to achieve SDG 2 ('End hunger, achieve food security and improved nutrition, and promote sustainable agriculture') mentions nutrition actions.

This chapter argues that the failure of global actors to adapt to new forms of food and nutrition insecurity beyond mal- or under-nutrition has led to a set of policy and programmatic responses that not only fail to address the problem, but may in fact exacerbate it. In order to make this point, the chapter examines the shortcomings and problems associated with existing food and nutrition policy and programming at three different scales. First, it examines some of the shortcomings and inadequacies of current, dominant international discourses and policy models on food and nutrition security. Specifically, it will show how: (1) the framing of food and nutrition insecurity by global development agencies and national governments has failed to adjust to the changing nature of malnutrition in the global south; (2) the current siloed approaches to address malnutrition cannot address the systemic nature of the problem; and (3) the way in which private sector actors have been able to position themselves as 'partners in development' and frame the development agenda has hindered attempts to mitigate food and nutrition insecurity.

Second, the chapter will, using the case of South Africa, explore how this global agenda and policy models interact with national policy formulation and implementation. This section again highlights shortcomings and problems with the framing at the national scale. Situating the work in South Africa is useful, as the country's population is vulnerable to all three kinds of malnutrition as described by Gómez et al. (2013): undernourishment, micronutrient deficiencies and over-nutrition manifest in overweight and obesity (Shisana et al., 2013). In addition, South African retailers and companies are playing an important role in shaping the food systems in the rest of the African continent, and so the changes evident in the South African food system – and therefore diets – may be viewed as projections of future African realities (see e.g. Thow et al., 2015).

Third, the chapter, drawing on research carried out in Cape Town, explores the lived experiences of children of the food system to highlight the weaknesses of existing framings of the food security problem. Given the focus on child nutrition within the global food and nutrition security agenda and SDG indicators, this study of how children actually access food and what drives their consumption plays an important role in highlighting the weaknesses of assumptions underlying existing approaches. The data presented do not originate from conventional case studies. Instead they have their genesis in a series of projects and fieldwork reflections on work conducted under the auspices of the African Food Security Urban Network (AFSUN) in Cape Town and earlier work conducted on education funded by the Oppenheimer Foundation.

The chapter highlights the gaps in current approaches to address food and nutrition insecurity, and argues that food is best understood as a social and economic practice which people use to 'plug' underlying gaps in local economic, spatial and social systems. It therefore concludes that food policy cannot be effective if it does not consider the interactions of multiple processes and domains in shaping consumption and developing inter-sectoral policies. The chapter argues that there is a need to shift the food and nutrition security agenda towards greater consideration of the health implications of the current food system's transformation trajectories. This call for re-calibration provides greater scope for connection between global health research and food security research.

The changing face of food and nutrition insecurity

Within the Global South, the nutrition challenge has largely been framed as one of hunger and acute malnutrition (see e.g. the first MDG, the second SDG and the FAO's State of Food Insecurity in the World series). This is often contrasted with the high levels of obesity and overweight in the Global North to make a political point about inequality and waste in the food system (Patel, 2008). However, it is increasingly apparent that this dichotomy of one billion hungry and one billion obese (Gustafson, n.d.) is a gross over-simplification and that the nature of malnutrition in the Global South is changing (Popkin *et al.*, 2012). A joint WHO/FAO report noted in 2003 that, 'Given the rapidity with which traditional diets and lifestyles are changing in many developing countries, it is not surprising that food insecurity and undernutrition persist in the same countries where chronic diseases are emerging as a major epidemic (WHO/'FAO. 2003, 8). It is common to have both obesity and malnutrition present in the same household, and even in the same individuals (Doak *et al.*, 2005). Households in the Global South now experience the double burden of disease, affected both by traditional diseases of poverty and diseases of affluence, including diabetes, hypertension and other diet-related diseases.

A number of studies have highlighted the dramatic rise of obesity rates globally, particularly in the Global South. Obesity rates before the 1980s were generally below 10 per cent, but, since then, rates have doubled and even tripled in many countries (Cecchini *et al.*, 2010, 1778). Ng and colleagues' (2014) review of 1749 surveys, studies and reports found that increases in obesity in developed countries had attenuated in the past decade, but that obesity rates in developing countries, where almost two-thirds of the world's obese population live, continue to increase (Ng *et al.*, 2014, 777). It was estimated that in 2010 overweight and obesity caused 3.4 million deaths, 3.9 per cent of life lost, and 3.8 per cent of disability-adjusted life-years (DALYs) worldwide (Lim *et al.*, 2012 in Ng *et al.*, 2014, 767).

South Africa typifies this changing food and nutrition insecurity profile. The most recent large-scale national assessment of food security, the South African National Health and Nutrition Examination Survey (SANHANES) using the Community Childhood Hunger Identification Project index (CCHIP) found that only 45.6 per cent of South Africans could be classified as food secure while the other 28.3 per cent were at risk of hunger and 26 per cent actually experienced hunger (Shisana *et al.*, 2013). The SANHANES report compared other large-scale data sets and found that although levels of food security had improved since the 1990s, these levels had plateaued, suggesting persistent moderate and severe food insecurity.

However, as elsewhere, this data obscures a changing malnutrition profile. Although food-insecure households continue to be malnourished in terms of essential nutrients for health and development, they are also now characterised by increasing obesity. National surveys have found obesity rates of over 50 per cent for women and 30 per cent for men (Shisana *et al.*, 2013). The SANHANES survey found obesity and overweight in children to be most prevalent in urban areas. The SANHANES figures were compared to the 2006 Health of the Nation Study, and it was found that levels of both overweight and obesity within children had increased significantly over the seven years in question (Shisana *et al.*, 2013, 209). There is increased presence of diseases associated with obesity: coronary heart disease, diabetes mellitus and hypertension.

There are many contributing factors to this global and local rise in obesity, including lifestyle changes and foetal nutrition, with early nutritional deficits followed by later excesses (Popkin *et al.*, 2012, 6–7). However, the most apparent shifts are the increased food energy supply and the globalisation of food supply, increasing the availability of obesogenic ultra-processed foods (Vandevijvere *et al.*, 2015, 446). While earlier work on nutrition transition identified changes in consumption as being driven in part by increased disposable income in developing countries (Popkin, 1999, 2003), more recent work has highlighted the fact that it is lower income households who are most exposed to foods that are high in energy but nutritionally compromised. Wealthier households are equally exposed to these foods, but are able to afford to buy higher quality foods. Wiggin and Keats' (2015) analysis of food pricing in Brazil, China, Mexico and Korea found that fruit and vegetable prices had risen by 55 to 91 per cent between 1990 and 2012, but that the prices of four of the six processed foods tracked had shown price falls since 1990. In South Africa, a study of the availability and cost of healthier food choices of commonly consumed foods found that the cost of healthier options was always more expensive than the 'normal' option. The price differences ranged from 11 per cent (high-fat vs. low-fat minced beef) to 58 per cent (brick margarine vs. low-fat margarine) (Temple *et al.*, 2006, 2011). Otero and colleagues (2015) argue that this food inequality must be understood as part of a wider political economy of food, which is characterised by trade liberalisation and other state and supra-state regulatory structures and legal frameworks that favour large corporations, such as the food processors and agribusiness multinationals. They term the resultant prevalence of highly processed, nutrient-poor foods the 'neoliberal diet'.

Policy responses to obesity often focus on nutrition education to help consumers make better choices. These efforts have largely ignored the systemic drivers of food choice; as Drewnowski and Darmon (2005, 266S) ask: 'Does the obesity problem lie with fast-food outlets and vending machines, or are there broader social issues that have to do with the falling value of the minimum wage, the lack of health and family benefits, and declining neighbourhood resources?' In the North American and British context, the question of physical and economic accessibility of healthy and less healthy foods has gained considerable traction through research on food deserts (see e.g. Shaw, 2006; Cannuscio *et al.*, 2010). The complex relationships between space, retail and food choice in South Africa are described in Battersby and Peyton (2014), who challenge the logic of supermarket expansion necessarily having food security benefits for the poor.

The nutrition transition and food desert literatures suggest that food insecurity and poor diet cannot be addressed by poverty alleviation strategies and nutrition education programmes alone. Both food insecurity and poor diet need to be understood in the context of the wider food system and related spatial systems, and in the way food connects to wider spatial, economic and social practices. However, as the Foresight Report on Obesity in the United Kingdom notes, although the complexity and interrelationships of the obesity system 'make a compelling case for the futility of isolated initiatives. . . . There are, as yet, no concerted strategies or policy models that adequately address the problem (Butland *et al.*, 2007, 10). It is evident that despite this acknowledgement, little progress has been made globally (Popkin and Bellagio Meeting Group, 2013, Roberto *et al.*, 2015).

Problems of global food and nutrition security discourses and policies

Current, global approaches to food and nutrition fail to adequately address these new food and nutrition realities, and may in fact exacerbate the trend towards obesity and diseases of diet. There are three main reasons for this failure, which this section explores in turn: outdated diagnosis of the problem, short-term oriented and disconnected responses, and an uncritical approach to the private sector's role in the food system.

Old diagnoses for new diseases

Approaches to food and nutrition insecurity continue to consider hunger and hunger-based malnutrition as the main or only problem to be addressed. The WHO/FAO argued that the treatment of under-nutrition and chronic diseases as two totally separate problems has 'obstructed effective action to curb the advancing epidemic of chronic diseases' (WHO/FAO, 2003, 9). Despite this being acknowledged over a decade ago, the framing of food and nutrition security in the South remains resolutely focused on hunger and under-nutrition, as evidenced by the targets and indicators of the new food and nutrition security SDG. This global agenda may be attributed to a large degree to the power of the MDGs in shaping the global and local responses to development challenges generally, and a particular role in shaping the food response.

One of the reasons for the success of MDGs in shaping the global development agenda was their ability to distil complex challenges to a small number of readily understandable targets and indicators (Higgins, 2013). The problem is that these targets and indicators that were meant to serve as proxies for complex social problems have taken on a life of their own and are now used as planning targets rather than proxies (Fukuda-Parr and Orr, 2014, 147). So, within the MDGs, the global food and nutrition agenda came to be distilled down to MDG Target 1C's injunction to 'halve the proportion of people suffering from hunger'. This target hollowed out earlier goals to address food and nutrition, such as those of the 1996 FAO's World Food Summit (WFS) and the 1992 International Conference on Food (ICN) (Pogge, 2004). These viewed food and nutrition insecurity as systemic and as requiring approaches that would address the structural drivers of food insecurity, including unemployment, gender inequality, unequal access to productive assets and unequal trade (see e.g. FAO, 1996). The condensing of a wider set of food and nutrition concerns to a single issue – hunger, rather than the quality of food or the sustainability of the food system – has led to the marginalisation of debates about the political economy of food (McMichael and Schneider, 2011).

Given that the MDGs are set to be replaced by the SDGs, it is worth briefly considering whether the SDGs are likely to shift the global discourse and practice regarding food and nutrition insecurity. Goal 2 of the SDGs, 'End hunger, achieve food security and improved nutrition and promote sustainable agriculture', does take a broader stance on food and nutrition security, but still fails to acknowledge the nutrition challenges associated with the rapid nutrition transition underway in the Global South. In the most recent available list of proposed indicators (dated 12 June 2015: SDSN, 2015), there is no indicator addressing obesity as a marker of a form of malnutrition for Target 2.2; however, earlier lists did (Action Against Hunger, 2015; FAO, 2015). This inclusion and then omission suggests that there is some appreciation of the fact that the problem is not simply scarcity, but that this is a minority view. This inclusion and then omission may be attributed to the powerful voices of Big Food protecting their business interests (see Brownell (2012) for previous examples of Big Food's influence in the health arena). Goal 3 seeks to ensure healthy lives and promote well-being at all ages. Within this goal there is a focus on addressing non-communicable diseases, with a potential focus on diet-related disease, but it is not clear how the goals interact. It is likely that the problem of over-nutrition will continue to be omitted from the global food and nutrition security agenda.

Indicator-led, siloed approaches

The MDGs played an important role in shaping the way in which the problem of food and nutrition security has been understood (what Porter would term their 'knowledge effect' (Porter, 2012 in Fukuda-Parr and Orr, 2014)). In addition, they have played an important role in shaping the types of policies and programmes that have emerged to address the problems identified (what Porter would term their 'governance effect').

It has been argued that the MDGs lacked a recognisable theory of change (Haddad, 2013), and that their target and indicator structure led to the emergence of short-term, quick-fix solutions that were designed to meet the achievement of particular indicators, rather than addressing the broader development challenges for which the indicators served as proxies (Fukuda-Parr and Orr. 2014).

In the case of food and nutrition security, the governance effect has been to generate a set of policy and programmatic responses at the global and national scales that are based on the 'twin-track' approach of:

(a) direct interventions and social investments to address the immediate needs of the poor and hungry (food aid, social safety nets, and so on) and (b) development programmes to enhance the performance of the productive sectors (especially to promote agriculture and rural development), create employment and increase the value of assets held by the poor.

(CFS, 2006, 16 in Crush and Frayne, 2011, 529)

This approach neither addresses the systemic issues within the food system nor the changing nature of malnutrition. Within this framing, obesity and other diet-related diseases are viewed as resulting from poor individual choice-making, necessitating a focus on nutrition education.

An uncritical approach to the role of the private sector

A consequence of the framing of the problem and the lack of a clear theory of change has enabled a number of large, private sector-driven international initiatives to position themselves as 'partners-in-development', working towards ending hunger and malnutrition. These include the Alliance for a Green Revolution in Africa (AGRA), Scaling-Up Nutrition (SUN) and the New Alliance for Food Security and Nutrition (Fukuda-Parr and Orr, 2014). This has replaced the earlier objective of a systemic approach with a large-scale (often unsustainable) agriculture and nutrition supplementation approach, which positions the private sector as 'partners in development'.

The relative power of the private sector in developing food and nutrition security programmes may be attributable in part to the deregulation and liberalisation of food markets during the 1980s and 1990s (Otero *et al*., 2015). This liberalisation of food markets was a central component of the Structural Adjustment Programmes that transformed the relationships between the state and private sector in the Global South (Briggs and Yeboah, 2001). The relative power afforded to the private sector and its ability to position itself as a vital contributor to the global development agenda has been widely questioned (Vandemoortele, 2009). Concerns have been raised about the way in which transnational corporations exert pressure on national government and the negative impact they have had on the diets of the poor (Moodie *et al*., 2013).

The uncritical embrace of the private sector by major development agencies, legitimised by the UN's favouring of public–private partnerships in the delivery of the SDGs (Ki-Moon, 2014), has reinforced the misdiagnosis of the food and nutrition security problem and has taken the development pathways in directions that will hasten the increase of diet-related non-communicable diseases.

Translating global trends to local realities: South Africa

It is essential to understand how these global development agendas interact with national and local policy formulation and implementation. The study of a situation in a particular country provides a mechanism to examine the critical gaps between the imagined problem and solutions and the nuanced lived experience of the problem.

Following the global lead, in South Africa, food and nutrition security has persistently been framed as a problem of hunger and under-nutrition, despite clear evidence of nutrition transition in the country. As in the global case, there has been a general failure to act upon food and nutrition security as a systemic challenge and a persistently siloed approach to generating solutions. In South Africa there are two major policy structures in place to address food insecurity and malnutrition: the Integrated Nutrition Programme (INP) and the Integrated Food Security Strategy (IFSS).[1]

The Department of Health's Integrated Nutrition Programme was designed to encourage and support programmes that were integrated, sustainable and community driven. However, while there were attempts within the first iteration of the INP framework to have community-based nutrition projects that would encourage 'multisectoral government support to communities to "solve" their own nutritional problems' (Labadarios *et al.*, 2005, 102), these were removed from later INP objectives. The projects that were trialled were generally not successful, as a result of unrealistic objectives and lack of appropriate resources. So, while they were omitted to encourage better use of limited resources, it has written the local food system and food economies out of the INP, as resources have been re-focused on single department, single objective projects. This absence is a critical limitation.

While the logic of locating an 'integrated' programme within one department is clear, it limits the conceptualisation of the nutrition problem and the kinds of responses possible (Chopra *et al.*, 2009). Due in part to this location and the programmatic focus of the Department of Health, there is an absence of focus on the role of the market in shaping nutritional outcomes.

The same lack of integration and cross-departmental engagement has hampered the 2002 Integrated Food Security Strategy (IFSS), which was introduced to integrate previously disparate food security policies and programmes. Although the programme has wide-ranging objectives, the actual programmatic outcomes of the IFSS have been limited and have tended towards production-based interventions, due to its location within the Department of Agriculture (now the Department of Agriculture, Forestry and Fisheries). Although hampered by technical and capacity challenges (Drimie and Ruysenaar, 2010), even if the IFSS had functioned as intended and had achieved cross-departmental integration, its conceptualisation of food insecurity as predominantly rural and hunger-based would have limited its ability to alleviate food insecurity.

Further to the INP and IFSS, the Child Support Grant (and other social grants) is a programme that may be viewed, indirectly, as a food security programme (Patel *et al.*, 2012). However, viewing the Child Support Grant as a food security initiative reduces food insecurity to being primarily a problem of insufficient income. In addition, it assumes that children's food consumption is determined by an adult provider. As will be illustrated in this chapter, this is not the case for many children. The Social Grants do not interact directly with the other food and nutrition programming.

Why does this siloed approach persist in South Africa? In part it may be attributed to the current indicator-led development process that is by necessity short term and results-oriented (Fukuda-Parr and Orr, 2014, 154). This approach lends itself to single department-driven programmes with single objectives. However, in South Africa, it is clear that there have been attempts to achieve multi-sectoral, multi-departmental responses. The failure of these programmes to achieve their aims and their reversion to single department-led programmes may be attributed to the challenges of institutional capacity and budgeting processes which make cross-departmental programming difficult to sustain (Chopra *et al.*, 2009; Drimie and Ruysenaar 2010). This natural tendency towards working within existing departmental structures is reinforced by reporting structures which focus on progress towards specific outcomes – a process reinforced by the current global development agenda.

The relatively uncritical approach towards the private sector within global development practice is magnified in South Africa, where the deregulation of markets and liberalisation of trade was a deliberate policy in the 1990s to dismantle the apartheid agriculture and trade system (Kirsten and Van Zyl, 1996). This has been identified by the Competition Commission as having led to uncompetitive pricing, which impacts upon the welfare of poorer households (Competition Commission, 2008). The South African food system is now one of the most consolidated and corporate-driven in the world (Greenberg, 2010; Igumbor *et al.*, 2012).

Despite these concerns, both the INP and IFSS have 'blind spots' with regard to the role of markets in food security and nutrition, and the possibility of interventions into the structure of the market. The state has instead tended to implement only 'second-class' interventions that seek to mitigate the negative impacts of the prevailing food system, rather than directly engaging the largely private sector-driven structural problems of the food system (Kirsten, 2012). Within the South African system, the major producers and retailers have been particularly effective in positioning themselves as modernisers, agents of local economic development, and as providing equal access to goods and services historically reserved for whites (Battersby and Peyton, 2014). The state therefore often views these actors as core partners in development, even disbursing social grants through supermarkets. The unwillingness of the state to acknowledge the role of the private sector in generating the conditions under which food and nutrition insecurity flourish fundamentally hinders efforts to address the problem.

Three sites of food consumption

Focusing the gaze on the lived experience of children and their geographies of food consumption further illustrates and complicates the limitations of the dominant framings and approaches to food and nutrition insecurity. The daily lives of children in urban areas engage the food environment at multiple points which shape their foodways.[2] This chapter presents three key food moments for children: the school, the journey to and from school, and the home. They highlight the multiple ways in which the intentions of the INP, the IFSS and Child Support are compromised through the lived experience of children in the food system. Food is effectively a fix to address gaps in the economic, spatial and social system. As each site is introduced, the ways in which present and past non-food-related policy structures impact upon foodways is discussed.

The school

The school is a key site for INP interventions, both through the Primary School Nutrition Programme and through nutrition education. There has been research on some of the challenges associated with school feeding reach (Poswell and Leibbrandt, 2006), nutritional adequacy (Clacherty *et al.*, 2006) and even conflicting messages on nutrition communicated to children through the types of food they consumed (Child Health Unit, 1997).

While the direct nutrition programmes have been extensively researched, what is less well understood is the role of the school as a source of food outside of these programmes (Temple *et al.*, 2006). Children obtain food at school from a number of sources. These sources are driven largely by the economic contexts of schools and, as will be demonstrated, the kinds of food sold often provide contradictory messages to those of nutrition education and the feeding scheme. If food and nutrition programmes are to be improved, it is essential to understand the economic, social and spatial relationships that form children's foodways.

Within the school environment, the most direct, non-programmatic source of food is the tuck shop, a food retail outlet within the school grounds. Research conducted in a range of schools in Cape Town found that 69.3 per cent of sampled pupils bought food at school on the day prior to their interview. Of these, 79.7 per cent bought this food at the school's tuck shop (Temple *et al.*, 2006, 254). As will be discussed in the section on the journey to and from school, these purchases are informed in part by the long journeys many children undertake to school, which impacts upon their ability to eat breakfast at home or to bring lunches from home. However, it is essential to understand the tuck shop in the context of the wider economy of the school.

Although basic education receives the largest portion of the national budget, it is widely acknowledged that this funding is not sufficient to adequately fund schools (Lemon and Battersby-Lennard, 2009b). The provincial education department has a formula by which it calculates the number of teachers per school based on enrolment. These teachers are then paid by the state. These staffing costs amount to some 90 per cent of the provincial education budget (Karlsson, 2002).

From the remaining 10 per cent, a 'provincial allocation' is allocated with which schools are meant to meet their operational needs, including maintenance, utility bills, stationery, textbooks, etc. These provincial allocations are allocated on a pro-poor basis in an attempt to address historical inequities in the education system. Despite these attempts to preferentially fund lower income schools, schools still reported substantial funding shortfalls. Schools therefore employ a number of fundraising strategies to address their budget shortfalls, including generating income from the school tuck shop (Lemon and Battersby-Lennard, 2009a, 86). Schools appear to use pupil-focused fundraising to leverage fee equivalents from children at non-fee-paying schools.

In interviews conducted with school principals by the author in 2005, the tuck shop was identified as a consistent revenue stream for the school. In one school, the annual provincial allocation was R147,000[3] per annum and the tuck shop brought in R25,000 per annum. This school also generated R50,000 from a food fair and flea market event and an additional R15,000 from an annual market day at school in which pupils are encouraged to cook food and bring it into school to sell to their classmates. Given the importance of the tuck shop as a fundraiser, schools actively encouraged their pupils to buy from it. In another school the prize for an internal school competition was a set of vouchers for the tuck shop.

While some schools have taken decisions to address the nutritional quality of foods sold in the tuck shop, the majority of schools sell popular, highly processed, high-fat, high-sugar foods like chips, pies and carbonated soft drinks (Temple *et al.*, 2006; Stupar *et al.*, 2012). The decision on what the tuck shop should stock does not rest with the school. The tuck shop, as a non-pedagogic function, is the responsibility of the School Governing Body (SGB), which is tasked in the South African Schools Act to 'take all reasonable measures within its means to supplement the resources supplied by the State in order to improve the quality of education provided by the school to all learners at the school' (Department of Education, 1996, 26 in Karlsson, 2002, 331). As such, there is no obligation on the part of the tuck shop to adhere to nutritional guidelines, but simply to generate revenue.

The SGB's tuck shop stocking decisions are therefore driven by both their income-generation mandate and the desires of the wider parent body. In more middle-income areas, the tuck shops have responded to concerns about food and pupil health and behaviour. In lower income areas, a different set of concerns drive stocking: affordability and providing economic opportunities for parents, lack of proper facilities to prepare and store healthier foods, and a lack of time and of manpower to produce healthier foods (Battersby, 2002; Marraccini *et al.*, 2012). This is further evidence of the way in which food options reflect structural inequality.

The economic realities of the school therefore undermine the nutrition messages that are part of the core curriculum. Nutrition education messages are compromised in the very environment in which they are being transmitted. In their work, Temple *et al.* (2006) asked pupils to distinguish between healthy and unhealthy foods. Although pupils were able to easily identify six of the nine foods as healthy or unhealthy, almost 40 per cent incorrectly identified Coca-Cola as healthy. Almost 50 per cent identified samosas and pies as healthy (Temple *et al.*, 2006, 256). The mis-identification of Coca-Cola as healthy may be the consequence of the advertising presence that the product has in many low-income schools and local retail. The mis-identification of pies and samosas may be the consequence of these being home-cooked products and thus viewed as wholesome. The fact that these products are sold in the tuck shop compounds nutrition confusion.

In many schools, parents and other local traders sell food to children through the school fence. The foods sold in this manner are predominantly low-cost, high-energy foods. The school is therefore not just a site of education, but also of economic opportunity for community members. This activity places the child at the heart of the market structure. In some cases teachers will sell food to supplement income. In this case, the child is again being used to offset funding limitations within the school environment. The role of teachers in this kind of food retail may directly undermine their role as nutrition educators.

The multiple economic and social realities of the school directly and indirectly challenge the viability of school-based nutrition programmes.

The journey

The second key food site is the journey from home to school and back. Under apartheid, pupils were only allowed to attend schools designated for their race group and schools were differentially funded according to race, with white schools occupying the most privileged position. After the opening of schools to all races in 1990, pupils began to travel out of their residential areas to attend historically advantaged schools (Soudien, 2004). Given the legacy of the Group Areas Act, many of these pupils undergo long journeys to school each day. These long journeys to school have been identified as a crucial constraint upon children's experiences of schooling (Battersby, 2002; Stupar 2012). In work conducted in ten schools in Cape Town, it was found that although many pupils did not have excessively long journeys, they did have very early starts to their days, with more than half of the sampled pupils leaving home before 7 a.m. (Lemon and Battersby-Lennard, 2011, 17). These journey lengths and early starts impact upon the food habits of children.

In research on evaluating school feeding schemes and food insecurity in a primary school populated by children from low-income areas in Cape Town, it was found that over 63 per cent of pupils stated that they skipped meals and that the most frequent meal skipped was breakfast. When asked why they missed meals, 25 per cent stated that they missed meals because of time constraints and just 6 per cent identified not enough money or not enough food[4] (Watson, 2009, 52). In Stupar and colleagues' (2012) work with secondary schools, pupils identified breakfast as an important meal, but one that they frequently skipped because of the demands of leaving the house early to get to school on time.

As a consequence of missing breakfast because of travel time, pupils in both Watson's (2009) and Stupar et al.'s (2012) research were given money to buy food during the day, either at school or on the journey. This is not unique to South Africa. Research in Ibadan, Nigeria found that 98 per cent of schoolchildren bought their breakfast on the street (Children of the Tropics, 1994 in Ruel et al., 1998, 14).

The time pressures of the school journey coupled with the school's food environment shape children's food choice. In addition, informal food trade locates itself relative to the paths that children take through the city on the journey from home to school and back. Spazas[5] and street traders often operate close to schools in order to capture passing trade from pupils. While conducting site visits for AFSUN research, the author visited a number of house shops located near schools. After school and during break periods, these shops were occupied by a constant stream of children buying snacks. An estimated three-quarters of stock consisted of sweets, chips and soft drinks. Research on Spazas across South Africa found that 56 per cent of customers were children (Ligthelm, 2005, 211). Recent research in Avian Park, a low-income area in Worcester in the Western Cape, found that 100 per cent of spazas sold chips, sweets and carbonated soft drinks, but only 67 per cent sold potatoes, 58 per cent sold onions, 17 per cent sold tomatoes and none sold green vegetables (Roos, 2012, 43). These businesses are often survivalist in orientation, meaning that they have low profit margins and the longevity of their business is precarious. These businesses are often highly dependent on sales to children to maintain a regular income.

Informal food retail also proliferates around transport hubs (Battersby, 2012). These traders are not as dependent on sales to children and youth as the spazas – as their client base also includes adults commuting to and from work on public transport, but their location and sustainability is dependent on the flows of people buying food as they move through the city on a daily basis. These flows and purchasing patterns are the out-workings of spatial mismatches between residential and employment opportunities and residential and retail opportunities (Zager, 2011; Battersby, 2011b).

The mismatch between home and school/work geographies creates a particular form of time–space constraint. The informal food retail sector has been able to respond in order to overcome this time–space constraint, but in doing so increases exposure to highly processed foods.

In the USA there have been a series of local food ordinances to prevent the new location of fast-food retailers and to ban the location of mobile food vendors near schools (NPLAN, 2008). This has also been taken up in various cities in the Philippines (see e.g. City of General Santos, 2013). The application of this kind of zoning regulation may not be viable in a city like Cape Town given the levels of informality in the food system. In addition, the importance of these traders as the primary source of food for low-income households would mean that this form of regulation may significantly impact upon the food security of the poor and remove essential sources of livelihoods for many (Battersby, 2011b).

What remains as an ongoing challenge is the fact that the day-to-day sustainability of this vital source of food is generated through the sale of nutritionally poor food to children. This chapter does not have an easy answer to this conundrum, but seeks only to flag it as a pernicious problem that demands further research and policy focus.

The home

The final location for discussion is the home, which is generally assumed to be the primary site of consumption for children. It is also assumed that children's consumption patterns are determined by adults in the home. The disbursement of the Child Support Grant to mothers as a means to support child nutrition is based on this assumption. While there is evidence that the grant has had a positive impact on child nutrition (Patel *et al.*, 2012), it should not be assumed that the home is necessarily the main site of consumption for children.

This chapter has already indicated that the school and the school journey are important sources of food where money is provided for food by parents, but the parents have no direct role in the food choices made by children. Even within the home environment, children's consumption patterns are not simply determined by food provided by parents at meal times. Children are actively engaged in the local food economy through the social processes of home. The use of food in these processes is incidental to the ultimate purpose of engagements, but serves to undermine nutritional messages and compromise the diets of children. As with the site of the school, children's engagements with the food economy in the home are initiated by adults in response to the wider economic and spatial context.

Children are used extensively both by parents and neighbours to help carry shopping. This activity is often incentivised with a few Rand to buy some sweets or chips. While this may seem removed from questions of the wider urban food system, it is a direct outcome of the inequities in the system. Shopping habits are curtailed by formal retail location and product size. When low-income shoppers do buy from supermarkets, it is in bulk that is hard to carry alone and often involves the use of public transport. It is possible to take an additional, smaller, unregistered taxi from the bus stop or taxi rank to the house, but this adds additional cost to the shopping trip that may already have had extra fares charged for the space taken up by shopping (Battersby, 2015). Shoppers therefore often use children to help carry the shopping home for a small tip. This activity encourages consumption of junk food by children and may be understood to be the result of the spatial inequities in food retail.

Given the time–space constraints described earlier, parents often arrive home after the supermarkets have closed. They therefore send children to buy food at the local spazas when they get home, again incentivised by a small tip used at the spaza. Children are therefore an essential part of the social process of food within the household and their roles in overcoming time–space constraints are compensated with resources which lead to increased consumption of junk food. Therefore, while adults may seek to provide nutritious food for their children and use state-provided grants to prioritise food for those children, their efforts are inadvertently compromised by the lived reality of food access in low-income urban areas.

There is a third form of social practice through which parents encourage poor dietary habits in an attempt to manage neighbourhood-scale challenges. Working in Manenberg, a low-income area of Cape Town with a history of gangsterism, Cooke (2012) has found that parents will use spazas as a form of safe space for their children on weekends and during school holidays. Some of the larger spazas have coin-operated video games or a pool table. Parents give their children a small amount of money to buy food from these traders in order to legitimise their presence so that they can play the games. In this way, parents have some peace of mind that their children are not going to be caught up in gangsterism. Places like Manenberg are under-resourced in terms of community centres and safe public spaces; the spaza environment therefore becomes a safe haven for children. This kind of long-term exposure of children to the products for sale by these traders, and their association with games and safety, potentially undermine the messages of formal nutrition education.

Children's food consumption is shaped both by the ways in which households attempt to navigate the food system and how they maintain safe environments for their children. As with the school, and the journey to and from school, food is used within the home to address gaps in the economic, spatial and social systems in which these households operate. In all of these cases, food is incidental to the wider processes at play, but the kinds of food economy that have emerged compromise children's food security, nutrition and understanding of nutrition.

As is evident from these examples, there are fundamental mismatches between the way in which the food and nutrition challenge has been framed and acted upon and the lived reality of food and nutrition insecurity. These findings indicate that there is a need to consider how the food system interacts with a range of other systems and how food has multiple meanings and uses within these systems. While it is unrealistic to expect policy to respond to this level of nuance, there is a need to find ways to reframe the problem, and to generate programmes and policies that engage several departments to address the transversal nature of the problem. It is further essential for the assumptions about the role of the private sector as an agent of development to be interrogated by the state.

Conclusion

The new Sustainable Development Goals, which are set to profoundly influence policy and programme development at the global and national scales, fail to acknowledge the health and development challenges associated with rapidly changing food consumption patterns in the developing world. The dominant framing of nutrition challenges remains that of under-nutrition. This chapter has argued that, while under-nutrition remains a critical health and development challenge, the focus on it as the sole nutrition problem has the potential to exacerbate the rapid rise in obesity and associated diseases.

The food-related SDGs have been informed by the global food security literature, which has been dominated by a discourse that equates food insecurity with hunger and malnutrition. This then proposes solutions based on increased production and social safety nets. Where obesity is acknowledged, it is often understood as being driven by poor food choices, and therefore proposes nutrition education. The absence of focus on obesity and the nutrition transition in the SDGs may also be attributed to the relative absence of focus on this issue within the global health literature, which has until recently had a bias towards infectious diseases. Although obesity is increasingly an object of study, this disciplinary shift did not make a contribution to the SDGs. There remains a disconnect between the global food security and global health literatures which has led to the failure of the SDGs to acknowledge the emerging realities of food and nutrition security. This disconnect is also likely to lead to the continued neglect of the drivers and impacts of the nutrition transition at the global, national and local scales.

This chapter has argued that policies and programmes that respond to changing food consumption patterns, which are leading to the shift in nutrition-related disease profiles, are required. It is not enough, however, that these focus on poverty alleviation and nutrition education to help people make better choices. Rather, this chapter has argued that food and nutrition insecurity needs to be viewed as a food system issue requiring a multi-sectoral set of policy responses. Such a set of policy responses requires one to understand the drivers of policy at these scales. The chapter therefore considered the ways in which the global policy agenda has been interpreted at the national scale, and how that national scale policy agenda relates to the actual drivers of food choice. To do so, the chapter presented data on the lived experience of food choice by children in Cape Town, South Africa. These data illustrate that food choices need to be understood in the wider spatial, social and economic contexts of the food environment. Through focusing on three sites of food engagement – the home, the school and the journey – the chapter illustrates the multiple ways in which food choice is mediated by economic, social and spatial processes. Food is used by a range of actors, such as the school and the family, to meet a set of broader non-food-related objectives. The ways in which these objectives shape food choice need far greater interrogation.

This chapter therefore argues that national and global food policies and strategies need to better acknowledge the systemic drivers of food insecurity and inadequate nutrition. Many of the authors previously advocating for this have taken a political economy of food perspective and have focused their critique at the global scale (see e.g. Patel, 2008; McMichael, 2009). Others from a public health perspective have argued for approaches that address the food environment, food system and behaviour change communication in an integrated manner (Hawkes *et al.*, 2013). I argue for something slightly different, namely a greater consideration of how food choice is mediated by the interactions between the food system and other spatial, economic and political systems. The work presented in this chapter suggests that there is a need for greater levels of cross-departmental integration within food policy.

However, in order to achieve this there is a need to work towards disrupting the current development narrative of food and nutrition insecurity to expose the systemic drivers of food and nutrition insecurity. This will require a shift in research focus within food security studies in the Global South to acknowledge the nutrition transition, as well as continued research within global health studies on obesity and diet-related NCDs. Finally, it will require fine-grained transdisciplinary research engaging the social, economic, political and spatial drivers of food consumption, as well as research on the impacts of existing food and health policies on food consumption. Without such research, the impacts of the nutrition transition will continue to be neglected and food policies that accelerate this transition will continue to be the norm.

Notes

1 The IFSS is set to be replaced by the new National Food and Nutrition Security Policy.
2 This chapter uses the term 'foodways' as described by Cannuscio *et al.* (2010, 382): 'Foodways are the processes involved in the growth, purchase, preparation, consumption, sharing – or absence – of food within communities.'
3 At the time of research the Rand to pound sterling exchange rate was approximately 11.6:1.
4 Thirty-eight per cent gave no answer to this question.
5 Small shops operated within houses.

References

Action Against Hunger (2015) *Joint Statement on the Need for an Indicator on Childhood Wasting in the Sustainable Development Goals.* Available at http://www.actionagainsthunger.org.uk/publication/joint-statement-need-indicator-childhood-wasting-sustainable-development-goals.

Battersby, J. (2002) *A Question of Marginalization: Coloured Identities and Education in the Western Cape, South Africa.* Unpublished D.Phil. thesis, School of Geography, Oxford University.

Battersby, J. (2011a) The state of urban food insecurity in Cape Town. *Urban Food Security Series No. 11,* African Food Security Urban Network, Queen's University, Canada.

Battersby, J. (2011b) Urban food insecurity in Cape Town, South Africa: an alternative approach to food access. *Development Southern Africa* 28(4): 545–561.

Battersby, J. (2012) Beyond the food desert: finding ways to speak about urban food security in South Africa. *Geografiska Annaler, Series B Human Geography* 94(2)?

Battersby, J. (2015) Food security as a lens on the lived experience of poverty in Philippi. In Brown-Luthango, M. (ed.) *State/Society Synergy in Philippi, Cape Town.* African Centre for Cities, University of Cape Town, pp. 94–117.

Battersby, J. and Peyton, S. (2014) The geography of supermarkets in Cape Town: supermarket expansion and food access. *Urban Forum* 25(2): 153–164.

Briggs, J. and Yeboah, I.A.E. (2001) Structural adjustment and the contemporary sub-Saharan African city. *Area* 33(1): 18–26.

Brownell, K. (2012) Thinking forward: the quicksand of appeasing the food industry. *PLoS Med* 9(7): e1001254, doi: 10.1371/journal.pmed.1001254.

Butland, B., Jebb, S., Kopelman, P., McPherson, K., Thomas, S., Mardell, J. and Parry, V. (2007) *Foresight: Tackling Obesity: Future Choices – Project Report.* London: Government Office for Science.

Cannuscio, C.C., Weiss, E.E. and Asch, D.A. (2010) The contribution of urban foodways to health disparities. *Journal of Urban Health* 87(3): 381–393.

Cecchini, M., Sassi, F. and Lauer, J.A. (2010) Tackling of unhealthy diets, physical inactivity, and obesity: health effects and cost-effectiveness. *The Lancet* 376(10): 1775–1784.

Child Health Unit (1997) *Evaluation of South Africa's Primary School Nutrition Programme.* Durban: Health Systems Trust.

Chopra, M., Whitten, C. and Drimie, S. (2009) Combating malnutrition in South Africa. *GAIN Working Paper No.1,* Global Alliance for Improved Nutrition.

City of Cape Town (2007) *Five Year Plan for Cape Town: Integrated Development Plan (IDP): 2007/8-2011/2012.* City of Cape Town.

City of General Santos (2013) An ordinance providing for a comprehensive policy for the respect, promotion, fulfillment and protection of children's rights, enhancement of support system and mechanism, and for other purposes, Ordinance No. 07 Series of 2013. Available at http://spgensantos.ph/2013/11/ordinance-07-series-of-2013/.

Clacherty, A., Mabogoane, M. and Pelo, T. (2006) *South African School Nutrition Programme: Formative Evaluation Report*. Report Commissioned by DPRU, UCT. Appendix B to Poswell, L. and Leibbrandt, M. *Report 2 on the National School Feeding Scheme: Evaluation Methodologies*. Development Policy.

CMC (Cape Metropolitan Council) (1996) *Metropolitan Spatial Development Framework: Technical Report*. Cape Town: CMC.

Competition Commission (2008) Competition Commission focus on agriculture and food value chains. *Competition News* 29: 1–4.

Cooke, K. (2012) personal communication.

Crush, J.S. and Frayne, G.B. (2011) Urban food insecurity and the new international food security agenda. *Development Southern Africa* 28: 527–544.

Department of Agriculture (2002) *Integrated Food Security Strategy for South Africa*. Pretoria: Government Printer.

Department of Health (2002) *Integrated Nutrition Plan: Strategic Plan 2002/2003 to 2006/2007*. Nutrition and Provincial Nutrition Units, Department of Health.

Doak, C.M., Adair, L.S., Bentley, M., Monteiro, C. and Popkin, B.M. (2005) The dual burden household and the nutrition transition paradox. *International Journal of Obesity* 29(1): 129–136.

Drewnowski, A. and Darmon, N. (2005) The economics of obesity: dietary energy density and energy cost. *American Journal of Clinical Nutrition* 82(Suppl.): 265s–73s.

Drimie, S. and Ruysenaar, S. (2010) The Integrated Food Security Strategy of South Africa: an institutional analysis. *Agrekon* 49(3): 316–337.

FAO (1996) Rome Declaration on World Food Security. Available at http://www.fao.org/docrep/003//w3613e/w3613e00.htm.

FAO (2015) Indicators for the post-2015 Sustainable Development Agenda Joint Proposal of the Rome Based Agencies (RBAs) of indicators for GOAL 2: End hunger, achieve food security and improved nutrition and promote sustainable agriculture. Draft 25, February. Available at http://unstats.un.org/unsd/post-2015/activities/egm-on-indicator-framework/docs/Goal%202%20joint%20proposal_final_draft_CC.pdf.

Fukuda-Parr, S. and Orr, A. (2014) The MDG Hunger Target and the Competing Frameworks of Food Security. *Journal of Human Development and Capabilities: A Multi-Disciplinary Journal for People-Centered Development* 15(2–3): 147–160.

Gómez, M.I., Barrett, C.B. and Raney, T. (2013) Post-green revolution food systems and the triple burden of malnutrition. *Food Policy* 42: 129–138.

Greenberg, S. (2010) *Contesting the Food System in South Africa: Issues and Opportunities* (No. 42). Institute for Poverty, Land and Agrarian Studies, University of the Western Cape.

Gustafson, E. (n.d.) About 30 Project. Available at http://ellengustafson.com/30-project/.

Haddad, L. (2013) How should nutrition be positioned in the post-2015 agenda? *Food Policy* 43: 231–352.

Haddad, L.J., Hawkes, C., Achadi, E., Ahuja, A., Ag Bendech, M., Bhatia, K. and Flores-Ayala, R. (2015) *Global Nutrition Report 2015: Actions and Accountability to Advance Nutrition and Sustainable Development*. International Food Policy Resources Institute.

Hawkes, C., Jewell, J. and Allen, K. (2013) A food policy package for healthy diets and the prevention of obesity and diet-related non-communicable disease: The NOURISHING framework. *Obesity Reviews* 14(Suppl. 2): 159–168.

Higgins, K. (2013) The power of global goals: Reflections on the MDGs. North South Institute Policy Brief.

Igumbor, E., Sanders, D., Puoane, T., Tsolekile, L., Schwarz, C., Purdy, C., Swart, R., Durão S. and Hawkes, C. (2012) 'Big Food,' the consumer food environment, health, and the policy response in South Africa. *PLoS Medicine* 9(7).

Karlsson, J. (2002) The role of democratic governing bodies in South African schools. *Comparative Education* 38(3): 327–336.

Ki-Moon, B. (2014) *The Road to Dignity by 2030: Ending Poverty, Transforming All Lives and Protecting the Planet*. Synthesis report of the Secretary-General on the post-2015 Sustainable Development Agenda.

Kirsten, J. (2012) The political economy of food price policy in South Africa. Working Paper No. 2012–102. UNU-WIDER, Helsinki.

Kirsten, J. and Van Zyl, J. (1996) The contemporary agriculture policy environment: undoing the legacy of the past. In *Agricultural Land Reform in South Africa*. Cape Town: Oxford University Press.

Labadarios, D., Steyn, N.P. and Maunder, M. (2005) The National Food Consumption Survey (NFCS): South Africa, 1999. *Public Health Nutrition* 8(5): 533–543.

Lemon, A. and Battersby-Lennard, J. (2009a) Emerging geographies of school provision in Cape Town, South Africa. *Geography* 94(2): 79–87.

Lemon, A. and Battersby-Lennard, J. (2009b) Overcoming the apartheid legacy in Cape Town schools. *The Geographical Review* 99(4): 517–538.

Lemon, A. and Battersby-Lennard, J. (2011) Studying together, living apart: emerging geographies of school attendance in Cape Town, South Africa. *African Affairs* 110(438): 97–120.

Ligthelm, A.A. (2005) Informal retailing through home-based micro-enterprises: the role of spaza shops. *Development Southern Africa* 22(2): 199–214.

Marraccini, T., Meltzer, S., Bourne, L. and Draper, C.E. (2012) A qualitative evaluation of exposure to and perceptions of the Woolworths Healthy Tuck Shop Guide in Cape Town, South Africa. *Childhood Obesity* 8(4): 349–377.

McMichael, P. (2009) A food regime analysis of the 'world food crisis'. *Agriculture and Human Values* 26: 281–295.

McMichael, P. and Schneider, M. (2011) Food security politics and the Millennium Development Goals. *Third World Quarterly* 32(1): 119–139.

Moodie, R., Stuckler, D. and Monteiro, C. (2013) Profits and pandemics: prevention of harmful effects of tobacco, alcohol, and ultra-processed food and drink industries. *The Lancet* 381: 670–679.

Ng, M., Fleming, T. and Robinson, M. (2014) Global, regional, and national prevalence of overweight and obesity in children and adults during 1980–2013: a systematic analysis for the Global Burden of Disease Study 2013. *The Lancet* 384: 766–781.

NPLAN (National Policy and Legal Analysis Network) (2008) *Model Healthy Food Ordinance: Creating a Health Food Zone Around Schools by Regulating the Location of Fast Food Restaurants (and Mobile Food Vendors)*. Oakland, CA: NPLAN.

Otero, G., Pechlaner, G., Liberman, G. and Gürcan, E.C. (2015) Food security and inequality: measuring the risk of exposure to the neoliberal diet. Simons Papers in Security and Development, No. 42/2015. School for International Studies, Simon Fraser University, Vancouver, March.

Patel, L., Hochfield, T., Moodley, J. and Mutwell, R. (2012) The gender dynamics and impact of the Child Support Grant in Doornkop, Soweto. Centre for Social Development Research Report, University of Johannesburg.

Patel, R. (2008) *Stuff and Starved: The Hidden Battle for the World Food System*. New York: Melville House.

Pogge, T. (2004) The First United Nations Millennium Development Goal: a cause for celebration? *Journal of Human Development: A Multi-Disciplinary Journal for People-Centered Development* 5(3): 377–397.

Popkin, B.M. (1999) Urbanization, lifestyle changes and the nutrition transition. *World Development* 27(11): 1905–1916.

Popkin, B.M. (2003) The nutrition transition in the developing world. *Development Policy Review* 21(5–6): 581–597.

Popkin, B.M. and Bellagio Meeting Group (2013) Bellagio Declaration 2013. *Obesity Reviews* 14: 9–10.

Popkin, B.M., Adair, L.S. and Ng, S.W. (2012) Global nutrition transition and the pandemic of obesity in developing countries. *Nutrition Reviews* 70(1): 3–21.

Poswell, L. and Leibbrandt, M. (2006) *Report 1 on the National School Feeding Scheme: Targeting Criteria and Appropriateness*. Development Policy Research Unit and Southern Africa Labour Research Unit, University of Cape Town.

Reubi, D., Herrick, C. and Brown, T. (2016) The politics of non-communicable diseases in the global South. *Health & Place* 39: 179–187

Roberto, C.A., Swinburn, B., Hawkes, C., Huang, T.T-K., Costa, S.A., Zwicker, L., Cawley, J.H. and Brownwell, K.D. (2015) Patchy progress on obesity prevention: emerging examples, entrenched barriers, and new thinking. *The Lancet* 385: 2400–2409.

Roos, J.A. (2012) *Food System Analysis and the Development of a System Dynamics Approach to Improve Food Security for a Vulnerable Community in the Breede River Region, Western Cape Province, South Africa*. Unpublished Master's thesis, Department of Engineering Management, Stellenbosch University.

Ruel, M.T., Haddad, L. and Garrett, J.L. (1998) Some urban facts of life: implications for research and policy. *World Development* 27(11): 1917–1938.

SDSN (2015) Indicators and a monitoring framework for the Sustainable Development Goals: Launching a data revolution for the SDGs. *Sustainable Development Solutions Network: Paris, New York, New Delhi*, 12. Available at http://unsdsn.org/resources/publications/indicators/.

Shaw, H.J. (2006) Food deserts: towards the development of a classification. *Geografiska Annaler: Series B, Human Geography* 88(2): 231–247.

Shisana, O., Labadarios, D. and Rehle, T. (2013) *South African National Health and Nutrition Examination Survey (SANHANES-1)*. Cape Town: HSRC Press.

Soudien, C. (2004) Constituting the class: an analysis of the process of 'integration' in South African schools. In Chisholm, L. (ed.) *Education and Social Change in South Africa*. Pretoria: HSRC Press, pp. 89–114.

Stupar, D., Eide, W.B, Bourne, L., Hendricks, M., Iverson, P.O. and Wandel, M. (2012) The nutrition transition and the human right to food for adolescents in the Cape Metropolitan Area: implications for nutrition policy. *Food Policy* 37(3): 199–205.

Temple, N.J., Steyn, N.P., Myburgh, N.G. and Nel, J.H. (2006) Food items consumed by students attending schools in different socio-economic areas in Cape Town, South Africa. *Nutrition* 22(3): 252–258.

Temple, N.J., Steyn, N.P., Fourie, J. and De Villiers, A. (2011) Price and availability of healthy food: A study in rural South Africa. *Nutrition* 27(1): 55–58.

Thow, A.M., Sanders, D. and Drury, E. (2015) Regional trade and the nutrition transition: opportunities to strengthen NCD prevention policy in the Southern African Development Community. *Global Health Action* 8: 28338.

Turok, I. (2001) Persistent polarisation post-*Apartheid*? Progress towards urban integration in Cape Town. *Urban Studies* 38(13): 2349–2377.

Vandemoortele, J. (2009) The MDG conundrum: meeting the targets without missing the point. *Development Policy Review* 27: 355–371.

Vandevijvere, S., Chow, C.C. and Hall, K.D. (2015) Increased food energy supply as a major driver of the obesity epidemic: a global analysis. *Bulletin of the World Health Organization* 93: 446–456.

Watson, K. (2009) *Food Security and Dietary Diversity for Learners at Observatory Junior Primary School in Cape Town, South Africa.* Unpublished Honours thesis, Department of Environmental and Geographical Science, University of Cape Town.

WCED (Western Cape Education Department) (2007) *R50 Million Feeding Scheme Benefits Two Hundred Thousand Learners.* Available at http://www.capegateway.gov.za/eng/pubs/news/2007/mar/153763.

WHO/FAO (2003) Diet, nutrition and the prevention of chronic diseases: a report of a joint WHO/FAO Join Consultation, WHO Technical Report Series No. 916. Geneva, Switzerland.

Wiggin, S. and Keats, S. (2015) The rising cost of a healthy diet: changing relative prices of food in high-income and emerging economies. *ODI Report May 2015*. London: ODI.

Zager, K. (2011) *Commutes, Constraints and Food: The Geography of Choice*. Unpublished Honours thesis, Department of Environmental and Geographical Science, University of Cape Town.

12 Structural violence, capabilities and the experiential politics of alcohol regulation

Clare Herrick

Introduction

In South Africa, alcohol and its multiple harms represent a significant and multi-dimensional urban governance problem. Liquor consumption contributes to the country's substantial double burden of infectious and non-communicable disease (Parry *et al.*, 2011), violence, injury (Seedat *et al.*, 2009) and HIV/AIDS (Chersich and Rees, 2010). More than this, though, 'the harmful use of alcohol inflicts significant social and economic losses on individuals and society at large', and thus 'has to be addressed to ensure sustained social and economic development throughout the world' (WHO, 2014: vii). Alcohol is thus rising up the global health agenda thanks to this strategic and semantic elision of development threat and its categorisation as one of the four modifiable risk factors for the worldwide NCD burden. This has led to a new voluntary target for a 10 per cent per capita reduction in harmful consumption by 2025 (ibid.). On the ground, however, there still seems to be a significant gap between efforts to regulate alcohol and its consumption and attention to 'the many political and social determinants of health that make people vulnerable to disease and injury' (Biehl and Petryna, 2013: 3). This upstream perspective is central to the analysis of how, in the urban contexts explored in this chapter, alcohol can be implicated in a 'pathogenic social spiral' in which already risky lives can beget further risk-taking (Nguyen and Peschard, 2003: 464). This 'spiral' forms part of a broader landscape of what Paul Farmer (2004) terms 'structural violence' or those 'social arrangements that put individuals and populations in harm's way' (Farmer *et al.*, 2006: e448) and that are usually 'beyond [their] control' (Nguyen and Peschard, 2003: e449).

Structural violence, Farmer argues, stymies the exercise of individual and collective agency, thus reinforcing the multiple inequalities that are both its cause and effect (2004: 307). In this chapter therefore, alcohol is taken as an example through which to explore the effects of structural violence on everyday lives, not least for the ways in which it speaks directly to the kinds of individual and collective vulnerabilities – or what Sen (1999) has termed 'unfreedoms' – that are so often absent from global health's programmatic mindset. Within the context of development and public health policies in South Africa, alcohol is a particularly fraught object of governance, as it has long offered a means for individuals to realise greater freedoms through its small-scale retailing, but also through its genesis of spaces of socialisation, self-presentation and leisure. On the flip side, alcohol's negative externalities may be rendered more pernicious by many South Africans' lack of substantive freedoms (e.g. low life expectancies, HIV, unemployment). In this sense and in Sen's language, the everyday experiences of alcohol and its consumption may undermine people's 'functioning' or their ability to lead lives of value. Structural violence and the Capabilities Approach, as well as emergent concerns with the nature of 'structural vulnerability' (Quesada *et al.*, 2011), further highlight the impact of alcohol on poor communities as a clear issue of social justice (Venkatapuram, 2009). Alcohol has yet to be explicitly examined in relation to structural violence, despite its sale and consumption in South Africa invoking the same issues of rights, power and agency under conditions of inequity that motivate calls for a 'biosocial' approach to affliction (Farmer, 2004: 19; see also Gandy, 2005).

To explore these ideas, this chapter offers three arguments. First, rather than evidence of individual deviance or 'cultural obstacles' (Biehl and Petryna, 2013: 15), risky alcohol consumption in the poor urban communities studied emerges as a form of coping, escapism and pleasure-seeking under situations of structural violence. These include gender and socio-economic inequality, residential segregation, unemployment and persistent inequities in law enforcement. Second, drinking practices and their consequences *contribute to* and *reinforce* broader conditions of structural violence which can have further complex, intended and unintended impacts. And third, these *impacts* (e.g. violence, crime, injury, poor health) and their *settings* (e.g. townships, informal settlements, unlicensed drinking venues or 'shebeens') have tended to be the central object of political intervention, rather than the upstream structural conditions that engender them. From a sustainable development perspective, this approach may ultimately be ineffective in reducing risk and vulnerability, facilitating coping and, therefore, enhancing freedoms. To explore these contentions I turn first to the intersections of structural violence, vulnerabilities and the Capabilities Approach to theorise the complex set of problems posed by alcohol and its regulation in Cape Town, before offering a brief methodological note. I then analyse the findings of a series of focus groups according to themes that respond to the chapter's three arguments: the factors that drive drinking; the experiences and harms of alcohol, and respondents' suggestions for how best to unravel the pathogenic social spiral perpetuated by liquor. In exploring respondents' embodied encounters with liquor and how they reflect (and are reflective of) the broader inequities that pattern daily life and life chances, I hope to uncover how suffering unfolds in relation to alcohol use and abuse and, therefore, contribute new empirical and geographical dimensions to both the study of structural violence and the politics of alcohol regulation in the context of shifting global health agendas.

Alcohol, structural violence, vulnerabilities and capabilities in South Africa

Over the past decade, Michael Marmot and colleagues have argued for a shift in attention from the aetiology of disease to the 'more fundamental structures of social hierarchy and the socially determined conditions in which people grow, live, work, and age' (Marmot, 2007: 1153). Amartya Sen's Capabilities Approach has been central to work on the social determinants of health in its concern with the causes and consequences of the inequitable distribution of poor health. Here, health represents a 'meta-capability ... to achieve a cluster of capabilities to be and do things that reflect a life worthy of equal human dignity' (Venkatapuram, 2012: 9). This holistic perspective is valuable (if under-explored) with respect to the study of behavioural risks such as drinking alcohol, for which acute and chronic health outcomes are set alongside equally pernicious social and economic ones (e.g. absenteeism, violence and crime), which are often the more powerful policy motivators. However, when capability deprivation is deemed to emerge from 'the lack of opportunities to choose from and a poorly developed opportunity to choose' (Leßmann, 2011: 457), there needs to be greater recognition of how and why people's choices are often preconfigured by the distal pathogenic effects of inequality. In turn, this deeply problematises the assumption of individual 'choice' (e.g. to consume or sell liquor) and individual agency that tends to characterise neoliberal health policy (Leßmann, 2011).

In South Africa, alcohol is conceptualised as a problem along two primary axes: (1) how, where, when and by whom it is retailed; and (2) the nature and consequences of its consumption. The contemporary urban retail landscape of liquor and its regulation is a clear legacy of colonial and apartheid restrictions over the right to buy and consume 'white liquor' among Africans (Mager, 2004; Rogerson and Hart, 1986). As Wilfried Schärf has argued, not only did 'the state's liquor interests [form] an integral part of the functioning and success of apartheid policy' (1985a: 53), but the distribution of liquor among non-whites was 'a conscious instrument of class control' (1985a: 57). This socio-spatial legacy lives on in Cape Town as 'previously advantaged' neighbourhoods continue to hold the monopoly of liquor licences. Past inequalities in economic, social and political rights to drink have produced the social and spatial 'fix' of South Africa's vast illegal liquor retailing sector. These township shebeens (unlicensed and therefore illegal bars) are typically small-scale, survivalist and located in residential areas. Their numbers also dwarf the formal trade. The South African state has long grappled with the 'shebeen problem' (Rogerson, 1992) and the 2012 Western Cape Liquor Act represents the Provincial government's most recent attempt to mitigate and manage the multiple risks the sector is argued to pose to health and human life. This management strategy has primarily been through 'zero tolerance' police raids of unlicensed premises, seizing alcohol and fining shebeeners found to be in possession of more than 150 litres of alcohol. These endeavours have met with mixed reactions: from welcome relief, to anger, alienation and confusion on the other (Faull, 2013). In early 2014, a new consultation process for the Act's amendment began after acknowledgements that the 150-litre rule had made raiding shebeens (which rarely store such volumes) unlawful and securing a conviction impossible. In a twist that manifestly highlights the socio-economic disparities and tensions of South African life, the proposed amendments would not only grant the police extended powers to inspect and close shebeens without warrants and sell any confiscated liquor at state-run auctions, but would also secure the rights of 'bona-fide wine collectors storing more than 150 litres'. The politics of liquor and its control run deep in South Africa, a point brought home by the focus group findings explored below.

A brief methodological note

Focus groups were undertaken in three case study sites in Cape Town: Salt River; Freedom Park and Philippi. The three sites are representative, in different ways, of some of the broad human, social and economic development challenges facing the city: poverty; inequality; unemployment; poor health, and inadequate infrastructure. Salt River is located on the edge of the Central Business District and was originally a coloured community. More recently it has become home to a significant influx of pan-African immigrants as well as a growing number of pioneer gentrifiers drawn to the area's affordable housing stock and its burgeoning array of cafés and restaurants, amid significant numbers of homeless. Philippi is a relatively new black township built on once-rural land that now houses approximately 200,000 people. The area still has an agricultural periphery, but has recently come under pressure to turn over this land for urban expansion. This pressure compounds current problems of inadequate service delivery (housing, transport, sanitation) facing the community. Freedom Park is, by contrast, a small upgraded community that sits on the former site of a coloured squatter settlement. Its residents may now have formal housing and (limited) services, but they also suffer significant problems of domestic violence and drug abuse.

Focus groups are a particularly valuable method for approaching the sensitive topic of alcohol consumption/harms, as they can explore individual and collective values, attitudes and beliefs, and how these are corroborated or contested within and by the group dynamic (Kidd and Parshall, 2000). Their ability to uncover the context or 'situatedness' of experience is particularly pertinent to the study of alcohol given that drinking is intricately linked to the multi-scalar ecologies of place: the availability of alcohol; the nature of access; local cultures of drinking; social norms; community awareness and support; economic opportunities; recreation and leisure; and policing (Jayne *et al.*, 2008a, 2008b). To explore these issues, the facilitator's schedule of questions was kept consistent across the sites and explored: where people drank in the local area; what they drank; when they drank; the motives for, experiences of and consequences of drinking; how much money was spent, and what respondents felt should be done to reduce alcohol consumption and its harms.

Eight groups were convened in total: four split by age and gender in Philippi, members of a church group and community policing forum in Salt River, and two mixed-age female groups in Freedom Park.[1] The composition of these groups reflects some of the challenges faced in recruiting participants in each of the sites (Lawhon et al. 2014) as well as the stigma and fear attached to discussing alcohol in a culture where the majority of people are actually teetotal. After all groups were completed, the facilitators transcribed the audio recording in its original language (Xhosa and Afrikaans) and then translated this transcription into English for inductive qualitative content analysis (Hsieh and Shannon, 2005). This approach seeks themes, meanings and contexts to build a picture of participants' 'emplaced everyday experiences', as well as deeper insight into how they 'understand and frame [such] experiences' (Wiles *et al.*, 2005: 97–98) with reference to broader conditions of structural violence.

Experiencing, mitigating and managing structural violence

The drivers of drinking

In order to explore the experiences of alcohol, it is fundamental to understand *why* people drink. Across all three sites, respondents identified the main underlying drivers of consumption as personal stress and unemployment. Thus, when asked the question, 'Why do people in your community drink?', a respondent from Freedom Park replied that people drink as they have 'too many worries. Financial worries come first . . . joblessness, that's my problem. I live from day to day' (FP1). This view of the causal influences of stress, poverty and unemployment was reiterated by two members of the second focus group in Freedom Park:

> 1: Stress plays a big role. It's almost like there's no way out, and then you drink because of it, but the next day you wake up with that same stress, and then you go back to the bottle again. So that's also a big problem in our community.
> 2: Poverty also plays a big role in it, and unemployment.
>
> (FP2)

It is important to note that people drink to escape the stresses caused by poverty and unemployment, but that these are then magnified by the cost of drinking. In turn, this compounds stress, ensuring that the cycle of *needing to drink* remains intact (Mulia *et al.*, 2008). It is interesting that the ascription of drinking to life's quotidian stresses was more common among older respondents, especially in Philippi. For example, the older male group concurred that 'when you have financial problems you tend to drink thinking that your problems will disappear or will be lighter [but] alcohol wastes money – the only people who are benefiting are those who sell alcohol' (POM). Among this group, alcohol was viewed as an effective (although short-term) and socially normalised distraction from everyday problems. By contrast, while the group of young men from Philippi did not mention stress per se, they did ascribe drinking to the boredom of being jobless and a lack of alternative leisure activities. The group of older women discussed family dynamics and the pressures of children's expectations of parents as a source of stress in which 'some [parents] are getting strangled by their children for money. That is why many parents think, let me just drink' (POW). For the respondents in Philippi therefore, stress emerged in differentiated ways, with drink seen as a common solution to (or escape from) both the state of stress itself and stressful environments.

Respondents also cast the drivers of drinking as originating in childhood, whether through parents taking children to shebeens, sending them to fetch drinks, teenage socialisation or peer pressure. For respondents in Salt River and Freedom Park in particular (most likely reflecting the higher rates of foetal alcohol syndrome in these communities), there was a strong sense that many children could be born biologically addicted to drink, with attendant consequences for violence as learned behaviour. As one group member explained, 'when the parents are alcoholics the children automatically become alcoholics too. If you were a man that abused your wife while you were drinking, the children do the exact same, because that is their way of thinking' (FP2). Familial learning and influence was also felt to be notable when families contained 'a drinker'. For example, one respondent from Freedom Park explained how her father 'worked and he was a drinker'. More than this, she detailed how 'he was one of the people that get crazy when they drink. . . . He drank every day. Drinking was his hobby, get up and drink, go to bed and drink, every day.' The semantic bifurcation between 'drinkers' and 'non-drinkers' was often used as shorthand for an individual's moral status and for narrating individuals' changing relationships with alcohol through time. In addition, it helped people explain how certain life events or triggers – such as finding religion in the case of respondents from Freedom Park and the Salt River Church Group – spurred their moral salvation as they crossed over from 'drinker' to 'non-drinker'.

Young male respondents in Philippi held quite different views of the reasons for drinking initiation. As one respondent summed it up, 'some people drink because they think that they are flushing out their stress and problems by drinking, but most people want to be happy and have fun' (PYM). The young men, for example, were keen to discuss the micro-dynamics of the tavern as space for simple enjoyment, socialisation and pleasure, meeting people (particularly for many migrants from the Eastern Cape), making a name for oneself and asserting masculinity through consumption. As one group member recounted:

> I'm new in Philippi . . . I want to introduce myself at the shebeen. If I was not drinking people would not know me or I am not cool. It's a way of setting a statement, be acknowledged as a guy. . . . You will buy beers and share with others and chat and you will find out that you are from the Eastern Cape and also you find out that you are from the same *Majola* clan. When you are drunk you can speak with somebody that you never spoke to. Next time when you don't have the money he is the one who buys the liquor for you.
>
> (PYM)

This assertion of confident masculinity plays out in two ways within drinking spaces: through the type and volume of liquor consumed and through using liquor as a vehicle to secure the attention of women. The two are, however, inherently linked, as the purchase of an appropriately impressive volume of (premium brand) liquor can help secure female attention or at least sufficiently lessen inhibitions to make a move. The need to fit in with the activities of peers, ensure bragging rights, and establishing social norms and camaraderie drive a desire and need to drink. These kinds of social motivations mark out South African youth as strikingly similar to those in many other countries (Engels *et al.*, 2006; Kuntsche *et al.*, 2005). Equally significant, however, is that while the *causes* of drinking noted by respondents exhibit broad parallels with the findings from other qualitative surveys in a variety of countries, the *consequences* of these practices exhibit particularities that are inextricable from the quotidian physical and structural violence of South African society (Altbeker, 2007; Steinberg, 2008). These are explored below.

Consequences

Across the case study sites, respondents reported that alcohol drained financial resources, perpetuated food insecurity, caused family breakdown and initiated a spiral of debt with profound social consequences. Respondents were keen to share these experiences, which varied from killing people while driving drunk, to indecent exposure, being unable to go to work on Monday, missing trains to work, being arrested for evading train fares, being mugged, stabbed and getting fired. Several young men also flagged alcohol as a driver of unsafe sex, putting them at greater risk of contracting HIV. Another suggested that the cold temperature of drinks was inherently unhealthy, as it could *cause* TB. When asked where people got enough money to drink through whole weekends, respondents across all three sites suggested that many drinkers (as well as drug-takers in the case of Freedom Park) had turned to crime to finance their habits. The constant need for money (as well as for reciprocal acts of generosity to compensate for a lack of money) was also viewed as a major *driver* of interpersonal violence in communities. One young man in the Philippi group recounted an example of where drunkenness had led one man to stab another 'because of a cigarette'. Alcohol and its effects thus seep into the pores of everyday life in the case study communities, too often in the form of severe violence and trauma that compound more commonplace socio-environmental 'insults' (Quesada *et al.*, 2011). In one example, a resident told of being repeatedly woken by women screaming throughout the night:

> In the taverns they like things that make people cry till morning . . . when you wake up you don't sleep again because it sounds like things are making noise inside the house. . . . Once there was a corpse at this tavern in front of me, and that person didn't do anything.
>
> (POW)

The persistence of threat was, in this instance, compounded by the gruesome (but not uncommon) experience of witnessing a dead body about which nothing was done. In situations of violence, liquor was often seen as an excuse enabling the guilty to escape conviction. Thus, instead of drunkenness *aggravating* the crime, respondents suggested that inebriation often facilitated pleas of innocence if and when the case ever made it to the judicial system. This reinforced some respondents' overriding moral panic that alcohol was fuelling a culture of irresponsibility and immorality:

> Look how many of children are getting raped these days. What do they say? I was drunk. I didn't know what I was doing . . . I read now the other day about quite a few guys that got off free, there was not good evidence or whatever, they just say they were drunk they didn't know what they were doing.
>
> (SRCG)

Violence might be attributed to intoxication, but it was also ascribed to the effects of specific drink *types and venues*. For example, older women in Philippi suggested that 'the places with fights are the ones with jukeboxes' as they often had a more intoxicating mix of young male drinkers, women and glassware. By contrast, venues for traditional African beer drinkers were seen as more innocuous social spaces where 'they are sitting with their beer. . . . They have their conversation, nothing causes a fight' (POW). 'Problem' shebeens stopped many residents sleeping because of loud music, people standing and drinking near their houses and constant fears over personal safety. This severely compromised quality of life and well-being, especially for tired children unable to concentrate in school. This is a clear example of alcohol magnifying the structural violence perpetuated by already-existing inequalities in educational provision and quality – the inability of one Provincial education department to supply school textbooks, classroom over-crowding, schools without electricity and inadequate resources – hindering students' own abilities to achieve the qualifications needed to overcome South Africa's 'structural crisis of waged employment' (Barchiesi, 2007: 574).

One of the central themes brought up in focus group discussions was the changing gender dynamics of drinking and its consequences for cultural, family and economic life. Female drinkers were judged (most critically by other women) for failing in their maternal and marital duties, choosing alcohol over feeding their children and losing their self-respect. However, rather than question why changing community and individual circumstances may have catalysed women to turn to drink, respondents frequently cast them as immoral and guilty, especially when household or maternal duties were neglected. The group of older women in Philippi also reported their disgust at the growing number of women using men for alcohol and, in turn, using alcohol strategically to get men, without thought to the circumstances that may have precipitated these tactics. Within the masculinist culture of township life (Mager, 2010; Morrell *et al.*, 2012) where domestic violence is rife, drinking is a clear reflection of the multiple forms of violence exerted upon women's lives and bodies. In communities where rape is routinely underreported and a patriarchal society tends to pre-assume a women's guilt, drinking is a double-edged sword. Women may have an equal right to drink, but in so doing it places them in situations where they could be blamed for being victims of violence as a 'socially endorsed punitive project' that 'inscribe[s] subordinate status' (Moffett, 2006: 129). Women are thus trapped: if they drink they are rendered vulnerable to the actions of men and the moral judgements of others in the community. Yet, even if they do not drink, they are vulnerable to the significant pressure on household resources and violence that too often stems from men drinking.

Stories such as the one below were thus common:

> He says to his wife here is the money for groceries, and this is for my beer. When his money's finished he comes back home and demands the grocery money. The wife tries to stop him explaining that I haven't bought the groceries. The wife is at the risk of being beaten up and being sworn at and told 'you are not working'.
>
> (POW)

Here, high rates of female unemployment and single female-headed households not only drive the stresses that provoke drinking as a coping mechanism, but also create a dependency on men that becomes dangerous when household resources get converted to liquor. Women are reluctant to leave their husbands or partners even in violent situations, as they are wholly dependent on their income for basic household provisions for themselves and their children (who are viewed as their responsibility). This has further consequences for the reduction of community capabilities and freedoms. For example, members of the church group in Salt River highlighted that the monopolisation of household resources by male drinkers had led at least one woman they knew to start a shebeen from her home so as to feed her family. Selling liquor to pay for the drinking habits of others is deeply ironic, but for many poor communities it is a crucial coping strategy that eases the impact of certain vulnerabilities at the direct expense of reinforcing others. Vulnerabilities are further compounded by the use of social grant, disability, child credit or pension money to pay for alcohol, creating cycles of poverty, debt and dependency. Alcohol also provides sociable spaces of escape from these lived experiences.

Unfurling the pathogenic social spiral

This final section explores respondents' ideas about how alcohol-related harms should best be addressed, and crucially, who should assume responsibility for these efforts. The 2012 Western Cape Liquor Act, for example, has been justified with respect to the province's high rates of alcohol-related crime, violence, injury and foetal alcohol syndrome. Yet despite the legislation's long period of drafting, debate and attendant media attention, very few focus group respondents were aware of the new legislation or its likely effect. Rather, they *experienced* the Act through the increasing frequency with which local shebeens were raided, patrons threatened or arrested and liquor confiscated. It is thus unsurprising that opinions among group members differed in the extent to which they believed alcohol should be subjected to the kinds of governmental control set out in recent WHO publications. In Freedom Park, for example, residents complained that the police are either slow to respond when called out, or never come at all. The inadequacies of post-apartheid policing in South Africa's poor neighbourhoods have been documented elsewhere (Altbeker, 2005, 2007; Lemanski, 2004; Steinberg, 2008), but it also represents a clear form of structural violence with profound implications for community trust and cohesion. Respondents voiced concerns that the police were not doing enough to enforce laws such as the minimum drinking age or opening hours, giving shebeeners little incentive to stick to the regulations. For the young women in Philippi, this was indicative of 'alcohol tampering with values' in which police inaction was part of a broader shift in collective rights, duties and responsibilities. An example of this came from the Salt River Church Group in which one respondent highlighted community fears about the potentially lethal consequences of intervening in alcohol-related incidents:

> If you see a couple fighting in the road because of alcohol, you can get killed. So many times I think that is why neighbours won't get involved. So many times a husband beats his wife up, or a mother and daughter beat each other to death in front of everybody, because the community won't get involved because if they do they can get killed.
>
> (SRCG)

There is no doubt that this situation would be ameliorated if group members had felt able to trust in the police to protect them, but many felt they were too embroiled in scams with corrupt shebeeners. As one older respondent from Philippi noted, 'the police do not do their job and they are not of great help, the shebeen owners give them alcohol so they keep quiet. Even volunteers helping the police tell us the police are coming' (POM). There was also a suggestion that some shebeeners used police raids to their advantage by tipping off the police about competitors, thus ensuring a short-lived advantage while the other shebeen was temporarily closed. This evokes an argument made by Schärf almost three decades ago when he contended that 'the initial illegality of selling liquor ... amplifies the illicit methods by which the business survives' (1985b: 100). By extension, these illicit methods magnify existing vulnerabilities in the communities under study, entrenching life's everyday dangers. Indeed, the intersection of the liquor trade, the state and the informal sector arguably still constitutes 'a powerful form of control over the working class' (1985b: 105). While we could replace 'working class' with 'poor' in this context, such forms of control nevertheless still comprise punitive limits on the freedoms available to respondents, with freedom of choice and mobility persistently compromised.

When pressed about solutions to the everyday violence of alcohol, one proffered suggestion was making alcohol less 'cheap for even the poor man' (SRCPF), echoing the WHO's stance that increased taxation should decrease demand. The Freedom Park focus group, however, questioned the utility of a price increase, with one member arguing convincingly that beer was already more expensive than bread, but many drinkers still chose the former over the latter. Increasing prices may also only perpetuate the often-violent gendered struggles over household resources documented here (see also Bähre, 2007). One point of agreement was the need for greater state investment or in Sen's language 'collective responsibility' for addiction treatment services and educational provision. In contrast to the public health dismissal of education as a tool of alcohol harm reduction (Craplet, 2006; Foxcroft, 2006; Rehm *et al.*, 2006), respondents in Freedom Park wanted to learn more about the health effects of drinking. However, they also recognised the significant community stigma attached to attending such events as 'people don't respond because it gets put in the local newspaper, and I think everybody reads the local newspaper' (FP1). One of the biggest barriers is the social normalisation of drinking which means that 'while [people have] got the money to spend, while they choose to live their lives the way they want to, there is very little you can do [as] people will always find a way' (SRCG). This determination to drink (Measham, 2006) was a marked characteristic of the respondents' everyday experience of alcohol and seemed to feed into a generalised feeling of the futility of harm reduction efforts. Such apathy could also, however, be read as a strong justification for the curtailment of *certain* freedoms not through more laws, but through the effective and equitable *enforcement* of the panoply of existing rules and regulations, without which there will be few deterrents to risk-taking.

Conclusion

In this chapter, I have followed three lines of inquiry. First, I have explored how, rather than evidence of wilful deviance, risky alcohol consumption represents a form of coping, escapism and pleasure under situations of structural violence. While it may be expected that respondents in the different sites would vary in their views of drinking and its harms, they concurred about the magnitude of the problems they faced, as well as their underlying causes and consequences to a striking degree. There was also, however, a degree of agreement that the socialisation afforded by and through drinking – in neighbourhoods with precious few alternative leisure activities – was in itself an important way of coping with the persistent challenges of urban life. The second argument concerns how drinking practices and their consequences *contribute to* and *reinforce* broader conditions of structural violence which, in turn, have further intended and unintended impacts. When alcohol is laid over situations of absolute as well as relative poverty, then the consequences of drinking are only magnified in their significance. Moreover, these effects are deeply and persistently unequal. As Nguyen and Peschard have forcefully argued, 'in every society misfortune is selective, affecting some but not others' (2003: 467). It may not be that effects are absent, but as one respondent suggested, 'in the poor areas you see the results, but in the rich areas you don't see it clearly, but it's there, sometimes even worse' (SRCPF). The irony and challenge for South African alcohol policy is that home-based shebeens and their allied services (e.g. takeaway food, security and car attendants) also offer a means to mitigate and manage some of alcohol's externalities through providing employment and offering places of socialisation away from the home. Thus, the question of how policy might respect the rights of the poor to choose and to consume, while protecting communities from harm, is evocative of the 'regulatory complexity' evinced by Valverde (1998: 10). This complexity is further entrenched by policy's tendency to tackle liquor's downstream effects by closing shebeens rather than the political sphere acting upon the very reasons why shebeens remain an omnipresent feature of South African life. To therefore reflect on the problematic of policy, I will dwell in more detail on the final line of argument: that alcohol-related harms (e.g. violence, crime, injury, disease) and their settings (e.g. townships, informal settlements, shebeens) have long been the central object of policy interventions, rather than the structural conditions that have engendered them.

To return to Sen, if the aim of development policy is to expand individuals' freedoms so that they can 'make choices that matter to them' (Alkire, 2005: 117), Famer's suggestion that conditions of structural violence fundamentally 'constrict' and 'curb' agency and, therefore, choice (2004: 272) is significant. Sen is far more circumspect about the value of choice and, as Alkire (2005: 121) explains, increased choice may not guarantee the enjoyment of more valuable freedoms. Yet, without adequate capabilities, the ability to make choices that 'matter' is restricted, compromising the broader goals of social justice within which both Sen's and Farmer's work is so embedded. Under conditions of deprivation or 'capability inadequacy' (Sen, 1999: 90), individuals are 'deprived not only in terms of wellbeing, but also in terms of the ability to lead responsible lives, which are contingent on having certain basic freedoms' (1999: 284). This is significant for alcohol control policies – and indeed for the other NCD behavioural risk factors – because responsibility for one's actions can only be realised through the very freedoms inhibited by structural violence. Public policy thus has a role in 'creating more opportunities for choice and for substantive decisions for individuals who can then act responsibly on that basis' (Sen, 1999: 284). Here, responsibilities are the shared domain of the social and the individual. For alcohol, not only may this mean the state assuming responsibility for the fair and equitable enforcement of liquor policy, but also for the provision of and support for alternative income sources, something that is entirely absent in the WHO's Global Alcohol Strategy. Thus the state may need to ensure training, access to capital and subsidised business premises. In turn, individuals will need to comply with regulations in the name of the common good. An understanding that matters of health are, more often than not, also matters of livelihoods in the Global South is essential to ensuring that global health aspirations are supported, rather than undermined, by national and local policies.

Notes

1   In the text, the groups are delineated as follows: Philippi young men (PYM); Philippi young women (PYM); Philippi older women (POW); Philippi older men (POM); Freedom Park (FP1 and FP2); Salt River Community Policing Forum (SRCPF); Salt River Church Group (SRCG).

References

Alkire, S. 2005. Why the capability approach? *Journal of Human Development* 6: 115–135.

Altbeker, A. 2005. *The Dirty Work of Democracy; A Year on the Streets with the SAPS* (Jonathon Ball Publishers, Johannesburg).

Altbeker, A. 2007. *A Country at War with Itself: South Africa's Crisis of Crime* (Jonathon Ball Publishers, Johannesburg).

Ataguba, J.E-O. and Alaba, O. 2012. "Explaining health inequalities in South Africa: A political economy perspective. *Development Southern Africa* 29: 756–764.

Babor, T., Caetano, R. and Casswell, S. 2010. *Alcohol: No Ordinary Commodity: Research and Public Policy* (Oxford University Press, Oxford).

Bähre, E. 2007. Reluctant solidarity: Death, urban poverty and neighbourly assistance in South Africa. *Ethnography* 8: 33–59.

Barchiesi, F. 2007. South African debates on the basic income grant: Wage labour and the post-apartheid social policy. *Journal of Southern African Studies* 33: 561–575.

Biehl, J. and Petryna, A. 2013. *When People Come First: Critical Studies in Global Health* (Princeton University Press, Princeton, NJ).

Chersich, M.F. and Rees, H.V. 2010. Causal links between binge drinking patterns, unsafe sex and HIV in South Africa: its time to intervene. *International Journal of STD & AIDS* 21: 2–7.

Craplet, M. 2006. Open letter to my friends and colleagues. *Addiction* 101: 450–452.

Cunningham, J.A., Sobell, L.C., Sobell, M.B., Agrawal, S. and Toneatto, T. 1993. Barriers to treatment: Why alcohol and drug abusers delay or never seek treatment. *Addictive Behaviors* 18: 347–353.

Engels, R.C.M.E., Scholte, R.H.J., van Lieshout, C.F.M., de Kemp, R. and Overbeek, G. 2006. Peer group reputation and smoking and alcohol consumption in early adolescence. *Addictive Behaviors* 31: 440–449.

Farmer, P. 1996. Social inequalities and emerging infectious diseases. *Emerging Infectious Diseases* 2: 259–269.

Farmer, P. 2004. An anthropology of structural violence. *Current Anthropology* 45: 305–325.

Farmer, P. 2005. *Pathologies of Power: Health, Human Rights and the New War on the Poor* (University of California Press, Berkeley).

Farmer, P.E., Nizeye, B., Stulac, S. and Keshavjee, S. 2006. Structural violence and clinical medicine. *PLoS Med* 3: e449.

Farmer, P., Kleinman, A., Kim, J. and Basilico, M. 2013. *Reimaging Global Health: An Introduction* (University of California Press, Berkeley).

Faull, A. 2013. Policing taverns and shebeens: Observation, experience and discourse. *South African Crime Quarterly* 36: 35–48.

Foxcroft, D. 2006. Alcohol education: Absence of evidence or evidence of absence. *Addiction* 101: 1057–1059.

Gandy, M. 2005. Deadly alliances: Death, disease, and the global politics of public health. *PLoS Med* 2: e4. doi:10.1371/journal.pmed.0020004.

Hsieh, H-F. and Shannon, S.E. 2005. Three approaches to qualitative content analysis. *Qualitative Health Research* 15: 1277–1288.

Jayne, M., Valentine, G. and Holloway, S.L. 2008a. Geographies of alcohol, drinking and drunkenness: A review of progress. *Progress in Human Geography* 32(2): 247–263.

Jayne, M., Valentine, G. and Holloway, S.L. 2008b. Fluid boundaries — British binge drinking and European civility: Alcohol and the production and consumption of public space. *Space and Polity* 12(1): 81–100.

Kidd, P.S. and Parshall, M.B. 2000. Getting the focus and the group: Enhancing analytical rigor in focus group research. *Qualitative Health Research* 10: 293–308.

Kuntsche, E., Knibbe, R., Gmel, G. and Engels, R. 2005. Why do young people drink? A review of drinking motives. *Clinical Psychology Review* 25: 841–861.

Lawhon, M., Herrick, C., and Daya S. 2014. Researching sensitive topics in African cities: reflections on alcohol research in Cape Town. South African Geographical Journal 96(1):15–30.

Lemanski, C. 2004. A new apartheid? The spatial implications of fear of crime in Cape Town, South Africa. *Environment and Urbanization* 16: 101–112.

Leßmann, O. 2011. Freedom of choice and poverty alleviation. *Review of Social Economy* 69: 439–463.

Mager, A. 1999. The first decade of 'European beer' in apartheid South Africa: The state, the brewers and the drinking public, 1962–72. *The Journal of African History* 40: 367–388.

Mager, A. 2004. 'White liquor hits black livers': Meanings of excessive liquor consumption in South Africa in the second half of the twentieth century. *Social Science & Medicine* 59: 735–751.

Mager, A. 2005. 'One beer, one goal, one nation, one soul': South African breweries, heritage, masculinity and nationalism 1960–1999. *Past and Present* 188: 163–194.

Mager, A. 2010. *Beer, Sociability, and Masculinity and South Africa* (Indiana University Press, Bloomington).

Marmot, M. 2007. Achieving health equity: From root causes to fair outcomes. *The Lancet* 370: 1153–1163.

Measham, F. 2006. The new policy mix: Alcohol, harm minimisation, and determined drunkenness in contemporary society. *International Journal of Drug Policy* 17: 258–268.

Moffett, H. 2006. 'These women, they force us to rape them': Rape as narrative of social control in post-apartheid South Africa. *Journal of Southern African Studies* 32: 129–144.

Morrell, R., Jewkes, R. and Lindegger, G. 2012. Hegemonic masculinity/masculinities in South Africa: Culture, power, and gender politics. *Men and Masculinities* 15: 11–30.

Mulia, N., Schmidt, L., Bond, J., Jacobs, L. and Korcha, R. 2008. Stress, social support and problem drinking among women in poverty. *Addiction* 103: 1283–1293.

Nguyen, V-K. and Peschard, K. 2003. Anthropology, inequality, and disease: A review. *Annual Review of Anthropology* 32: 447–474.

Parry C.D.H. 2005. South Africa: Alcohol today. *Addiction* 100: 426–429.

Parry, C.D., Patra, J. and Rehm, J. 2011. Alcohol consumption and non-communicable diseases: Epidemiology and policy implications. *Addiction* 106: 1718–1724.

Quesada, J., Hart, L.K. and Bourgois, P. 2011. Structural vulnerability and health: Latino migrant laborers in the United States. *Medical Anthropology* 30: 339–362.

Rehm, J., Babor, T. and Room, R. 2006. Education, persuasion and the reduction of alcohol-related harm: A reply to Craplet. *Addiction* 101: 452–453.

Rogerson, C. 1992. 'In their right place'. Beer halls in Johannesburg 1938–1962. *African Studies* 51: 95–122.

Rogerson, C. and Hart, D. 1986. The survival of the 'informal sector': The shebeens of black Johannesburg. *GeoJournal* 12: 153–166.

Ross, F. 2010. *Raw Life, New Hope: Decency, Housing and Everyday Life in a Post-Apartheid Community* (UCT Press, Cape Town).

Salecl, R. 2010. *Choice* (Profile Books, London).

Schärf, W. 1985a. Liquor, the state and urban blacks, in *Crime and Power in South Africa*, ed. D. Davis and M. Slabbert (David Phillip, Cape Town), pp. 48–59.

Schärf, W. 1985b. Shebeens in the Cape Peninsula, in *Crime and Power in South Africa*, ed. D. Davis and M. Slabbert (David Phillip, Cape Town), pp. 97–105.

Schwartz, B. 2004. *The Paradox of Choice: Why Less is More* (Harper Collins, London).

Seedat, M., Van Niekerk, A., Jewkes, R., Suffla, S. and Ratele, K. 2009. Violence and injuries in South Africa: Prioritising an agenda for prevention. *The Lancet* 374: 1011–1022.

Sen, A. 1992. *Inequality Reexamined* (Harvard University Press, Cambridge, MA).

Sen, A. 1999. *Development as Freedom* (Oxford University Press, Oxford).

Sen, A. 2002. Why health equity? *Health Economics* 11: 659–666.

Stats, S.A. 2005. *Income and Expenditure Survey*. Available at http://www.statssa.gov.za/ies/docs/P01002005.pdf.

Steinberg, J. 2008. *Thin Blue: The Unwritten Rules of Policing South Africa* (Jonathon Ball Publishers, Jeppestown).

Steinberg, J. 2009. Perpetually half-formed – State and non-state security in the work of Wilfried Scharf. *South African Journal of Criminal Justice* 162: 162–175.

Tsoeu, M. 2009. *A Value Chain Analysis of the Formal and the Informal Economy: A Case Study of South African Breweries and Shebeens in Soweto*. Faculty of Humanities, University of the Witwatersrand, Johannesburg.

Valverde, M. 1998. *Diseases of the Will: Alcohol and the Dilemmas of Freedom* (Cambridge University Press, Cambridge).

Venkatapuram, S. 2009. A bird's eye view. Two topics at the intersection of social determinants of health and social justice philosophy. *Public Health Ethics* 2: 224–234.

Venkatapuram, S. 2012. Health, vital goals and central human capabilities. *Bioethics* no no.

Wiles, J.L., Rosenberg, M.W. and Kearns, R.A. 2005. Narrative analysis as a strategy for understanding interview talk in geographic research. *Area* 37: 89–99.

Willis, J. 2005. Drinking power: Alcohol and history in Africa. *History Compass* 3: 1–13.

World Health Organisation. 2008. *Closing the Gap in a Generation: Health Equity through Action on the Social Determinants of Health* (ed. WHO, Geneva).

World Health Organisation. 2014. *Global Status Report on Alcohol and Health 2014* (WHO, Geneva).

Index

Page numbers in *italics* denote an illustration, **bold** indicates a table